Emerging Roles of Nanocarriers in Cancer Therapy

This book addresses the limitations of existing therapeutic approaches using nanoparticles. *Emerging Roles of Nanocarriers in Cancer Therapy* will further provide information for the development of successful cancer nanomedicine therapies.

Features

- Explains different types of nanoparticles, targeting mechanisms, and approved nanotherapeutics for oncological implications in cancer treatment.
- Covers in detail the characteristics of various nanotechnology-based drug delivery systems.
- Discusses passive and active cellular targeting, ligand-based targeting of nanoparticles, and strategies to improve nanoparticle-cellular membrane interaction.
- Presents the application of nanotherapeutics, current challenges, and prospects, and describes the path of future research.
- Highlights smart strategies for improving the clinical impact of cancer nanomedicine.

The text is primarily written for graduate students and academic researchers in the fields of biotechnology, nanotechnology, drug delivery, pharmaceutical science, and pharmacology.

Emerging Roles of Nanocarriers in Cancer Therapy

Rishabha Malviya, Arun Kumar Singh, and Sonali Sundram

CRC Press
Taylor & Francis Group
Boca Raton London New York

CRC Press is an imprint of the
Taylor & Francis Group, an **informa** business

Design cover image: Shutterstock – image number 2049407213

First edition published 2025
by CRC Press
2385 NW Executive Center Drive, Suite 320, Boca Raton FL 33431

and by CRC Press
4 Park Square, Milton Park, Abingdon, Oxon, OX14 4RN

CRC Press is an imprint of Taylor & Francis Group, LLC

ISBN: 9781032583525 (hbk)
ISBN: 9781032586748 (pbk)
ISBN: 9781003451020 (ebk)

DOI: 10.1201/9781003451020

Typeset in Times
by Newgen Publishing UK

Contents

Foreword

I am delighted to introduce the outstanding collection *Emerging Roles of Nanocarriers in Cancer Therapy* authored by Drs. Rishabha Malviya, Arun Kumar Singh, and Sonali Sundram. This book provides an authoritative and comprehensive overview of the cutting-edge field of nanomedicine and its revolutionary potential for the treatment of cancer.

Affecting millions of people worldwide, cancer continues to be one of the major healthcare challenges. Nanomedicine has emerged as a promising treatment in the race for improved and tailored therapies. With its capacity to modify molecules at the nanoscale, nanotechnology presents unique prospects to transform cancer therapies.

This book takes readers on an informative overview of the most recent developments, prospects, and cancer treatment options with nanomedicine. A prominent group of specialists led by Dr. Malviya has been brought together to lend their knowledge and understanding to the range of subjects addressed in this book.

An introduction to nanomedicine sets the stage for later chapters of the book, which explore well-known nanoparticle platforms like liposomes, polymeric micelles, and dendrimers. These chapters highlight new opportunities in nanomedicine for improved tumor treatment in addition to examining the special qualities and benefits of these delivery systems.

The chapters explore the diversity of cancer-targeted therapy, nanotechnology-enabled chemotherapy, and innovative approaches used to increase the clinical impact of nanomedicine. These chapters include insightful discussions of the most recent findings and innovations influencing the field, from examining the promise of polymer–drug conjugates for combination therapy to reviewing the developments in nanoparticle-mediated cancer immunotherapy.

The book also discusses the use of polymeric micelles for effective and targeted cancer therapy, the synergistic advantages of combining nanomedicine with hyperbaric oxygen therapy, and the delivery of siRNA medicines for cancer treatment. Additionally, it highlights the value of cellular targeting and techniques to strengthen nanoparticle–cellular interactions for better therapeutic effects.

For scientists, doctors, researchers, and students interested in cutting-edge cancer treatment, *Emerging Roles of Nanocarriers in Cancer Therapy* is a vital resource for individuals who want to stay up to date on the most recent developments and accomplishments in nanomedicine. This book is an invaluable resource due to its multidisciplinary approach and the extensive depth of knowledge offered by the contributing writers.

I appreciate Dr. Rishabha Malviya and his team for their outstanding job in putting together this important book. The book shows their dedication to developing nanomedicine and their commitment to encouraging collaboration and knowledge sharing.

I encourage you to read *Emerging Roles of Nanocarriers in Cancer Therapy* from beginning to end and learn more about the revolutionary potential of nanotechnology in the battle against cancer. Let us work together to make cancer therapy more patient-centric, effective, and targeted in the future by embracing the exciting possibilities provided by nanomedicine.

Best wishes,

Dr. Rajendra Singh
Former Associate Director
The Defence Research and Development Organisation, Govt of India
Research Advisor
Galgotias University, India

Preface

The understanding of nanomedicine has undergone considerable advances recently, redefining the way researchers approach cancer therapies. The combination of nanotechnology and medicine has created new opportunities for effective and focused cancer treatment, giving both patients and medical professionals a lot of hope.

This book, *Emerging Roles of Nanocarriers in Cancer Therapy*, explores the most recent developments, prospects, and difficulties in the field of nanomedicine as they apply to the treatment of cancer. It examines the many nanoparticle platforms that have already proven to be effective at delivering therapeutic compounds to the target site.

The interesting field of nanomedicine and its potential uses in cancer treatment are introduced to readers in Chapter 1.

The application of nanotechnology in cancer chemotherapy is the primary focus of Chapter 2. It looks at several nanoparticle delivery systems, such as liposomes, polymer–drug conjugates, micelles, and dendrimers, which have shown significant progress in delivering chemotherapeutic medicines with greater efficacy and fewer adverse effects.

The book significantly explores the use of nanomedicine in targeted cancer therapy in Chapter 3. It focuses on how conjugated nanoparticles can be used to target cancer and how they may navigate challenges related to tumor treatment.

Intelligent methods for enhancing the clinical effectiveness of cancer nanomedicine are addressed in Chapter 4. It explores methods for immunomodulation, drug selection, combination therapy, and patient classification that can improve the effectiveness of nanomedicine.

In Chapter 5, the progress of nanoparticle-mediated cancer immunotherapy is highlighted. It offers an in-depth investigation of the various types of immunostimulatory nanoparticles and investigates methods for their optimization.

The exploration of polymer–drug conjugates in Chapter 6 offers novel prospects for drug combination therapy in the treatment of cancer. It examines the prospect of combination medicine, concentrating on preclinical research and the difficulties involved in employing polymer–drug conjugates.

The concept of nanoparticles for siRNA drug delivery in cancer research and therapeutic applications is explored in Chapter 7. It covers the benefits and drawbacks of siRNA delivery for the treatment of cancer, the characteristics of siRNA nanocarriers, and numerous methods for introducing siRNA therapeutics into cancer cells.

Hyperbaric oxygen treatment (HBOT) and nanomedicine utilize coordination are discussed in Chapter 8. It gives an extensive overview of HBOT and its uses in various cancer therapy.

In Chapter 9, the concept of combination nanomedicine is explored, with a special emphasis on the co-delivery of multimodal medicines for effective, targeted, and secure cancer treatment.

The multifunctional properties of polymeric micellar nanomedicine in cancer therapy are further discussed in Chapter 10.

The last chapter, Chapter 11, focuses on the use of nanoparticles to target cancer cells. The strategies used to enhance nanoparticle uptake and cellular membrane interaction are discussed along with aspects affecting nanoparticle–cellular interactions and passive and active cellular targeting techniques.

We invite you to learn more about the most recent studies, scientific developments, and cutting-edge cancer prevention and treatment methods by utilizing the amazing field of nanomedicine.

Authors

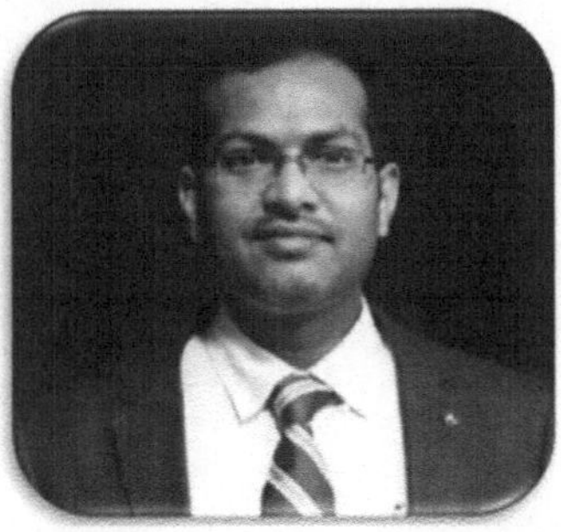

Dr. Rishabha Malviya earned a BPharm degree from Uttar Pradesh Technical University and an MPharm (pharmaceutics) degree from Gautam Buddha Technical University, Lucknow Uttar Pradesh. His PhD (pharmacy) work was in the area of novel formulation development techniques. He has more than 12.5 years of research experience and is presently working for the past eight years as an associate professor in the Department of Pharmacy, School of Medical and Allied Sciences, Galgotias University. Dr. Malviya's areas of interest include formulation optimization, nanoformulation, targeted drug delivery, localized drug delivery, and characterization of natural polymers as pharmaceutical excipients. He has authored more than 200 research/review papers for national/international journals of repute. He has 58 patents (19 grants, 38 published, 1 filed) and publications in reputed national and international journals with a more than 225 cumulative impact factor. Dr. Malviya is editing 60 books and has authored 125 book chapters. He is a reviewer/editor/editorial board member of more than 50 national and international journals of repute.

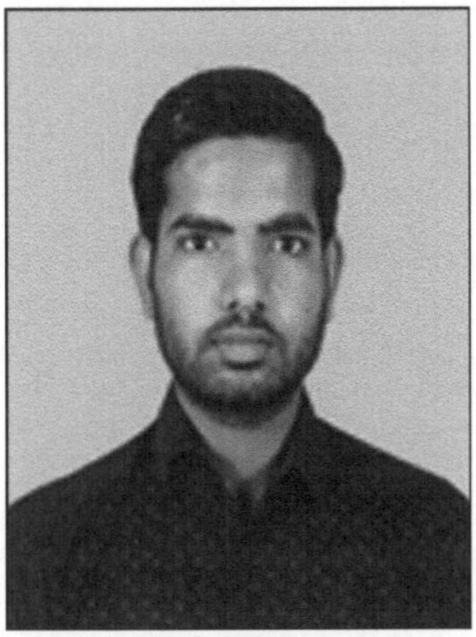

Arun Kumar Singh earned his BPharm and MPharm degrees from Galgotias University, India. He has authored four books and three book chapters and has published manuscripts with reputed publishers such as *Biochimica et Biophysica Acta (BBA) – Reviews on Cancer* (impact factor 11.414), *Journal of Controlled Release* (impact factor 11.467), *Current Cancer Therapy Reviews* (Scopus), *Recent Advances in Food, Nutrition & Agriculture* (Scopus), *Recent Patents on Anti-Cancer Drug Discovery* (impact factor 3.038), *Current Cancer Drug Targets* (impact factor 2.907), and many more.

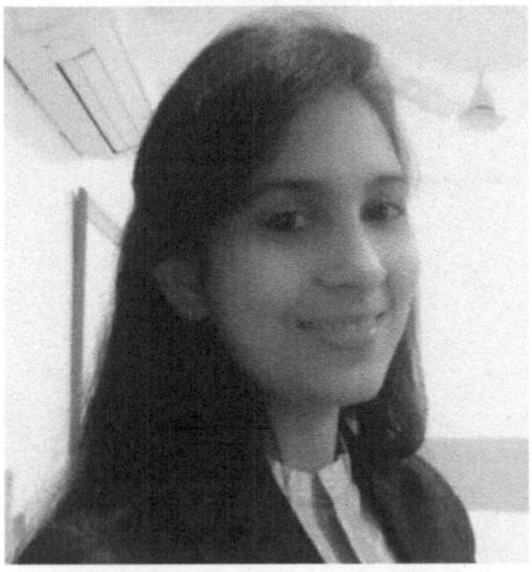

Prof. Sonali Sundram earned her BPharm and MPharm (pharmacology) degrees from AKTU, Lucknow. She worked as a research scientist for an ICMR project at King George's Medical University, Lucknow. Afterward, she joined BBDNIIT, and is currently working at Galgotias University, Greater Noida, India. Her PhD (pharmacy) work was in the area of neurodegeneration and nanoformulation. Dr. Sundram's areas of interest are: neurodegeneration, clinical research, and artificial intelligence. She is editing more than 25 books and 45 book chapters. She has attended and organized more than 15 national and international seminars/conferences/workshops. She has more than eight national and international patents to her credit. Dr. Sundram has published six SCI-indexed manuscripts (cumulative impact factor 20.71) with reputed international publishers and delivered oral presentations at international conferences throughout varying European countries.

Introduction

This informative and comprehensive book, *Emerging Roles of Nanocarriers in Cancer Therapy*, explores the fast-developing discipline of nanomedicine along with how it is used to treat cancer. It provides an in-depth analysis of the trends, prospects, and difficulties associated with using nanotechnology to improve cancer therapies.

This text covers a wide range of issues, from fresh perspectives in nanomedicine for improved tumor treatment to proven nanoparticle platforms like liposomes, polymeric micelles, and dendrimers.

The book's chapters are carefully arranged to lead readers through several aspects of nanomedicine in cancer therapy. Readers obtain a fundamental understanding of nanomedicine and its potential in cancer treatment after reading the initial chapter. The chapters focus on particular topics, including cancer-targeted therapy, nanotechnology-enabled chemotherapy, and innovative strategies to increase the therapeutic impact of nanomedicine.

In addition, the book highlights recent advances in nanoparticle-mediated cancer immunotherapy, emphasizing the use of a variety of nanoparticles and methods for enhancing their immunostimulatory capabilities. Additionally, it explores the promising prospects of polymer–drug conjugates for combination therapy and discusses the difficulties involved in their production and clinical use.

Furthermore, readers will learn about the practical application of polymeric micelles for effective and targeted cancer therapy as well as the function of nanocarriers in the delivery of siRNA therapeutics for cancer treatment. A chapter on the cellular targeting of nanoparticles is included in the book's final component, and it highlights its importance in enhancing cellular uptake and interactions for improved therapeutic effects.

For academics, scientists, doctors, and students looking for in-depth information on the most recent developments in nanomedicine for cancer treatment, *Emerging Roles of Nanocarriers in Cancer Therapy* is an excellent resource. It brings together the most recent scientific discoveries, technical innovations, and useful insights to promote additional innovation and advancement in this rapidly transforming industry.

Explore the countless opportunities that nanotechnology has for revolutionizing cancer therapeutics until you commence on this journey through the worldwide field of nanomedicine. Let us work together to develop more efficient, focused, and individualized strategies to fight this terrible disease.

1 Nanomedicine as Cancer Therapeutics
Current Trends and Opportunities

1.1 INTRODUCTION

Considering the millions of deaths caused by cancer annually, it remains a serious public health concern [1]. The Greek physician Hippocrates is credited with coining the term "cancer" because of the finger-like projections that grow from it that resemble crabs. Nevertheless, these traditional methods of treatment come with unpleasant side effects, poor targeting, and pain. Nanomedicines are becoming a more popular option because of their low toxicity, bioavailability, and targeting capabilities. Both active and passive mechanisms are used by nanoparticles to target cancer cells. Many nanotherapeutics have been developed since the FDA approved Doxil®, and some of them have been approved for use in the treatment of cancer. Not only are liposomes, solid lipid nanoparticles, polymeric nanoparticles, and nanoemulsions being researched and used in practice but there are even more recent methods involving extracellular vesicles (EVs) and thermal nanomaterials [2]. The cell-killing specificity, which was created to prevent the toxicities related to more traditional chemotherapeutics, boosted antitumor activity. HER2 was shown to be overexpressed in one-quarter of breast tumors, leading to the development of trastuzumab (Herceptin), which is a recombinant monoclonal antibody that binds to the extracellular domain of HER2.

It has been shown time and time again that the new chemotherapeutics have improved patient survival, but they are yet hampered by a variety of biological hurdles that impede effective drug distribution after systemic injection. The non-specific dispersion of new and classic chemotherapeutics means that only a tiny percentage of medications can reach the tumor. The reticuloendothelial system (RES), a mechanism of monocytes as well as macrophages that clears foreign substances, has long been recognized to sequester injected materials [3]. Due to their inherent toxicity, drugs build up in healthy organs, with a fine line between tolerability and serious morbidity, like the case of doxorubicin, a type of DNA intercalator that induces cardiotoxicity [4]. Tumors have aberrant blood flow, interstitial pressure gradients, as well as cellular-nuclear membrane traversals, to mention just a few. Anticancer medications have limited curative potential due to the combination of these variables, necessitating the development of new delivery methods. In the 1960s and 1970s, liposomes as well as polymer-drug conjugates were created to adapt Paul Ehrlich's "magic bullet" notion for chemotherapy [5]. Nanomedicine is a multidisciplinary area that tries to enhance the delivery of chemotherapeutics by using nanoscale (1–100 nm) structures [6]. These carriers' primary function is to aid in the solubilization of drugs and to guard against their deterioration. As a consequence of tumor blood vessel leakiness, the increased permeation and retention (EPR) effect allows medications to agglomerate in tumors via nanoscale size range plus the ubiquitous existence of poly(ethylene glycol) (PEG) onto their surface [7]. In healthy organs, lower sequestration rates

DOI: 10.1201/9781003451020-1

are associated with increased accumulation and retention, but in malignancies, greater accumulation and retention are associated with reduced side effects [8].

In several significant cases, the promise of nanomedicine in enhancing cancer treatment has started to be realized clinically. 2008 was the first clinical trial of a systemically administered nanoparticle carrying siRNA in people with solid tumors, which was carried out by a Davis-led team. It was shown that at therapeutically relevant concentrations, nanoparticles made up of a linear polymer (CDP), anti-R2 siRNA, and transferrin (Tf) protein-targeting ligands, could be accumulated in tumor cells. To put it another way: using the technology, researchers discovered that siRNA can target particular genes in the human genome [9].

1.2 THERANOSTIC APPROACHES OF NANOPARTICLES FOR CANCER

1.2.1 Liposomal Delivery

The most researched nanodrug delivery vehicle, liposomes, are spherically shaped vesicles made up of one or more phospholipid bilayers. The main advantages of liposomes over conventional drug delivery methods are their targeted delivery, high biocompatibility, biodegradability, ease of functionalization, low toxicity, enhanced therapeutic indices, and improved sustained release of the drug they carry. The studies of liposome composition have grown in scope as a result of the quick development of nanotechnology. Long-circulating PEGylated liposomes, ligand-functionalized liposomes, stimuli-responsive liposomes, and advanced cell membrane-coated biomimetic nanocarriers are just a few examples of the molecular diversity of liposome composition that gives their drug delivery distinct physiological functions [10–13]. Many liposomal doxorubicin formulations are presently being tested in clinical studies, with the help of doxorubicin liposomes. It contains the RAF antisense oligonucleotide that suppresses c-raf, which is responsible for resistance to radiation and chemotherapy [14]. Four of the twelve patients tested in a phase I research of patients having advanced solid tumors that were receiving radiation therapy had partial responses. Three of the five monitored patients had suppressed C-raf-1 mRNA, while four of the five had inhibited Raf-1 protein [15,16].

1.2.2 Polymer Micelles Delivery

A variety of medicinal substances Figure 1.1 have been transported by polymeric micelles, which are nanoscale assemblies of amphiphilic polymers with a core–shell composition. Their ability to solubilize drugs that are poorly soluble in water, their biocompatibility, and their enhanced permeability and retention (EPR) ability to accumulate in tumors have all drawn attention to them. Furthermore, a further modification can give the micelles additional functionality. For instance, targeted ligand-modified micelle surfaces enable improved tumor accumulation and precise targeting. When stimuli-sensitive groups are introduced, the drug is released in response to changes in the surrounding environment [17–19]. Clinical trials of a polymeric micelle, NC-6004, which incorporates cisplatin, were recently conducted in patients with various solid tumors. Micelles were well accepted by patients, as shown by the fact that seven of the 17 patients treated had stable illnesses. Patients having metastatic breast cancer were examined in phase II clinical research using GenexolPM, a PEG-PLA micelle comprising paclitaxel [20]. After giving 300 mg m^2 to 41 patients once every 3 weeks, the overall rate of response was 58.5%, with 19 partial and five full responses.

1.2.3 Dendrimer Delivery

Surgery, chemotherapy, and radiation therapy are the primary treatments for cancer, a condition that is one of the leading causes of death in the world. Nanomaterials are being used more frequently as

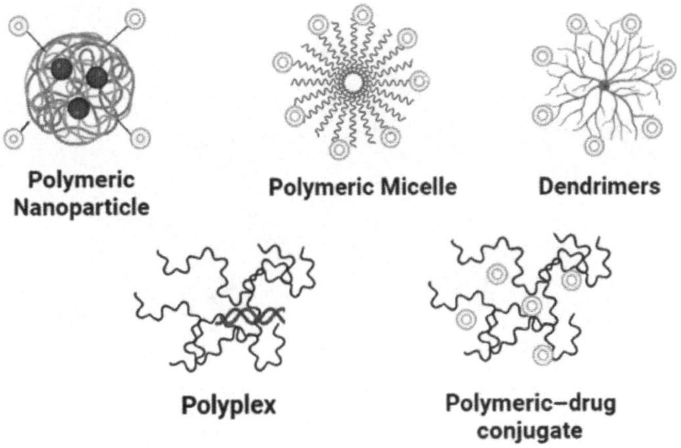

FIGURE 1.1 Nanoparticle platforms for the delivery of anticancer drugs. (Created with Biorenders.com.)

the structures for anticancer therapies because these treatment modalities are intrusive and can have serious negative effects on organisms. One kind of nanomaterial with special qualities is dendrimers; their synthesis can be manipulated to produce compounds with specific features. These polymeric molecules are utilized in the targeted distribution of certain pharmacological substances for cancer diagnosis and treatment. When it comes to anticancer therapy, dendrimers can accomplish multiple goals at once. These include directing the release of anticancer agents within the tumor microenvironment, focusing on tumor cells to prevent harm to healthy tissue, and combining anticancer strategies based on the administration of anticancer molecules to increase their effectiveness through photothermal therapy or photodynamic therapy [21–23]. Customizable dendrimer release profiles may be achieved by precise dendrimer depolymerization. Polyamidoamine (PAMAM) dendrimers may be changed to strengthen their biocompatibility or enhance tumor targeting by attaching ligands to them. In preclinical research, dendrimers are showing great promise for cancer treatment. In a recent work employing polylysine dendrimers, a5b1 integrin activation was targeted using polylysine dendrimers [23]. Yao and coworkers showed that the PHSCN peptide, which binds to activated a5b1, was 700- to 1100-fold more effective than the free peptide in preventing MDA-MB-231 tumor extravasation in mice's lungs, as revealed by Yao and colleagues. Following metastasis, the PHSCN dendrimer decreased the number of formed lung colonies [24]. Figure 1.1 depicts nanoparticle platforms for the delivery of anticancer drugs.

1.3 NOVEL TECHNIQUES FOR CANCER THERAPY IN NANOMEDICINE

1.3.1 Active Targeting Techniques

The so-called active targeting can even boost drug efficiency after it has accumulated in the tumor area. This is accomplished by decorating the surfaces of the nanocarriers with ligands that attach to receptors that are overexpressed on the tumor cells. This tactic will increase the nanocarriers' affinities for the cancer cell surface, enhancing drug penetration. The earliest indication of this phenomenon was put forth in 1980 when antibodies were grafted onto the surface of liposomes. Other ligand types, such as peptides, nucleic acids, and aptamers, were then added. The transferrin receptors (TfR) and nicotinic acetylcholine receptors, which permit access to the environment of brain tumors, are two examples of classical targets. This instance involves vascular targeting or the targeting of endothelial cells. Transferrin ligands were grafted on solid lipid nanoparticles (SNPs), micelles, dendrimers, and superparamagnetic iron oxide nanoparticles (SPIONPs) and applied to

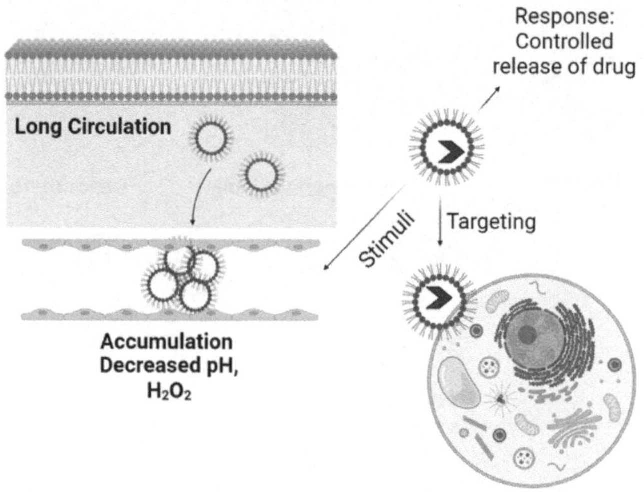

FIGURE 1.2 Improved tumor treatment using nanomedicine. (Created with Biorenders.com.)

target gliomas for drug delivery or biomedical imaging [25]. Compared to non-targeted controls, the PEGylated folate-functionalized dendrimers showed a considerable (about 40%) decrease in tumor development following two injections (days 0 and 7) over 20 days. However, trastuzumab may also be utilized as a targeting moiety in treating cancer. Anti-HER2 F5 antibody-functionalized liposomes have recently been developed for the treatment of BT-474 breast cancers [26]. After 53 days of therapy, anti-HER2-targeted liposomes outperformed non-targeted liposomes by a factor of over two and free topotecan by a factor of over five after intravenous injections of 5 mg kg liposomes on days 14, 18 as well as 21 after tumor implantation. One of the most common targets for angiogenesis is the transmembrane protein avb3, which is overexpressed in blood vessels that are in the process of angiogenesis. Active targeting of nanoparticles may be possible with the help of the (cRGD) peptide, which binds strongly to the Avb3 integrin [27]. The cRGD-targeting ligand was recently proven to be functionalized on doxorubicin PEG-PLA polymer micelles by Nasongkla and colleagues. Compared to non-targeted micelles, avb3-overexpressing SLK endothelial cells absorbed micelles more efficiently [28]. Tumor tissue was more successfully targeted and accumulated by cRGD-labeled micelles with superparamagnetic iron oxide nanoparticles in mice with A549 lung tumors, as shown by improved MRI imaging contrast [29]. Figure 1.2 represents new opportunities for improved tumor treatment in nanomedicine.

1.3.2 Controlled Release Strategies

Often referred to as "nanogels," hydrophilic polymers that have undergone physical or chemical crosslinking are used to create nanoscale dimension hydrogel particles. In recent times, nanogels have been utilized in diverse domains such as chemical and biochemical sensing, tissue engineering, cancer imaging, and diagnostics, particularly for drug delivery. When compared to current nanocarriers, therapeutic delivery with nanogels offers the following advantages: the drug has several advantages over liposomes and micelles, including (i) a high loading capacity; (ii) greater storage stability; (iii) controlled and sustained drug release; (iv) ease of synthesis; (v) response to external stimuli; and (vi) low inherent toxicity. When nanogels are in high-water aqueous media, they behave like soft materials. Cysteine has been used as a crosslinker in the synthesis of protease, redox, and pH-responsive PEGylated poly(methacrylic acid) PMAA nanohydrogels for the targeted delivery of anticancer drugs [30]. Only around 5% of the drug was released at pH 7.4 in the initial 24 hours, compared to 100% at pH 5.0. It was discovered that B16F10 as well as OVCAR-3 ovarian cancer cells responded more favorably *in vitro* to pH-sensitive micelles, which is probably because more acidic organelles were released. Furthermore, mice with B16F10 tumors were injected on days 3 and 6, and 8 days later, pH-sensitive micelles showed a greater than two-fold difference in tumor development decrease compared to PBS as well as free doxorubicin controls. The utilization of ultrasound to stimulate the release of therapeutic compounds from nanoparticles is gaining traction (Figure 1.2). When ultrasound breaks down polymers, increases local temperatures, and permeabilizes cell walls, the process is activated [31]. It has recently been established that ultrasound-triggered medication release from liposomes *in vivo* may be used to treat cancer patients [32].

After injecting J6456 lymphoma mice with liposomes, a low-frequency ultrasound was administered one hour later. The results showed that approximately 70% of cisplatin was released when ultrasonography was employed, compared to about 3% when ultrasound was not used. The levels of cisplatin in tumors that received ultrasound were roughly three times greater than in tumors that did not receive ultrasound. The liposomes were introduced intravenously into mouse C-26 colon cancers in the footpad and then irradiated with ultrasonography 24 hours later [33]. After 29 days, researchers found that mice given cisplatin-containing liposomes with ultrasound had considerably less tumor development in the footpad than mice given free cisplatin or ultrasound.

Tumors may be able to release drugs if their temperature is raised by external factors. Due to hydrophobic effects, nanoparticle instability occurs above the critical solution temperature (LCST) for polymers like pNIPAM, which have a lower critical solution temperature (LCST). Poly(2-[2-ethoxy]ethoxyethyl vinyl ether [EOEOVE], a copolymer having an LCST of 40C, was used by Kono and colleagues to generate thermosensitive doxorubicin liposomes [34]. Temperature-sensitive liposomes release doxorubicin at a rate of 10% per minute at 37°C, according to the results. Within the first 10 minutes of heating to 45°C, almost all of the medication was released. Following intravenous injection of the temperature-sensitive liposomes, tumors in mice containing subcutaneous C-26 colon tumor cells were subjected to heating at 45°C for 10 minutes at various intervals. Ten days later, a ten-fold change in tumor size was observed in response to elevated temperatures of 3, 6, and 12 hours following injection of liposomes.

1.3.3 Multistage Delivery Technique

The biological complexity of tumors and the constraints in the design of functional nanosized delivery systems make the development of conventional tumor-targeted drug delivery systems based on the EPR effect and receptor-mediated endocytosis extremely difficult. Tumor therapy and imaging have recently seen the emergence of multistage drug delivery systems (Ms-DDS), which are activated by a variety of distinct stimuli present in the tumor microenvironment. Ms-DDS can modify their physicochemical properties (e.g., size, hydrophobicity, or zeta potential) in response to variations in the intracellular environment, tumor microenvironment, and physiological blood circulation. This allows for effective endosomal escape, deeper tumor penetration, and timely drug release. These mechanisms allow Ms-DDS to deliver the greatest amount of medication to therapeutic targets, such as cells, tumor tissues, and subcellular organelles, and to ultimately show the highest level of therapeutic efficacy [35,36].

The reasoning for the technique is based on the knowledge of "oncophysics" and the necessity to overcome biobarriers in cancer treatment [37]. Drug-containing nanostructures will be encapsulated in mesoporous silicon particles (MSP), which will secure as well as transport them till they identify plus dock with tumor vasculature. As a result, the platform separates the many steps involved in delivering the medicine from the injection site to the tumor. MSNs are also incredibly biocompatible and biodegradable. The US Food and Drug Administration (USFDA) classifies them as "Generally Recognized as Safe" (GRAS). In simulated bodily fluid, cells, and the body itself, MSNs can completely degrade in as little as one month. Together with apparent ionic corrosion, hydrolysis, and dissolution of the silica framework are caused by water molecules and contribute to the degradation of mesoporous silica. The process of degradation is accelerated by the ionic exchange that takes place between the superficial mesoporous silica and the degradation medium, while the superficial silanol groups of the silica actively participate in the formation of a hydrogen bond with water. MSNs are resistant to a range of stresses, including thermal, mechanical, and pH stresses. To create formulations with on-command drug release that can deliver antitumor drugs selectively, MSNs can be modified with various gatekeeper molecules, such as inorganic, organic, self-gated drug molecules, and biological membranes, depending on the pore system and surface modification [36,38]. To boost tumor accumulation, they may be functionalized with PEG and other targeting moieties because of their enormous size and silicon chemistry's ability to encapsulate huge amounts of nanoparticles. In mice, there is no aggregation after intravenous administration, resulting in a reduced risk of thrombosis. A broad variety of nanoparticles may also be used in the second step of the process. PEG-FITC-single-walled carbon nanotubes (SWNTs), as well as quantum dots (QDs), were both loaded into MSP at the same time to demonstrate the point. It was discovered that SWNTs were located everywhere over the MSP, while QDs were found to be more concentrated in the center of the particle, even though they were co-localized inside a single MSP. Among the many advantages of the multistage strategy to drug administration is its capacity to significantly modify the pharmacokinetics of injectables, which is observable. MSPs were rationally created with appropriate shapes and sizes to optimize localization inside tumor vasculature while limiting RES absorption utilizing an integrated strategy integrating into silico mathematical modeling with *in vitro* along with *in vivo* research. This was accomplished by computationally compartmentalizing the MSP's vascular trip into three primary extents: (i) margination dynamics; (ii) firm adhesion; and (iii) regulation of internalization [39]. Researchers discovered that non-spherical particles into circulation travel laterally inside the blood flow utilizing a parallel-plate flow chamber having hydrodynamically regulated injection of varied particle shapes. As a result, nanoparticles are more likely than spherical ones to engage with blood artery walls, which makes it easier for them to attach to particular vascular targets. Platelet-like oblate-spherical particles, which have the same number of binding sites as spherical particles, tend to cling more strongly to vessel walls when flow is present. Particles administered intravenously into animals with MDA-MB-231 breast cancers have varied *in vivo* fates, according to research on *in vivo* biodistribution. Compared to spherical, discoidal, and cylindrical particles, hemispherical particles accumulated the most malignancies. These results on hemodynamic characteristics and biodistribution support the accumulation of MSP in tumor-associated arteries and highlight the relevance of considering certain geometrical structures of nanocarriers for medication delivery applications, which are site-specific when considered together Efficacy is determined by cellular interactions once particles have reached the tumor vascular and microenvironment. *In vitro* research was conducted to examine the effects of particle surface charge, opsonization, as well as inflammation on vascular endothelial cell adhesion [40].

MSP, both positively (oxidized) and negatively (APTES-modified) charged, may be quickly absorbed by endothelial cells by macropinocytosis and phagocytosis, respectively [41]. APTES-modified MSP was also shown to be more readily absorbed by endothelial cells after serum opsonization. Maximizing cell-killing effects with MSP requires an appropriate release of the therapeutic payload. Because the release of the second-phase nanoparticles from the MSP depends on the biological degradation of porous multistage particles within physiological conditions, researchers have discovered that they may manipulate the release kinetics of the MSP by adjusting the porosity of the MSP [42]. Extremely porous multistage particles break down in hours as opposed to particles that have little porosity, which take days to do so, allowing for the long-term release of payload. A contributing cause to degradation was also found to be MSP surface functionalization. In the second stage of drug administration, liposomes expressing siRNA targeting EphA2, an oncogenic tyrosine kinase receptor, were employed in a mouse model of ovarian cancer (SKOV3ip1). Simultaneous release of siRNA was achieved by loading liposomes into MSP [43]. For 3 weeks, mice received 5 lg EphA2-siRNA in intravenous siRNA-liposome injections twice a week for intravenous

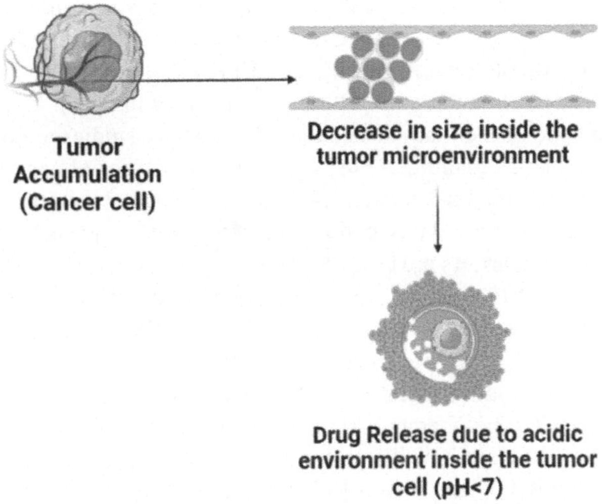

FIGURE 1.3 Destruction of cancer cells by nanoparticles. (Created with Biorenders.com.)

administration. An injection of 15 lg of EphA2-siRNA-liposomes at a dose of 15 lg EphA2 was given to a second group. After a single dose of the multistage delivery method, the SKOV3ip1 tumor EphA2 protein was silenced for 3 weeks, which resulted in an increased therapeutic response. There was a substantial reduction in tumor weight when EphA2-siRNA-liposomes were used in combination with non-silencing control siRNA-liposome and multistage non-silencing control-liposome treatments, respectively. Note that the single injection of EphA2-siRNA-liposomes had an anticancer effect similar to six repeated intravenous injections of the same substance. Resulting in improved biodistribution of the encapsulated liposomal siRNA formulations and continual release of these liposomes at the cancer site.

Recently, MRI contrast chemicals were enclosed in MSP and their magnetic properties were researched to create a theranostic nanoplatform, which combines therapeutic as well as imaging components into a single construct [44].

The T1 contrast agent, gadolinium, was encapsulated in MSP in many formulations, including Magnevist (Bayer Schering Pharma, Berlin, Germany), gadofullerenes, and gadonanotubes. Greater longitudinal proton relaxivity, which is directly related to greater image contrast, was demonstrated by the gadolinium-loaded MSP. These relaxivity values, which in some cases were 4–50 times greater than those of commercial formulations, were most likely brought on by the gadolinium getting nanoconfined and clustering within the MSP all through the research. Multistage delivery holds great promise for more effective cancer treatment and diagnosis, according to preliminary findings. Figure 1.3 depicts a nanoparticle representation of cancer cells being destroyed.

1.4 CHALLENGES AND FUTURE OPPORTUNITIES OF NANOMEDICINE IN CANCER TREATMENT

The use of nanotechnology for cancer diagnosis and treatment is still in its early stages of development, despite the rapid and extensive nature of nanotechnology research. The development of nanoparticles is fraught with difficulties that severely restrict their applicability in clinical settings. First, the EPR effect is the basis for passive tumor targeting in all commercially available cancer nanomedicines [45]. However, tumor heterogeneity affects the EPR effect itself, leading to variability between and even within patients. Furthermore, some research indicates that the EPR effect is more pronounced in smaller animals than in humans, which could skew the results regarding the effectiveness of a specific treatment. With the goal of achieving better clinical results, nanocarriers with enhanced tumor-targeting potentials were developed in an attempt to address the problem encountered by first-generation nanomedicines (i.e., EPR-based). Second, not all of the materials used to make nanocarriers have undergone extensive human testing [46]. Determining biocompatibility may therefore be one of the main difficulties. Our toxicity studies are designed primarily for materials that are used in large quantities. But because the properties of nanoparticles differ greatly from those of the corresponding bulk matter, standard toxicological profiling may not be adequate to determine or assess their toxicity. Thus, before conducting clinical trials for nanomedicines, long-term toxicity studies of nanocarriers are crucial.

Furthermore, a variety of techniques can be employed to synthesize nanocarriers, contingent upon the nature of the nanomaterials and the targeted properties of the nanocarriers. To achieve nanoformulation with desired reproducibility, many, if not all, of these techniques require close monitoring of various formulation parameters because small changes in these parameters can have a significant impact on the characteristics of nanocarriers. Among these, membrane extrusion, high-pressure homogenization, microfluidizer technology, and supercritical fluid technology have adequate scale-up capabilities [47]. However, it is still unlikely that these methods will be used to create multifunctional (surface-functionalized or TME-responsive, for example) nanocarriers on a large scale. Furthermore, repeatability and drug loading capacities need to be improved even more. Not to mention, the inability of experimental animal tumor models to accurately replicate the tumors found in human clinical cancer greatly impedes the clinical translation of nanomedicines. Because their experimental models closely resemble human tumors, great care must be taken in selecting which ones to use for evaluating the pharmacokinetics and efficacy of nanomedicines [48].

1.5 CONCLUSION

Cancer continues to be a significant public health concern, as it is responsible for millions of deaths each year. There are negative side effects, poor targeting, and pain associated with traditional treatments. Nanomedicines, which include liposomes, solid lipid nanoparticles, polymeric nanoparticles, and nanoemulsions, are gaining popularity as a result of their low toxicity, bioavailability, and the ability to target specific areas of the body. High biocompatibility, biodegradability, and low toxicity are some of the benefits that liposomes offer in terms of targeted delivery. The ability of polymeric micelles to solubilize drugs, as well as their ability to enhance permeability and retention in tumors, is currently being investigated. As a result of their potential to direct anticancer agents within the microenvironment of the tumor, nanoparticles are increasingly being utilized in the treatment of cancer. This is done with the intention of concentrating on tumor cells while minimizing damage to healthy tissue. Some of the nanomaterials that are utilized in the treatment of cancer include dendrimers, active targeting techniques, and controlled release strategies. In addition, multistage drug delivery systems, also known as Ms-DDS, are currently being developed in order to maximize the localization and absorption of RES.

REFERENCES

1. Torre LA, Siegel RL, Ward EM, Jemal A. Global cancer incidence and mortality rates and trends—an update. *Cancer Epidemiol. Biomark. Prev.* 2016; 25(1): 16–27.
2. Faguet GB. A brief history of cancer: age-old milestones underlying our current knowledge database: a brief history of cancer. *Int. J. Cancer* 2015; 136(9): 2022–36.
3. Peer D, Karp JM, Hong S, Farokhzad OC, Margalit R, Langer R. Nanocarriers as an emerging platform for cancer therapy. *Nat. Nanotechnol.* 2007; 2: 751–60.
4. Olson RD, Mushlin PS. Doxorubicin cardiotoxicity: analysis of prevailing hypotheses. *FASEB J.* 1990; 4: 3076–86.

5. Strebhardt K, Ullrich A. Paul Ehrlich's magic bullet concept: 100 years of progress. *Nat. Rev.* 2008; 8: 473–80.
6. Duncan R. The dawning era of polymer therapeutics. *Nat. Rev. Drug Discov.* 2003; 2: 347–60.
7. Ferrari M. Cancer nanotechnology: opportunities and challenges. *Nat. Rev.* 2005; 5: 161–71.
8. Maeda H. The enhanced permeability and retention (EPR) effect in tumor vasculature: the key role of tumor-selective macromolecular drug targeting. *Adv. Enzyme Regul.* 2001; 41: 189–207.
9. Davis ME, Zuckerman JE, Choi CH, et al. Evidence of RNAi in humans from systemically administered siRNA via targeted nanoparticles. *Nature.* 2010; 464: 1067–70.
10. Torchilin VP. Recent advances with liposomes as pharmaceutical carriers. *Nat. Rev. Drug Discov.* 2005; 4: 145–60.
11. Nakhaei P, Margiana R, Bokov DO, Abdelbasset WK, Jadidi Kouhbanani MA, Varma RS, Marofi F, Jarahian M, Beheshtkhoo N. Liposomes: structure, biomedical applications, and stability parameters with emphasis on cholesterol. *Front. Bioeng. Biotechnol.* 2021; 9: 705886.
12. Nsairat H, Khater D, Sayed U, Odeh F, Al Bawab A, Alshaer W. Liposomes: structure, composition, types, and clinical applications. *Heliyon.* 2022; 8: e09394.
13. Sahoo SK, Labhasetwar V. Nanotech approaches to drug delivery and imaging. *Drug Discov. Today.* 2003; 8: 1112–1120.
14. Hamilton A, Biganzoli L, Coleman R, et al. EORTC 10968: a phase I clinical and pharmacokinetic study of polyethylene glycol liposomal doxorubicin (Caelyx, Doxil) at a 6-week interval in patients with metastatic breast cancer. *Eur. Organ. Res. Treatment Cancer: Ann. Oncol.* 2002; 13: 910–8.
15. Northfelt DW, Dezube BJ, Thommes JA, et al. Efficacy of pegylatedliposomal doxorubicin in the treatment of AIDS-related Kaposi's sarcoma after failure of standard chemotherapy. *J. Clin. Oncol.* 1997; 15: 653–9.
16. Dritschilo A, Huang CH, Rudin CM, et al. Phase I study of liposomeencapsulated c-raf antisense oligodeoxyribonucleotide infusion in combination with radiation therapy in patients with advanced malignancies. *Clin. Cancer Res.* 2006; 12: 1251–9.
17. Oerlemans C, Bult W, Bos M, Storm G, Nijsen JFW, Hennink WE. Polymeric micelles in anticancer therapy: targeting, imaging and triggered release. *Pharmaceut. Res.* 2010; 27: 2569–89.
18. Huang Y, Jiang K, Zhang X, Chung EJ. The effect of size, charge, and peptide ligand length on kidney targeting by small, organic nanoparticles. *Bioeng. Transl. Med.* 2020; 5: e10173.
19. Ghezzi M, Pescina S, Padula C, Santi P, Del Favero E, Cantù L, Nicoli S. Polymeric micelles in drug delivery: an insight of the techniques for their characterization and assessment in biorelevant conditions. *J. Control. Release.* 2021; 332: 312–36.
20. Lee KS, Chung HC, Im SA, et al. Multicenter phase II trial of Genexol-PM, a Cremophor-free, polymeric micelle formulation of paclitaxel, in patients with metastatic breast cancer. *Breast Cancer Res. Treat.* 2008; 108: 241–50.
21. Bober Z, Bartusik-Aebisher D, Aebisher D. Application of dendrimers in anticancer diagnostics and therapy. *Molecules.* 2022; 27: 3237.
22. Fass L. Imaging and cancer: a review. *Mol. Oncol.* 2008; 2: 115–52.
23. Wolinsky JB, Grinstaff MW. Therapeutic and diagnostic applications of dendrimers for cancer treatment. *Adv. Drug Deliv. Rev.* 2008; 60: 1037–55.
24. Yao H, Veine DM, Fay KS, Staszewski ED, Zeng ZZ, Livant DL. The PHSCN dendrimer as a more potent inhibitor of human breast cancer cell invasion, extravasation, and lung colony formation. *Breast Cancer Res. Treat.* 2011; 125: 363–75.
25. Attia MF, Anton N, Wallyn J, Omran Z, Vandamme TF. An overview of active and passive targeting strategies to improve the nanocarriers efficiency to tumour sites. *J. Pharm. Pharmacol.* 2019 Aug; 71(8): 1185–98.
26. Drummond DC, Noble CO, Guo Z, et al. Development of a highly stable and targetable nanoliposomal formulation of topotecan. *J Control Release* 2010; 141: 13–21.
27. Ruoslahti E. Specialization of tumour vasculature. *Nat. Rev.* 2002; 2: 83–90.
28. Nasongkla N, Shuai X, Ai H, et al. cRGD-functionalized polymer micelles for targeted doxorubicin delivery. *Angew Chem. Int. Ed. Engl.* 2004; 43: 6323–7.
29. Khemtong C, Kessinger CW, Ren J, et al. In vivo off-resonance saturation magnetic resonance imaging of alphavbeta3-targeted superparamagnetic nanoparticles. *Cancer Res.* 2009; 69: 1651–8.

30. Senapati S, Mahanta AK, Kumar S, Maiti P. Controlled drug delivery vehicles for cancer treatment and their performance. *Signal Transd. Target Ther.* 2018 Mar 16; 3(1): 7.
31. Mitragotri S. Healing sound: the use of ultrasound in drug delivery and other therapeutic applications. *Nat. Rev. Drug Discov.* 2005; 4: 255–60.
32. Schroeder A, Honen R, Turjeman K, Gabizon A, Kost J, Barenholz Y. Ultrasound triggered release of cisplatin from liposomes in murine tumors. *J. Control Release.* 2009; 137: 63–8.
33. Piskin E. Molecularly designed water soluble, intelligent, nanosize polymeric carriers. *Int. J. Pharm.* 2004; 277: 105–18.
34. Kono K, Ozawa T, Yoshida T, et al. Highly temperature-sensitive liposomes based on a thermosensitive block copolymer for tumor-specific chemotherapy. *Biomaterials.* 2010; 31: 7096–105.
35. Zhang B, Zhang Y, Liao Z, et al. UPA-sensitive ACPP-conjugated nanoparticles for multi-targeting therapy of brain glioma. *Biomaterials.* 2015; 36: 98–109.
36. Rastegari E, Hsiao Y-J, Lai W-Y, Lai Y-H, Yang T-C, Chen S-J, Huang P-I, Chiou S-H, Mou C-Y, Chien Y. An update on mesoporous silica nanoparticle applications in nanomedicine. *Pharmaceutics.* 2021; 13: 1067.
37. Ferrari M. Frontiers in cancer nanomedicine: directing mass transport through biological barriers. *Trends Biotechnol.* 2010; 28: 181–8.
38. Huang P, Lian D, Ma H, Gao N, Zhao L, Luan P, Zeng X. New advances in gated materials of mesoporous silica for drug controlled release. *Chin. Chem. Lett.* 2021; 32: 3696–704.
39. Decuzzi P, Ferrari M. Design maps for nanoparticles targeting the diseased microvasculature. *Biomaterials.* 2008; 29: 377–84.
40. Decuzzi P, Godin B, Tanaka T, et al. Size and shape effects in the biodistribution of intravascularly injected particles. *J. Control Release.* 2010; 141: 320–7.
41. Serda RE, Gu J, Bhavane RC, et al. The association of silicon microparticles with endothelial cells in drug delivery to the vasculature. *Biomaterials.* 2009; 30: 2440–8.
42. Godin B, Gu J, Serda RE, et al. Tailoring the degradation kinetics of mesoporous silicon structures through PEGylation. *J. Biomed. Mater. Res. A.* 2010; 94: 1236–43.
43. Tanaka T, Mangala LS, Vivas-Mejia PE, et al. Sustained small interfering RNA delivery by mesoporous silicon particles. *Cancer Res.* 2010; 70: 3687–96.
44. Ananta JS, Godin B, Sethi R, et al. Geometrical confinement of gadoliniumbased contrast agents in nanoporous particles enhances T(1) contrast. *Nat. Nanotechnol.* 2010; 5: 815–21.
45. Paliwal R, Babu RJ, Palakurthi S. Nanomedicine scale-up technologies: Feasibilities and challenges. *AAPS Pharm. Sci. Tech.* 2014; 15: 1527–34.
46. Falagan-Lotsch P, Grzincic EM, Murphy CJ. New advances in nanotechnology-based diagnosis and therapeutics for breast cancer: an assessment of active-targeting inorganic nanoplatforms. *Bioconjugate Chem.* 2017; 28: 135–52.
47. Shi J, Kantoff PW, Wooster R, Farokhzad OC. Cancer nanomedicine: progress, challenges and opportunities. *Nat. Rev. Cancer.* 2017; 17: 20–37.
48. Kemp JA, Kwon YJ. Cancer nanotechnology: current status and perspectives. *Nano Converg.* 2021; 8: 34. doi: 10.1186/s40580-021-00282-7

2 Technology Utilizing Nanoparticles in Treating Cancer

2.1 INTRODUCTION

A paradigm shift in the field of drug delivery for oncological interventions has been brought about by nanoparticles. To be more precise, lipid, polymeric, and liposome nanoparticles have all been carefully designed to encapsulate and aid in the delivery of chemotherapy drugs. By doing this, they have skillfully overcome obstacles related to drug solubility and systemic toxicity, thereby announcing the advent of several drug delivery systems based on nanoparticles that are presently advancing through different phases of clinical development [1].

The strategic incorporation of nanoparticles has greatly enhanced the integration of imaging methodologies into the fields of cancer diagnostics and therapeutic monitoring. These small structures can be used to track the spread of therapeutic agents in real-time and visualize neoplastic lesions instantly when they are carefully loaded with imaging moieties like gold nanoparticles and quantum dots [2]. Due to these surface alterations, the emerging nanomaterials exhibit distinct capabilities depending on inherent features including form and size (Figure 2.1).

Oncology has already begun to enjoy the advantages of revolutionary nanoscale technologies, and the area promises to profit significantly from breakthroughs in nanotechnology [3]. Advances in illness diagnosis, imaging, and treatment have resulted from these advancements. According to the National Cancer Institute (NCI), nanotechnology may revolutionize cancer detection, treatment, and prevention [4]. The development of novel nanotechnology platforms, government funding, as well as venture capital investment have all increased as an outcome of the growing fascination with nanotechnology for therapeutic purposes among academic and industrial researchers [5]. It has been possible for nanotechnology to tackle critical medical problems because of the financing and early clinical results that have been available. As a result of the early success of cancer, other medical issues, such as cardiovascular disease and vaccinations, have been influenced by nanotechnology [6].

Nanotechnology has a lot of promise to change the way medications are distributed. Clinical translation of several different nanoscale systems for drug delivery has already shown the influence, even if the full potential of these systems is yet to be achieved [7]. Small molecules (hydrophilic and/or hydrophobic), nucleic acids, peptides, and protein-based medicines may all be enveloped in nanoscale drug delivery vehicles [8]. Solubility and stability of the medications may be increased by encasing them in a nanocarrier, which allows us to reconsider promising drugs previously overlooked due to their substandard pharmacokinetics. Encapsulated molecules might be delivered by nanocarriers gradually and deliberately to maintain a drug concentration below a therapeutic window. Alternatively, they may be released in response to a stimulus unique to the delivery area [9]. Designing the nanocarrier's surface might change the biological distribution as well as lengthen

DOI: 10.1201/9781003451020-2

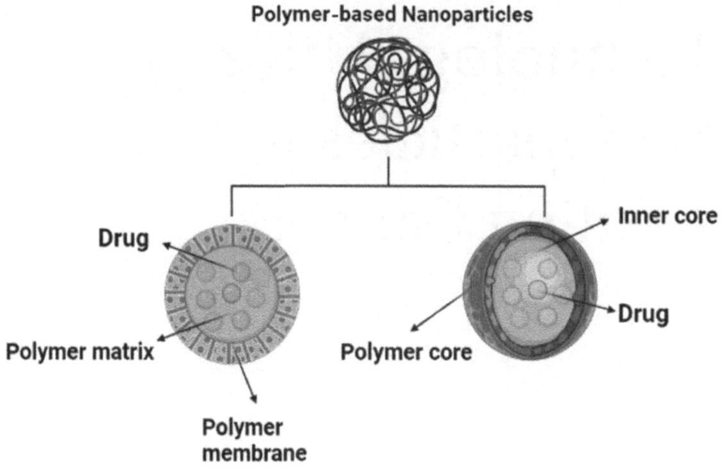

FIGURE 2.1 Structure of nanoparticle drug delivery system. (Created with Biorenders.com.)

the half-life of blood circulation, and attaching ligands that target the surface might increase the absorption by target tissues [10].

The diagnosis and treatment of cancer may be completely changed by nanotechnology. The potential to eradicate cancerous tumors with the least amount of harm to healthy tissue and organs is provided by the application of nanotechnology in cancer treatment. While some approaches have advanced to the preclinical or clinical trial stage, the majority of efforts to enhance cancer treatment through nanotechnology are still in the research or development stage. One treatment is targeted chemotherapy, which gives cancer tumors a dose of tumor necrosis factor-alpha (TNF), a substance that kills tumors [11]. TNF and polyethylene glycol that have been thiol-derivatized (PEG-THIOL) are attached to a gold nanoparticle to conceal the TNF-containing nanoparticle from the immune system. As a result, the nanoparticle is safe to travel through the circulation without being attacked. The CytImmune company developed this targeted chemotherapy technique to deliver TNF and other chemotherapy drugs to cancer tumors [12]. It is possible to use nanoparticle delivery systems to create new methods of medication delivery that might lead to new or complementary therapy options for illness [13].

The investigation of nanoparticle technology in the chapter will be primarily focused on the creation of nanocarrier systems to deliver drugs for tumor therapeutic applications (Figure 2.2). The presented class of nanoparticles includes a variety of distinct forms, such as polymeric nanoparticles, dendrimer nanoparticles, magnetic nanoparticles, nanoshells, and liposomes [14]. There will not be any mention of nucleic acid delivery methods, although they have already been widely described elsewhere.

The following section will cover both non-targeted as well as targeted nanocarriers for the treatment of cancer. For example, the FDA has authorized several first-generation nanocarriers for treatment, as well as several targeted nanocarriers that are now in clinical development. The chapter will concentrate on a variety of systems now undergoing clinical trials to clarify how nanocarrier systems are being created for clinical usage [15].

2.2 NOVEL APPROACHES OF NANOPARTICLES FOR DRUG DELIVERY

Initial reports of lipid vesicles from the 1960s led to the development of the term "liposomes," which were the first nanoscale drug delivery vehicles. As a result of these advancements, modern nanoparticle technologies are possible [16]. The first macromolecule delivery devices using controlled-release polymer polymers were disclosed in 1976 [17]. The first targeted liposome application was made in 1980 [18]. In the years 1990 and 1994, correspondingly, polyethylene glycol

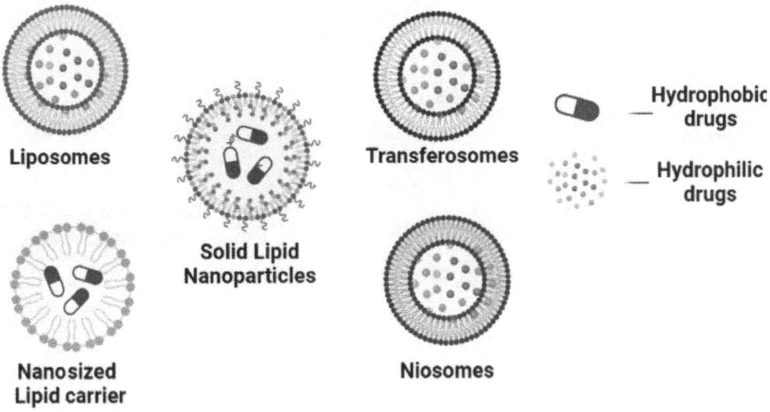

FIGURE 2.2 Various types of nanoparticulate system.

(PEG) was used for coating the surfaces of polymeric nanoparticles and liposomes, which resulted in longer circulation periods or "stealth" properties [19]. These developments led to the approval of Doxil, a doxorubicin-encapsulated vesicle system of administration that has been demonstrated to be a successful therapy for numerous types of cancer [20].

Since then, nanoparticles with several functions and "smart" qualities, such as the capacity to adapt to the environment, have been developed as a result of extensive study into their development [21]. There are now 361 clinical trials testing vesicle-based carriers, 208 clinical trials evaluating drug conjugates, and 70 clinical studies investigating nanoparticle carriers. Combination therapy and medications administered by different channels, such as the pulmonary and oral, are all part of the clinical studies [22].

Furthermore, the field of nanomedicine is a trailblazer in nanotechnology, focusing on the creation of potent methods for delivering specific biological compounds for therapeutic purposes and treating illnesses. With a few notable exceptions, injectables are the only way to administer biologics like therapeutic proteins, peptides, and antibodies. The development of painless injections, targeted therapy, and improved drug penetration of the blood–brain barrier (BBB) have all been accelerated by the use of nanodrug delivery. With the advent of liposome-mediated drug delivery methods and the encapsulation of medications like doxorubicin and CabiliviTM as nanosized drugs, researchers have advanced the applications of nanotechnology in medicine in this century. Promising outcomes are observed when lipid nanoparticles mediate synthetic compounds into nanodrugs [23]. Any drug delivery system's primary goal is to increase the effectiveness of treatments by regulating drug concentrations under the therapeutic window, minimizing cytotoxic effects, and enhancing patient compliance (Figure 2.3). As a result, treatment cycles may be kept as effective as possible while causing less harm to good cells and requiring less time to recover.

2.2.1 Liposomal Nanoparticles

Liposomes may increase the efficiency of treatment and improve drug delivery to brain tumors. By releasing their cargo in particular areas of the extravascular space and vasculature of the tumor, they carry out their therapeutic action. To deliver anticancer medications, liposomes can be directed to particular regions of the BBB or glioblastoma multiforme (GBM) tumors through targeted delivery [24, 25]. While hydrophobic molecules can be discovered in the hydrophobic regions of the lipid bilayer, hydrophilic substances can be located in the inner watery phase of the lipid bilayer [25]. By simply fusing easily accessible lipid molecules on the market, you can alter the charge on the surface, functionality, and size of the liposomes. DSPE (1,2-distearoylsn-glycero-3-phosphoethanolamine),

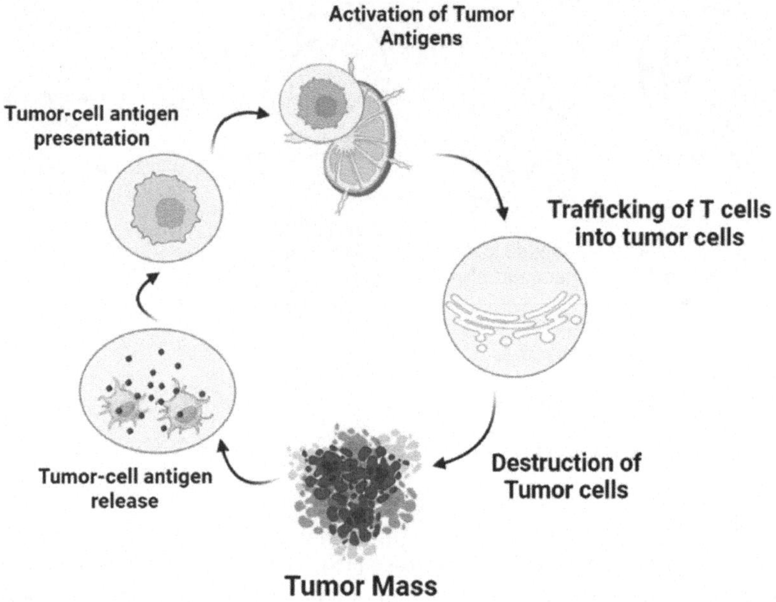

FIGURE 2.3 Cancer cell pathway.

HSPC (hydrogenated phosphatidylcholine derived by soybean lecithin), EggPG (egg yolk phosphatidylglycerol), and DSPC are among the lipids used in the creation of vesicular formulations. In comparison to alternate carriers, which necessitate several additional synthesis steps plus chemical modifications, resulting in a significant improvement. FDA-approved chemical 1,2-distearoyl-glycero-3-phosphocholine is normally present in human bodies [26, 27]. PEG, a substance that can be used to change the liposome's surface, can be used in the production of any of these lipids. Doxil, a pegylated liposome that is therapeutically utilized to treat various cancers, is an important development for liposomal drug delivery systems. The drug doxorubicin is loaded into Doxil, which has a loaded pegylated surface (2 kDa PEG chains), via diffusion of the drug with an ammonium salt gradient. The technique provides a long-term way of medication encapsulation in a crystal form along with little leakage. Doxil liposomes possess a surface charge of approximately 10 mV and a 2-year shelf life at 4°C [28]. Aphios Corp. recently made nanosomes (small liposomes, 100 nm) containing many drugs, including docetaxel, camptothecin, and bryostatin-1, as well as vitamin D analog for treating several types of tumors utilizing a production method based on the supercritical fluid procedure [29]. Novosom AG utilizes amphoteric liposomes as part of its nucleic acid delivery process. Variations in solution pH may affect the liposomal formulation's zeta potential. With endocytosis absorption occurring at an acidic pH, a charge switch allows nanocarriers to escape into the cytoplasm, where they may then deliver the therapeutic load [30].

Long circulating liposomes are one type of nanoparticle that makes use of the blood vessels' tendency to leak in tumor tissues. Liposomes can passively cross the capillary endothelial barrier and enter the interstitial space because tumor blood vessels have more fenestrations. Vascular endothelial cells are closely packed together with small para-cellular gaps ranging from 5 to 10 nm in normal non-tumor tissues. On the other hand, depending on the type of cancer, the distances between endothelial cells in tumor blood vessels can vary greatly, from 100 to 700 nm. Furthermore, solid tumors have an unorganized vascular architecture and an ineffective lymphatic system. The limited lymphatic drainage and leaky tumor vasculature combine to create an effect known as the enhanced permeability and retention (EPR) effect, which permits liposomes to passively accumulate and dispose of themselves inside the tumor site [31]. There are even severe side effects associated with liposomal formulations because of their accumulation in skin tissue. Though controlling the kinetics of long-term drug release using liposomal systems is a tough task, it is possible to create environmentally triggered release by introducing destabilizing lipids into the vesicle membrane or adding other ingredients like morpholine to the lipid formulation [32]. Lipid-based vesicles present several challenges in clinical trials for liposomal formulations alongside triggered drug release because they are unstable in the bloodstream, poorly soluble in lipid/surfactant solutions, and have a rapid, burst release of the drug. Currently, there are no approved or in-development liposomal formulations. However, LiPlasom Pharma has created non-targeted liposomes, which are intended to be destroyed by PLA2 as PLA2 is up-regulated in the cancer microenvironment [33]. Liposomes are a desirable drug delivery system because of their unique physicochemical characteristics, which enable them to overcome a range of obstacles and constraints. Numerous biomedical fields have been significantly impacted by the use of liposomes to enhance drug delivery. Research has demonstrated that liposomes can enhance the stability and biodistribution of medicinal agents, surmount restrictions on tissue and cellular uptake in target sites during *in vivo* testing, and mitigate systemic toxicity linked to non-encapsulated agents. But despite a great deal of preclinical research on liposomes, their clinical application has only made slow progress [34].

Multidrug delivery is also possible with the method. Azaya Therapeutics is investigating liposomal protein stabilization for the delivery of hydrophobic medicines like docetaxel for tumor treatment. Docetaxel is enclosed in a bilayer of liposomes and stabilized with the help of albumin to prevent quick drug leakage (ATI1123) [35]. According to effectiveness trials using human xenograft mouse models for pancreatic, prostate, as well as non-small-cell lung cancer (NSCL cancer), ATI-1123 was 90% more effective than docetaxel at the same doses (25 mg kg^1) in the PC3 tumor xenograft model. ATI-1123 has a slower plasma elimination time and better bioavailability than free docetaxel, which may explain this further [36].

2.2.2 Polymer–Drug Conjugated Nanoparticles

PDCs, or polymer-drug conjugates, have demonstrated great promise in improving the safety and effectiveness of cancer treatments. These conjugates result in better pharmacokinetics, regulated drug release, and targeted delivery to tumor tissues by combining the beneficial aspects of both polymers and pharmaceuticals. First, a discussion is held regarding the different types of polymers that are used in these conjugates. These include natural polymers like hyaluronic acid (HA) and synthetic polymers like poly(↗-caprolactone) (PCL), D-α-tocopheryl polyethylene glycol (TPGS), and polyethylene glycol (PEG). To achieve desired qualities like stability, biocompatibility, and controlled drug release, the polymer of choice is essential. The methods for conjugating drugs to polymers are then discussed. One such method is covalent bonding, which creates a stable bond between the drug and the polymer and ensures controlled release while reducing drug release too soon. By increasing the drug's circulation time, the use of polymers can promote enhanced drug accumulation within tumor tissues by the enhanced permeability and retention (EPR) effect [37, 38].

The HPMA backbone copolymer serves as the foundation for the drug, which is identical to Prolindac(AP5346), having platinum grafted onto its side chains via a chelator sensitive to pH for releasing of drugs in the tumor surroundings [39]. In preclinical models of numerous diseases, especially sarcoma M5076, multiple colon xenografts, as well as leukemia L1210 and 0157 hybridomas, which are platinum-resistant tumor xenografts, it is depicted that polymer-drug conjugates are more efficacious. Using a 25 kDa polymer chain, the oxaliplatin loading of the drug was lower than 10% (w/w) plus the drug release was sluggish [40]. Because of a higher intracellular amount of Pt, the polymer-drug conjugates significantly reduced tumor growth when administered once per week for 3 weeks. Platinum-resistant ovarian cancer responded to weekly injections of 640 mg Pt m^2 for

3 weeks in a clinical study in Europe [41]. Clinically, according to Access Pharmaceuticals Inc.'s phase II findings, 66% of ovarian cancer patients saw significant disease stabilization and little side effects [41].

By developing the conjugation of drugs to immunoglobulin, researchers introduced the significant phenomenon of PDCs and laid the foundation for conventionally targeted drug delivery systems. As a result, numerous PDC systems based on PVP of different antibiotic agents have been created to offer prolonged half-lives, selective targeting, and sustained release of medications into the bloodstream, including penicillin. Other researchers found that a wide variety of enzymes found in macromolecules' lysosomotropic and the lysosomal compartment of cells can break down PDCs. In 1975, Helmut Ringsdorf presented the basis of PDCs for targeted drug carriers based on the interpretation of these findings. Since then, the field of polymeric conjugates (PDCs) has experienced rapid growth, with almost a dozen polymeric conjugates advancing to clinical trial studies. The first generation of PDCs has also been used to treat diseases; one such application is the use of polyethylene glycol (PEG), which has been a PEGylated protein of bovine serum albumin conjugated [42–46].

2.2.3 Polymeric Nanoparticles

When compared to other types of NPs, polymeric NPs have distinct properties such as water solubility, biodegradability, nontoxicity, low cost, simple incorporation, and extended shelf life. These attributes are also dependent on the delivery system used. The term "shelf life" describes how long PNPs are reusable, safe for ingestion, or marketable. Furthermore, light, temperature, pH, NP size, and molecular weight are the most frequent variables that impact the stability of PNPs. By preventing instability in suspension, lyophilization has been utilized to improve PNPs' long-term stability for drug delivery implementations. Molecular imaging and freeze-drying, when combined with the right cryoprotectants, can also get around restrictions and increase shelf life [47]. Polymer-based controlled macromolecule release was proven by Langer and Folkman, paving the way for the creation of antiangiogenic drug delivery systems and cancer therapies. A renaissance in fascination with nanoparticles made of polymers along with their therapeutic potential resulted from Langer *et al.*'s description of PLA/PLGA and PEG block copolymer nanoparticles as "long-circulating nanoparticles" in 1994 [48]. In the 1990s, the approach of drug delivery using polymeric nanoparticles was infrequently employed, but approximately 200 papers utilizing the method were published in 2008.

They can be produced artificially or naturally, and they can be biodegradable or not. Polymeric nanoparticles provide tremendous versatility in design. PLA, dextran, and chitosan are some of the most often utilized polymers for nanoparticle production [49]. Metabolic processes normally remove and metabolize biodegradable polymer monomers, which are metabolized and excreted from the body. A polymer's dispersity index, molecular weight, hydrophobicity, as well as crystallinity characteristics can be changed to alter the way that it degrades and releases chemicals into the environment [50]. Medication delivery may be controlled due to the diffusion of the drug via the polymer matrix or actuated in reaction to the local environment. To stabilize nanoparticles, decrease hepatic absorption, and increase circulation half-life, hydrophilic polymers like PEG might be grafted, conjugated, or adsorb to their surfaces [51].

In different phases of preclinical and clinical research, many polymeric nanoparticles are presently available for use. Oral consumption of polymethacrylate nanocapsules loaded with drug (400 nm) encapsulated in 2–10-mm microspheres based on cellulose leads to absorption by M-cells as well as a drug blood bioavailability of less than 5%. Nanolymf Ltd. has developed microparticles containing nanocapsules that included pharmaceuticals, for instance. Particle form, size, and mechanical flexibility interact with cell membranes and regulate their internalization routes, as shown by Chu *et al.* "PRINT" technique (particle replication in non-wetting templates) has led to the preclinical development of polymeric for tumor treatment and various disorders [52].

2.2.4 Micelle-Based Nanoparticles

Micelles are multifunctional nanoscale structures made of molecules with amphiphilicity. The reasons behind their multifunctionality and possible applications in various clinical contexts include their small size, ability to encapsulate both hydrophilic and hydrophobic compounds, and ease of functionalization. Because they can transport hydrophobic anticancer medications to tumor sites, micelles have significant uses in cancer therapy. Applications that go beyond the administration of hydrophobic medications have been investigated recently [53]. Numerous studies have been conducted on the modification of the hydrophobicity, hydrophilicity, and stimuli-responsiveness of the corresponding micelles and polymers, as well as the surface modification of these entities using active targeting ligands. PM-based systems may hold the key to more effective treatments for solid tumors because they can optimize the system's thermodynamic and kinetic stability, control particle size, encapsulate large amounts of drugs, and decorate the particles' surfaces with ligands for active targeting. Furthermore, the delivery of genetic material as non-viral vectors through PM-based systems has resulted in the development of numerous formulations that are presently undergoing evaluation [54]. PDLLA (1.75 kDa) and mPEG (2 kDa) create the block copolymer known as "Genexol-PM," which forms micelles having an approximate size of 60 nm plus a paclitaxel loading of about 15% (weight for weight). Genexol-PM has a maximum tolerated dose (MTD) that is three times greater compared to Taxol's (20 mg kg^1), and one study reported that Genexol-PM's median lethal dosage (LD50) in Sprague-Dawley rats was 20 times greater than Taxol's. It is noteworthy to observe that both formulations' AUC values were the same. The Genexol-PM formulation caused paclitaxel to accumulate more significantly in organs like the liver and the tumor, which led to different tumor cytotoxicity and a reduction in tumor volume. The recommended dose for Genexol-MTD PMs was determined to be 300 mg m^2 according to the findings of a clinical phase I trial, even though Genexol-MTD PMs had almost twice the potency of Taxol (Kim and colleagues 2004). In clinical research conducted in Korea, the co-treatment of advanced NSCL with Genexol-PM and cisplatin was compared to a single-agent treatment (Kim and colleagues 2007a) [55]. The clinical phase II data depicted that with slightly lesser doses of cisplatin compared to the combination therapy of Taxol and cisplatin (60 mg m^2 vs. 75 mg m^2, respectively), 30% of the total patients showed a stable status of the disease, as well as 60% of the total patients, experienced an improved survival of a single year. Other companies, like Labopharm and Intezym, are trying to develop microparticle delivery methods using polyamino acids as well as synthetic polymers with diameters that range from 10 to 200 nm [56].

2.2.5 Dendrimer-Based Nanoparticles

Pharmacological compounds are carried by dendrimers to their unique properties. Encapsulation is done when the drug is contained within the dendrimer's cavities to produce a sustained release conjugate. Pharmaceutical substances are being utilized more and more as carriers for dendrimers. These substances can be encapsulated, or enclosed within the cavities of the dendrimer, or they can be placed on the surface of the dendrimer. With the three-dimensional dendrimer structure, a large range of medications can be used to create physiologically active drug conjugates. The ability of dendrimers to pass through the cell membrane has led to their use as non-viral gene transporters. New-generation vaccines can be made with dendrimers. Presently, the most promising fields in the fight against cancer are combination therapy and nanotechnology [57].

"Avidimers" are dendrimers that are functionalized with small targeting ligands and directed to the tumor vasculature using a PAMAM bioconjugation platform. "Avidimers" have been produced by Baker *et al.* [58]. A day later, various dendrimers (8% to 10% folate-targeted I.D./g of tissue for the target and non-targeted dendrimers, respectively) accumulated in a xenograft tumor model. Higher tumor accumulation was associated with slower tumor development, lower toxicity, as well as longer life spans as compared to a free drug of the same dose. Majorly, the latest investigations utilizing nanoparticles of transferrin-cyclodextrin-siRNA (CALAA-01) in animal models of human epithelial carcinoma depicted a decrease in the size of the tumor as well as differential distribution in cancerous cells. Preclinical information prompted CALAA-01's development to be expedited. After the release of the toxicological information regarding CALAA-01 (the initial targeted, nanoparticle platform based on the polymer for non-human primates) in April 2007, an experimental new drug application was made and human clinical studies for the treatment of solid tumors began in May 2008 [59].

2.2.6 Polymersomal Nanoparticles

For the past few decades, polymeric nanovesicles, also known as polymersomes, have been studied as a possible nanocarrier platform. Our basic understanding of how to modify physicochemical properties—such as size and shape, surface chemistry and functionalization, and membrane characteristics—has improved as a result of these studies. Beyond just drug delivery, polymersomes can be used for cancer treatment due to their high structural stability and versatile nature. To improve cancer immunotherapy, rational nanocarrier design enables spatiotemporal control over the activity of particular immune cell targets [60]. LNPs and polymersomes both have comparable levels of size control in the nanoscale range. However, in terms of shape, polymersomes are superior to LNPs because they can be kinetically trapped in a range of shapes, including discs, ellipsoids, and tubes, whereas LNPs are only able to maintain a spherical shape. It is possible to adjust the size and shape of polymersomes during or after the process of self-assembly, which has been thoroughly examined elsewhere [61]. Polymersomes are more stable and lateral fluid than liposomes, and the breakdown of the polymer chain as well as the instability of the shell layer trigger the release. White blood cells had affixed to and taken up polymersomes within ten hours after incubation in the circulation [62]. Following a single injection via intravenous route, polymersomes carrying 2.5 mg kg^1 of paclitaxel as well as doxorubicin, the maximally tolerated doses of each drug, were demonstrated to be efficacious in a breast cancer tumor xenograft model. The tumor size decreased five days following injection, as opposed to the free medication formulations [62].

2.2.7 Protein-Based Nanoparticles

The health of people has been seriously threatened by cancer. Protein nanoparticles are distinct among drug delivery vehicles due to their gentle and eco-friendly preparation techniques. Additionally, they inherit desirable properties like biocompatibility and biodegradability from natural proteins. As a result, they have found solutions to a few issues with inorganic nanocarriers, like their low biocompatibility. Additionally, protein nanoparticles' surface groups and cavities make it simple to modify the surface and load drugs. Furthermore, to create multifunctional theranostic platforms, protein nanoparticles can be mixed with inorganic nanoparticles or contrast agents. Albumin-based nanoparticles loaded with paclitaxel are one of the FDA-approved medications for clinically treating metastatic breast cancer, called Abraxane®. By preventing breast cancer cells from dividing, the medication can stop tumor growth. Additionally, by using albumin, the most abundant protein in humans, it is possible to prevent the hypersensitivity brought on by earlier drug solvents like Cremophor EL [63,64]. Also, in preclinical studies, the amount of paclitaxel attached to albumin was significantly increased in endothelial cells as well as the extravascular space (3–10 times). The observations suggest that whereas albumin may have intrinsic tumor-targeting properties, the effect of EPR may potentially contribute to tumor accumulation. The albumin-bound formulation of paclitaxel was found to be both more efficient and safe than the formulation of Taxol (260 mg/m^2 vs. 175 mg/m^2, correspondingly) [65]. Abraxane is nowadays being investigated as first-line treatment or as a complex with other different drugs (like rapamycin, verinostat, etc.) for treating metastatic breast cancer along with additional tumors, such as ovarian as well as prostate, that are responsive to taxane treatments. One drug being investigated as a platform for the administration of other water-insoluble substances, such as albumin, is rapamycin (2.5 mg ml^{-1}). An albumin-bound rapamycin (ABI-009) therapeutic research for non-hematologic malignancies has been going on since January 2008 [66].

2.2.8 Biological Nanoparticles

Bacteria are single-celled microorganisms, which include cytoplasmic components plus the hydrophobic molecules and hydrophilic molecules. They are an instance of a biological nanoparticle. EnGeneIC Pty Ltd has created a medication delivery device dubbed a "nanocell" that comprises anucleate globular bacteria (about 400 nm in diameter). Endogenous mutations and replication are prevented in the absence of DNA, as was first documented in 1967. According to a recent study, doxorubicin, paclitaxel, and siRNA, for instance, may be loaded into a nanocell via diffusion of drug in the bacteria under a few hours. Large animals like pigs and monkeys have not shown any harmful effects from repeated high-titer doses, although an immune response to lipopolysaccharide-containing carriers is a possibility (LPS) [67, 68].

2.2.9 Inorganic Nanoparticles

With their ability to target ligands to maximize therapeutic effect and reduce off-target side effects through drug adsorption and infiltration, inorganic nanoparticles for drug delivery in cancer treatment offer numerous potential benefits. While oncogene suppression, cancer cell signaling pathway inhibition, and cytotoxicity were the initial uses of inorganic nanoparticles as drug carriers, they have since been shown to have a variety of other therapeutic properties. The most promising cutting-edge approaches to cancer treatment are as synergistic drug delivery agents for the inhibition of cancer cell signaling pathways and as synergistic platforms for RNA interference (siRNA, miRNA, and shRNA) [69,70]. In clinical phase II research, nanoparticles of iron oxide covered with aminosilane (Nanotherm M01) are being used to induce hyperthermia and thermoablation for treating recurrent prostate cancer plus brain cancer in Germany. Phase I studies demonstrated that magnetic iron oxide nanoparticles may destroy prostate tumor cells locally. For 2 months, patients received weekly treatments of one hour of nanoparticle injection utilizing ultrasound guidance to target specific tumors [71]. It is possible to use magnetic fields (50 and 100 kHz) to create heat from tiny nanoparticles (20 nm) that can pass through tumors, infiltrate cancer cells, and heat a 20-cm-diameter circle of tissue. The authors did note some slight discomfort due to internal warmth, but no dose-limiting toxicities were noted. Gold-coated silica nanoparticles, which absorb the near-infrared laser radiation as well as change it to heat are being studied as a possible therapy for head as well as neck cancer [72]. Researchers discovered that nanoparticles employed in NIR thermal treatment caused irreparable harm to cancer tissue if heated to less than 40°C utilizing human breast cancer xenograft mice. The dispersed nature of nanoshells present inside the treated tumor volume was the cause of the significant temperature variance seen across treated animals (28–60°C). A few millimeters below the skin was where the temperature was highest, aside from that. Recently, the same 150-nm nanoparticles were used to treat brain tumors in an orthotopic canine model. Percutaneously infiltrated NIR fibers reached temperatures of 70°C in tumor tissues and 50°C in normal white and gray matter, killing tumors and causing significant damage to brain tissue not affected by the disease. It is expected to cause significant brain damage [73].

Gold nanoparticles' surface characteristics and capabilities have also been employed to deliver surface-bound medicines. For solid tumor treatment, CytImmune Sciences, Inc. has developed Aurimune(CYT-6091), an instance of tumor necrosis factor-alpha (TNF-alpha) coupled to gold nanoparticles coated with PEG (27 nm) [74]. To reduce systemic toxicities when used as an anticancer treatment, cytokines like TNF-alpha require a nanocarrier formulation. The SCK mammary tumor xenograft mouse model was used to test the effectiveness of nanoparticle formulations in slowing tumor development with local heating (42°C for 1 hour) [75]. However, the combination therapy demonstrated better effectiveness and a reduction in intratumor blood flow compared to single treatments. In breast tumor tissue sections, SEM micrographs of nanoparticles accumulating in contrast to healthy tissue suggested that the EPR effect may be responsible for their targeting. TNF plus paclitaxel or doxorubicin/interleukin-12 are only some of the many medication combinations presently under investigation. However, because of the surface adsorption density, the therapeutic agent's load is several hundred molecules, which may restrict its effectiveness [76]. Adair's team recently reported encapsulating organic substances in nanocomposite particles of calcium phosphate (27 nm) for imaging as well as delivery inside the cells. These biocompatible nanoparticles based on calcium phosphate may be used for controlling the release of chemicals in acidic tumor surroundings [77]. In *in vitro* studies using bovine endothelial cells, ceramide (Cer-6) treatment to human vesicular smooth muscular cells led to 100% suppression of cell growth [78]. A multitude of potential pathways exist within nanomedicine to address some of the drawbacks of traditional medicine. One such pathway is the improvement of cancer treatment's therapeutic efficacy through the benefits of (i) targeted delivery; (ii) drug stability; (iii) increased solubility; (iv) optimized half-life; (v) delivery of drugs responsive to stimuli; (vi) transportation of multiple therapeutic candidates; and (vii) circumvention of biological barriers. INPs, or inorganic nanoparticles, are becoming the main players in utilizing these tactics [79].

2.2.10 Hybridized Nanoparticles

Recently, two different forms of hybrid nanoparticles—solid liposomal nanoparticles and lipid-polymer nanoparticles—were created by fusing the advantages of existing systems with well-characterized characteristics. Hybrid nanoparticles have at minimum two distinct materials in their core as well as the corona. To generate a protective membrane (corona) like a liposome or micelle, metallic and polymeric components are coated with one or more lipid layers [80]. Hybrid nanoparticles for cancer treatment have been created by us and others. Based on studies in melanoma and Lewis lung carcinoma models, Sasisekharan and colleagues have shown that bi-phospholipid-coated PLGA-core nanoparticles can transport various medicines for the treatment of cancer [81]. Nanoparticles defined as "nanocells" are formed by combining doxorubicin with PLGA and combrestatin with phospholipids during the self-assembly process, resulting in nanoparticles with a doxorubicin concentration of 1% by weight and a combrestatin encapsulation effectiveness of 70% [82]. To reduce the density of the tumor's blood vessels, combrestatin was administered first. Doxorubicin was then released to destroy cancer cells [83]. The medications were delivered over 3 days at varied rates. Results demonstrated that tumor development was significantly slowed in both cancer models as a consequence of the EPR effect and that survival time was enhanced as a result. Cerulean Pharma is currently doing preclinical testing of its nanocell technology. Others showed combination therapy *in vitro* and *in vivo* using solid-lipid nanoparticles made from various polymers and formulas. An encapsulating technique for PEG liposomes comprising hydrophobic polymer core (PLA) was recently disclosed by Thevenot *et al.* [84]. Sterically stabilizing lipoparticles with excellent colloidal stability require PEG chain length, which was proven by using PEG (5 kDa) at a lipid content of 10%. PLA nanoparticles, with a diameter of 100 nm, self-assembled a single lipid layer on their hydrophobic surfaces [84]. The charge along with targeted ligand densities can be carefully modified by surface functionalization employing a variety of lipid components. This leads to the formulations of hybrid nanoparticles that are stable [85]. Because the layer of lipids on the exterior of the nanoparticles influenced the release kinetics of docetaxel, the drug's loading was raised to 8% of the total mass of the nanoparticles. The delivery of various drugs or radiation sensitizers, combination treatment methods like photothermal drug delivery, or the simultaneous administration of therapeutic pharmaceuticals plus imaging agents are just a few examples of the myriad cancer therapies that can now be combined [86].

2.3 TECHNIQUES FOR UTILIZING NANOPARTICLES FOR CANCER THERAPEUTICS

2.3.1 Nanoparticles For Cancer Metastasis

Metastasis is the main cause of cancer-related morbidity and death. It is the process by which cancer cells travel from the original tumor to nearby tissues and even distant organs. Cancer cells must separate from the original tumor, intravasate into the lymphatic and circulatory systems, elude the immune system, extravasate at distant capillary beds, invade, and multiply in distant organs to complete the metastatic cascade. There are currently several theories being put forth to try and explain where cancer metastasizes. These include the epithelial-mesenchymal transition, stem cell mutation accumulation, the facilitation of macrophages, and the origin of macrophages through transformation or fusion hybridization with neoplastic cells. Common macrophages share many characteristics with metastatic cancer cells [87, 88].

A deeper understanding of cancer biology, notably the function of the microenvironment, signaling pathways, and metastatic development, can be linked to advancements in cancer treatment. The epidermal growth factor receptor inhibitors, matrix metalloproteinases, transferases, and migration and angiogenesis have also been developed. Contrary to imatinib (a tyrosine kinase inhibitor for gastrointestinal stromal tumors), most contemporary therapies have only minimally increased life periods across several cancer types due to the intricacy of tumor growth, tumor makeup, blood vascular architecture, and drug resistance mechanisms [89]. The creation and assessment of prospective medication combinations have been made possible because of advances in the understanding of pharmacological action routes and cellular drug resistance mechanisms. Drug combinations are frequently tried to improve the effectiveness of the primary agent or to block alternate routes to prevent drug susceptibility to the primary agent. Combinations of medications have the significant advantage of preventing the occurrence of resistance to drugs during tumor treatment without aggravating the known side effects of individual agents [90]. Despite the widely accepted idea that cancer growth as well as metastasis are adaptive mechanisms, higher dosages of single drugs may in some situations prevent susceptibility processes *in vitro.* But in humans, multidrug regimens containing combined effects are depicted to be more efficacious, maybe because of the heterogeneity of the cells in the tumor along with the patient. Multidrug therapy necessitates laborious dose schedules. Using nanoparticle delivery techniques, both of these problems may be solved [91]. When compared to free delivery of drugs in both non-targeted as well as targeted delivery modes, nanoparticle administration of individual medications results in greater amounts of the drug in the tumor and permits bigger dosages. Without the need for complex multidrug regimens, there are numerous ways to combine multiple drugs into a single nanoparticle, improving patient compliance and lowering the likelihood of side effects.

2.3.2 Passive Targeting by Nanoparticles

The process of passive targeting enables the deposition of nanovectors in the tumor microenvironment because of unique features of the tumor environment that are absent from healthy tissues. In addition to characteristics of the nanoparticle itself, such as size, shape, and surface charge, factors related to the tumor microvasculature also influence the delivery of nanoparticles. To improve

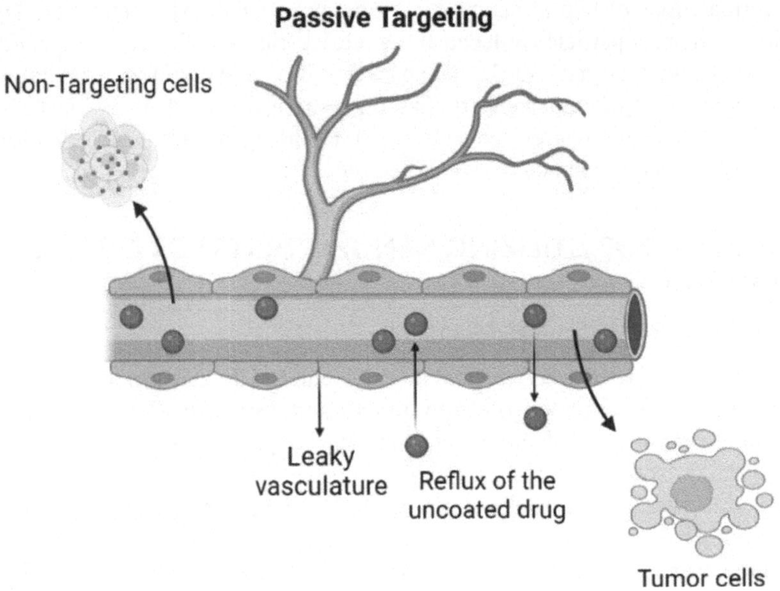

FIGURE 2.4 Illustration of "passive targeting" using enhanced permeability as well as retention (EPR).

the selective uptake of nanoparticles into the tumor cells, targeting strategies have advanced. The nanoreactor's surface has been coated with biorecognition molecules to specifically target markers that are overexpressed by cancerous cells (Figure 2.4) [92]. An increase in the intratumoral concentration of anticancer medications as a consequence of nanocarrier discharge is seen. Hydrophobic medications that are discharged into the environment are more likely to disperse and reach cancer cells, resulting in increased tumor cytotoxicity. As the tumor cell populations, antigen expression, microenvironment, density of the cell, and vascular density differ remarkably amongst malignancies and even under primary as well as secondary metastatic locales, nanoparticle biological distribution plus circulation length are essential properties for cancer treatment [93].

The most significant factors affecting the pharmacokinetic conduct of nanoparticles include their shape, surface charge, size, and stealth properties. Micelles, carriers based on proteins, liposomes, polymer-drug conjugates, plus other popular nanoparticle types have all received approval or are nearing the end of clinical trials [94]. Since postinjection time evaluations differ, it is challenging to compare the data for non-targeted nanoparticle accumulation in cancer xenograft mouse models. Polymer-drug conjugates, which range in size from 1 to 20 nm, with a half-life in human circulation that can range from hours to days, it depends upon the technique. Comparing the dextran-camptothecin (DE-310) formulation to the free drug formulation, clinical phase II testing revealed that DE-310 has the greatest human circulation half-life (300 hours) with no discernible toxicity [95]. However, in contrast to PEG-camptothecin alongside polyglutamate-camptothecin combinations (7,000 and 25 mg m^2, correspondingly), its dose regimen may limit its therapeutic efficacy [96]. These outcomes demonstrate that different polymer-drug conjugates have dramatically different pharmacokinetic features because the carriers have distinct loading profiles, release schedules, as well as molecular weights. Comparable half-lives in the circulation are shared by polymer-drug combinations like HPMA-drug combinations, polyglutamate-drug complexes, dextran-drug combinations, and pegylated medications like PEG-arginine deaminase (Hepacid, 7 days), as well as PEG-camptothecin (Prothecan, 40 hours). The maximum tolerated doses of larger nanoparticles, including micelles and liposomes, are higher, but their blood circulation half-life is shorter (2–50 hours) [97]. Two times as much HPMA-paclitaxel (PNU166945) as well as polyglutamate-paclitaxel (PNU166945) as Genexol-PM (Xyotax) is delivered [98]. Uncertainty remains regarding which factor is more crucial for optimal accumulation in malignant tissues: the circulation half-life or the maximum permissible dosage. For example, PEG-camptothecin conjugates along with polycyclodextrin-camptothecin micelles (IT-101) had very distinct drug accumulation in tumor xenograft specimens despite having identical circulatory half-lives [99]. However, it is probable that, as a result of the several xenograft models utilized. It is challenging to contrast the therapeutic effectiveness of diverse systems in humans with the variability of patients as well as stages of the disease. Clinical studies have shown that the physicochemical characteristics of the vehicle are related to nanoparticle biodistribution with circulation half-life [100]. The finding is supported by investigations on the circulatory half-life and *in vivo* biodistribution from animal models. The surface of nanoparticles may have PEG as well as other hydrophilic polymers grafted onto them for the formation of corona, which stabilizes the particle plus gives it the properties of "stealth" by restricting the absorption of protein and promoting its swift evacuation.

Recent studies have examined the surface properties of nanoparticles as well as their capacity to absorb blood proteins. The studied protein adsorption dynamics and composition about the particle size and hydrophobicity discovered that these factors influence the rate and composition of protein binding. According to the findings, albumin was more readily adsorbable to the surface of 200 nm nanoparticles than to those that were smaller (70 nm) [101]. With hydrophilic surfaces, hydrophilic nanoparticles greatly reduced protein adhesion. The curvature of smaller nanoparticles (70 nm) may diminish the protein adsorption of bigger proteins, according to one theory. Results reveal a rivalry between proteins, resulting in adsorption exchanges, despite their differing concentrations and affinity. Protein adsorption, as shown by Lundqvist *et al.*, is strongly influenced by the nanoparticles' size and charge [102]. The proteins discovered in the protein compositions attached to nanoparticles included lipoproteins, immunoglobulin, complement pathway proteins, as well as coagulation factor proteins. Initiation of complement, coagulation of blood, and capacities to absorb protein of hybrid nanoparticles along with accurate charge mediation have also been investigated [102].

Moreover, it is now commonly acknowledged that plastic nanoparticles (PNPs) pose a serious and growing risk to soil and aquatic environments. These particles, which are here defined as plastics with the largest dimension of less than 1000 nm, are released into the environment as primary products as well as through the breakdown of larger plastic waste. Given their small size, they have the potential to be very mobile, which raises questions about their potential global spread. Additionally, PNPs can adsorb a wide range of other pollutants, such as pesticides, heavy metals, and medications, which may increase the mobility of these dangerous substances. In the past few years, dozens of studies have been published that examine the toxicity of PNPs to various organisms, ranging from algae to humans, both with and without other adsorbed contaminants [103].

2.4 TARGETED NANOPARTICLES

One essential feature of nanocarriers for drug delivery is their ability to selectively target cancer cells, which increases therapeutic efficacy while shielding healthy cells from cytotoxicity. Several investigations have been conducted to investigate the targeting design of NP-based medications. Tumor biology and the relationship between nanocarriers and tumor cells must be understood before designing a nanocarrier system or attempting to target a tumor. The two main categories of targeting mechanisms are passive targeting and active targeting. One kind of serum glycoprotein that helps move iron into cells is called transferrin [104]. The majority of solid tumor cells overexpress transferrin receptors, whereas normal cells express only them at low levels. Thus, medications for the treatment of cancer are delivered using transferrin-conjugated NPs as an active targeting technique. Transferrin-modified NPs have been demonstrated to have improved intracellular drug delivery and higher cellular uptake efficiency when compared to unmodified NPs. Furthermore, data suggest that transferrin-conjugated polymeric nanoparticles are important in beating back chemotherapy that is resistant to drugs. The active targeting technique boosts cell uptake and tumor retention by utilizing associations among specific tissues or cellular surface antigens, along with the targeted ligand. Through conjugation procedures, the quantity of ligands on the surface of nanoparticles can be regulated [105]. The multivalent functioning on the outermost layer of nanoparticles gives adequate avidity in the case of weakly binding ligands. Antibodies, on the other hand, tend to be less appealing because of their greater stability, greater purity, simplicity of manufacture via synthetic pathways, and lack of immunogenicity. Receptor-mediated targeting may be accomplished in two ways [106]. Targeting the cancer microenvironment, particularly the extracellular matrix as well as receptors present on the surface of cancer blood vessel endothelial cells, may be a highly effective way to administer immune induction or antiangiogenic drugs (Figure 2.5).

The second tactic involves targeting cancer receptors on the cell surface with intracellular administration of lethal medicines or signal-pathway blockers. For efficient intracellular administration of therapeutic dosages, extracellular nanocarriers targeting transmembrane tumor antigens are frequently selectively taken up by cancer cells with the help of endocytosis mediated by receptors. It is unclear which strategy will have the greatest therapeutic effectiveness for treating tumor metastases, but the latest research using doxorubicin-delivery nanoparticles tailored to integrin receptors demonstrated positive results in primary and metastatic areas of human renal as well as pancreatic cancer animal xenograft models [107]. For both the main tumor and hepatic lymph node metastases, targeted nanoparticles demonstrated tumor accumulation and reduced tumor weight in response to treatment. Targeted nanoparticles have been created by us and others for a variety of cancers. Nucleic acid aptamer functionalized nanoparticles have been produced for regulated drug delivery. Due to their great degree of selectivity and affinity in attaching to certain targets, aptamers are being explored in clinical studies for a variety of reasons [108]. The blood–brain barrier (BBB) is unbroken during the early stages of brain tumor development and in the tumor's infiltration growth region. The blood–brain barrier (BBB) is a specialized system of capillary endothelial cells that is almost surrounded by astrocyte end feet and partially covered by pericytes and basement membrane. Its purpose is to block the passage of approximately 98% of small molecules and nearly 100% of large molecules, including recombinant proteins and genes, into the brain and tumor sites. The main obstacle to getting medication for brain tumors is the blood–brain barrier, which serves as a natural defense mechanism to shield the brain from dangerous substances in the bloodstream while providing the brain with the nutrition it needs to function properly.

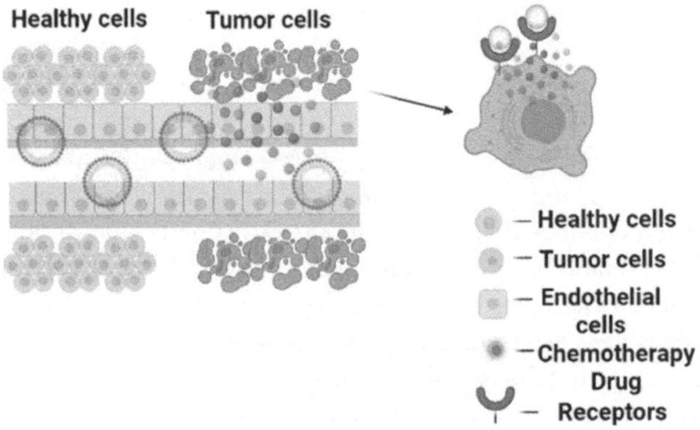

FIGURE 2.5 Illustration to show actively targeted delivery of functionalized nanoparticles to tumor cells.

2.5 ETHICAL CONSIDERATION OF NANOMEDICINE IN THE PHARMACEUTICAL INDUSTRY

Despite the fact that a sizable number of approved nanomedicines for biomedical applications have emerged in recent decades, these products' potential for greater influence in clinical practice has been limited by the absence of clear general protocols for preclinical development and characterization. Global regulatory trends have not yet been established, despite numerous attempts [109, 110]. The active principal ingredient (API) of nanomedicines determines the specifications that must be examined within the regulatory framework, according to regulators. The novel product must abide by the rules established for biological medicinal products and for new chemical entities (NCEs) when it comes to biological entities like proteins, peptides, or antibodies [111, 112]. Generally speaking, one of the obstacles to the regulation of nanomedicines is unquestionably connected to their unique qualities. Given the substantial body of evidence gathered for liposomes, polymer therapeutics, and other polymers (including polymeric micelles) as well as the regulatory concerns about their creation and development [113, 114], the clinical application of these intricate and sophisticated nanoproducts is heavily reliant on a thorough evaluation, characterization, and comprehension of key attributes. In actuality, their properties are easily modifiable through small adjustments to manufacturing procedures as well as minor adjustments to raw material composition. Additionally, although these modifications may only slightly affect the structure, they may have a substantial impact on the biological characteristics and biodistribution patterns [115–118].

Neverthless, the primary problem with regulating nanomedicines is that safety data from bulk materials—which do not exhibit the same pharmacodynamic and pharmacokinetic activity as nanomedicines—is used by regulatory agencies like the FDA. This means that once the nanomedicine has received marketing authorization, data on safety and efficacy will not accurately reflect what might actually happen when it is used in clinical settings. Because a nonnano version may meet regulatory requirements while a nanomedicine may not, this creates problems for developing regulations on the safety and efficacy parameters of nanomedicines [119]. The classification of nanomedicines is yet another extremely difficult task. They may be categorized as medical devices or medications, and different international regulators may have different opinions on this. Because a nanomedicine may be classified as a medical device in some countries and as a medicine in others, different countries may have different regulations that need to be followed. Because of this, different countries will have access to nanomedicines that may not have met regulatory requirements in another country due to differences in the specific safety and efficacy standards that must be met for the product to be sold. Another difficulty regulators confront is nanotoxicology and cellular response [120, 121]. Numerous ideas for realistic approaches to measuring nanotoxicity have been put forth. When it comes to measuring nanotoxicity, traditional toxicity measures—of which extensive animal testing for small drug molecules was once a common example—have been criticized for being impractical, too expensive, and unethical [122, 123].

An initial method for evaluating nanoparticles is through *in vitro* toxicity techniques. Compared to animal testing, it is a more cost- and time-effective method with greater control over the conditions of the experiment. But many of the widely used two-dimensional assays ignore the complexity of the human body, which employs complex metabolic processes, pathological reactions, and compensatory mechanisms to fight toxins. Furthermore, there is mounting proof that conventional assays for small compound *in vitro* testing are unsuitable for use with nanomaterials. Numerous nanoparticles interfere with the detection mechanism or interact with the reagents in *in vitro* assays, resulting in the generation of false positives or invalid data. Strong adsorption capacity, optical qualities, catalytic activity, acidity or alkalinity, magnetic properties, and dissolution are just a few examples of nanomaterial characteristics that may encourage interaction with *in vitro* testing reagents or measurements [124, 125].

2.6 CONCLUSION

Nanoparticles have revolutionized drug delivery for oncological interventions, with lipid, polymeric, and liposome nanoparticles designed to encapsulate and aid in chemotherapy drug delivery. These nanoparticles have overcome obstacles related to drug solubility and systemic toxicity, enhancing the integration of imaging methodologies into cancer diagnostics and therapeutic monitoring. Nanotechnology has the potential to change the way medications are distributed, with clinical translation of various nanoscale systems showing influence. The FDA has authorized several first-generation nanocarriers for treatment and targeted nanocarriers in clinical development. Nanomedicine is a pioneering field in nanotechnology, focusing on delivering specific biological compounds for therapeutic purposes and treating illnesses. Liposome-mediated drug delivery methods, polymer-drug conjugated nanoparticles, polymeric nanoparticles, dendrimer-based nanoparticles, and hybridized nanoparticles have improved cancer treatment efficacy through targeted delivery, drug stability, increased solubility, optimized half-life, drug responsiveness, and circumvention of biological barriers.

REFERENCES

1. Al-Jamal W, Kostarelos, K. Liposomes: from a clinically established drug delivery system to a nanoparticle platform for theranostic nanomedicine. *Acc Chem Res.* 2011;44:1094–1104.
2. Wen P, Ke W, Dirisala A, Toh K, Tanaka M, Li J. Stealth and pseudo-stealth nanocarriers. *Adv Drug Deliv Rev.* 2023;198:114895.
3. Mosleh-Shirazi S, Abbasi M, Moaddeli MR, Vaez A, Shafiee M, Kasaee SR, Amani AM, Hatam S. Nanotechnology advances in the detection and treatment of cancer: an overview. *Nanotheranostics.* 2022 Aug 21;6(4):400–423.
4. Dessale M, Mengistu G, Mengist HM. Nanotechnology: a promising approach for cancer diagnosis, therapeutics and theragnosis. *Int J Nanomedicine.* 2022 Aug 26;17:3735–3749.
5. Nance E. Careers in nanomedicine and drug delivery. *Adv Drug Deliv Rev.* 2019 Apr;144:180–189.
6. Jin C, Wang K, Oppong-Gyebi A, Hu J. Application of nanotechnology in cancer diagnosis and therapy – a mini-review. *Int J Med Sci.* 2020 Oct 18;17(18):2964–2973.
7. Afzal O, Altamimi ASA, Nadeem MS, Alzarea SI, Almalki WH, Tariq A, Mubeen B, Murtaza BN, Iftikhar S, Riaz N, Kazmi I. Nanoparticles in drug delivery: from history to therapeutic applications. *Nanomaterials (Basel).* 2022 Dec 19;12(24):4494.
8. Ristroph KD, Prud'homme RK. Hydrophobic ion pairing: encapsulating small molecules, peptides, and proteins into nanocarriers. *Nanoscale Adv.* 2019 Oct 1;1(11):4207–4237.
9. Lee JH, Yeo Y. Controlled drug release from pharmaceutical nanocarriers. *Chem Eng Sci.* 2015 Mar 24;125:75–84.
10. Din FU, Aman W, Ullah I, Qureshi OS, Mustapha O, Shafique S, Zeb A. Effective use of nanocarriers as drug delivery systems for the treatment of selected tumors. *Int J Nanomedicine.* 2017 Oct 5;12:7291–7309.
11. Santander-Ortega MJ, Jódar-Reyes AB, Csaba N, Bastos-González D, Ortega-Vinuesa JL. Colloidal stability of pluronic F68-coated PLGA nanoparticles: a variety of stabilisation mechanisms. *J Coll Interface Sci.* 2006;302(2): 522–529.
12. Al-Sharif M, Awen B, Molvi K. Nanotechnology in cancer therapy: a review. *J. Chem.* 2010;2(5):161–168.
13. De Jong WH, Borm PJ. Drug delivery and nanoparticles: applications and hazards. *Int J Nanomedicine.* 2008;3(2):133–149.
14. McMillan J, Batrakova E, Gendelman HE. Cell delivery of therapeutic nanoparticles. *Prog Mol Biol Transl Sci.* 2011;104:563–601.
15. Majumder J, Taratula O, Minko T. Nanocarrier-based systems for targeted and site specific therapeutic delivery. *Adv Drug Deliv Rev.* 2019 Apr;144:57–77.
16. Nsairat H, Khater D, Sayed U, Odeh F, Al Bawab A, Alshaer W. Liposomes: structure, composition, types, and clinical applications. *Heliyon.* 2022 May 13;8(5):e09394.

17. Kakkar A, Traverso G, Farokhzad OC, Weissleder R, Langer R. Evolution of macromolecular complexity in drug delivery systems. *Nat Rev Chem.* 2017 Aug;1(8):63.
18. Immordino ML, Dosio F, Cattel L. Stealth liposomes: review of the basic science, rationale, and clinical applications, existing and potential. *Int J Nanomedicine.* 2006;1(3):297–315.
19. Suk JS, Xu Q, Kim N, Hanes J, Ensign LM. PEGylation as a strategy for improving nanoparticle-based drug and gene delivery. *Adv Drug Deliv Rev.* 2016 Apr 1;99(Pt A):28–51.
20. Zhao N, Woodle MC, Mixson AJ. Advances in delivery systems for doxorubicin. *J Nanomed Nanotechnol.* 2018;9(5):519.
21. Murthy SK. Nanoparticles in modern medicine: state of the art and future challenges. *Int J Nanomedicine.* 2007;2(2):129–41.
22. Lajoie AC, Bonnet S, Provencher S. Combination therapy in pulmonary arterial hypertension: recent accomplishments and future challenges. *Pulm Circ.* 2017 Apr-Jun;7(2):312–325.
23. Bayda S, Adeel M, Tuccinardi T, Cordani M, Rizzolio F. The history of nanoscience and nanotechnology: from chemical–physical applications to nanomedicine. *Molecules.* 2019;25(1):112.
24. Li, XY, Zhao, Y, Sun, MG, Shi, JF, Ju, RJ, Zhang, CX, Li, XT, Zhao, WY, Mu, LM, Zeng, F, et al. Multifunctional liposomes loaded with paclitaxel and artemether for treatment of invasive brain glioma. *Biomaterials.* 2014;35: 5591–5604.
25. Chabner, BA, Roberts, TG. Chemotherapy and the war on cancer. *Nat Rev Cancer.* 2005;5:65–72
26. Le NTT, Cao VD, Nguyen TNQ, Le TTH, Tran TT, Hoang Thi TT. Soy lecithin-derived liposomal delivery systems: surface modification and current applications. *Int J Mol Sci.* 2019 Sep 23;20(19):4706.
27. van Hoogevest P, Wendel A. The use of natural and synthetic phospholipids as pharmaceutical excipients. *Eur J Lipid Sci Technol.* 2014 Sep;116(9):1088–1107.
28. Lombardo D, Kiselev MA. Methods of liposomes preparation: formation and control factors of versatile nanocarriers for biomedical and nanomedicine application. *Pharmaceutics.* 2022 Feb 28;14(3):543.
29. Russell LM, Hultz M, Searson PC. Leakage kinetics of the liposomal chemotherapeutic agent Doxil: the role of dissolution, protonation, and passive transport, and implications for mechanism of action. *J Control Release.* 2018 Jan 10;269:171–176.
30. Abbasi H, Kouchak M, Mirveis Z, Hajipour F, Khodarahmi M, Rahbar N, Handali S. What we need to know about liposomes as drug nanocarriers: an updated review. *Adv Pharm Bull.* 2023 Jan;13(1):7–23.
31. Al-Sharif M, Awen B, Molvi K. Nanotechnology in cancer therapy: a review. *J Chem.* 2010;2(5):161–168.
32. Fitzmaurice O, Bartkowski M, Giordani S. Molecular switches-tools for imparting control in drug delivery systems. *Front Chem.* 2022 Mar 31;10: 859450.
33. Jensen SS, Andresen TL, Davidsen J, Høyrup P, Shnyder SD, Bibby MC, Gill JH, Jørgensen K. Secretory phospholipase A2 as a tumor-specific trigger for targeted delivery of a novel class of liposomal prodrug anticancer etherlipids. *Mol Cancer Ther.* 2004 Nov;3(11):1451–1458.
34. Straubinger RM, Arnold RD, Zhou R, Mazurchuk R, Slack JE. Antivascular and antitumor activities of liposome-associated drugs. *Anticancer Res.* 2004;24:397–404.
35. Vakili-Ghartavol R, Rezayat SM, Faridi-Majidi R, Sadri K, Jaafari MR. Optimization of docetaxel loading conditions in liposomes: proposing potential products for metastatic breast carcinoma chemotherapy. *Sci Rep.* 2020 Mar 27;10(1):5569.
36. Mahalingam D, Nemunaitis JJ, Malik L, Sarantopoulos J, Weitman S, Sankhala K, Hart J, Kousba A, Gallegos NS, Anderson G, Charles J, Rogers JM, Senzer NN, Mita AC. Phase I study of intravenously administered ATI-1123, a liposomal docetaxel formulation in patients with advanced solid tumors. *Cancer ChemotherPharmacol.* 2014 Dec;74(6):1241–1250.
37. Liang T-J, Zhou Z-M, Cao Y-Q, Ma M-Z, Wang X-J, Jing K. Gemcitabine-based polymer-drug conjugate for enhanced anticancer effect in colon cancer. *Int J Pharm.* 2016;513:564–571.
38. Issarachot O, Suksiriworapong J, Takano M, Yumoto R, Junyaprasert VB. Folic acid-modified methotrexate-conjugated PEGylated poly(ε-caprolactone) nanoparticles for targeted delivery. *J. Nanoparticle Res.* 2014;16:2276.
39. Nowotnik DP, Cvitkovic E. ProLindac (AP5346): a review of the development of an HPMA DACH platinum polymer therapeutic. *Adv Drug Deliv Rev.* 2009 Nov 12;61(13):1214–1219.
40. Esim O, Bakirhan NK, Yildirim N, Sarper M, Savaser A, Ozkan SA, Ozkan Y. Development, optimization and in vitro evaluation of oxaliplatin loaded nanoparticles in non-small cell lung cancer. *Daru.* 2020 Dec;28(2):673–684.

41. Blagden SP, Cook AD, Poole C, Howells L, McNeish IA, Dean A, Kim JW, O'Donnell DM, Hook J, James EC, White IR, Perren T, Lord R, Dark G, Earl HM, Hall M, Kaplan R, Ledermann JA, Clamp AR. Weekly platinum-based chemotherapy versus 3-weekly platinum-based chemotherapy for newly diagnosed ovarian cancer (ICON8): quality-of-life results of a phase 3, randomised, controlled trial. Lancet Oncol. 2020 Jul;21(7):969–977.
42. Mathe G., Loc T.B., Bernard J. Effet sur la leucemie LI210 de la souris d'une combinaison par diazotation d'A-methopterine et de gamma-globulines de hamsters porteurs de cette leucemie par heterogreffe. *Comtes Rendus Hebd Seances AcadSci.* 1958;246:1626–1628.
43. Givental NI, Ushakov SN, Panarin EF, Popova GO. Experimental studies on penicillin polymer derivatives. *Antibiotiki.* 1965;10:701–706.
44. De Duve C, De Barsy T, Poole B, Trouet A, Tulkens P, Van Hoof FO. Lysosomotropic agents. *Biochem Pharmacol.* 1974;23:2495–2531. doi: 10.1016/0006-2952(74)90174-9.
45. Ringsdorf H. Structure and properties of pharmacologically active polymers. *J Polym Sci Polym Symp.* 1975;51:135–153.
46. Abuchowski A, McCoy JR, Palczuk NC, van Es T, Davis FF. Effect of covalent attachment of polyethylene glycol on immunogenicity and circulating life of bovine liver catalase. *J Biol Chem.* 1977;252:3582–3586.
47. Cajot S, Schol D, Danhier F, Préat V, De Pauw M-C G, Jérôme C. In vitro investigations of smart drug delivery systems based on redox-sensitive cross-linked micelles. *Macromol Biosci.* 2013;13(12):1661–1670.
48. Pridgen EM, Langer R, Farokhzad OC. Biodegradable, polymeric nanoparticle delivery systems for cancer therapy. *Nanomedicine (Lond).* 2007 Oct;2(5):669–680.
49. Zielińska A, Carreiró F, Oliveira AM, Neves A, Pires B, Venkatesh DN, Durazzo A, Lucarini M, Eder P, Silva AM, Santini A, Souto EB. Polymeric nanoparticles: production, characterization. *Toxicol Ecotoxicol Mol.* 2020 Aug 15;25(16):3731.
50. Makadia HK, Siegel SJ. Poly lactic-co-glycolic acid (PLGA) as biodegradable controlled drug delivery carrier. *Polymers (Basel).* 2011 Sep 1;3(3):1377–1397.
51. Suk JS, Xu Q, Kim N, Hanes J, Ensign LM. PEGylation as a strategy for improving nanoparticle-based drug and gene delivery. *Adv Drug Deliv Rev.* 2016 Apr 1;99(Pt A):28–51.
52. Chu KS, Finniss MC, Schorzman AN, Kuijer JL, Luft JC, Bowerman CJ, Napier ME, Haroon ZA, Zamboni WC, DeSimone JM. Particle replication in nonwetting templates nanoparticles with tumor selective alkyl silyl ether docetaxel prodrug reduces toxicity. *Nano Lett.* 2014 Mar 12;14(3):1472–1476.
53. Kataoka K, Harada A, Nagasaki Y. Block copolymer micelles for drug delivery: design, characterization and biological significance. *Adv Drug Deliv Rev.* 2001;47(1):113–131.
54. Oerlemans C, Bult W, Bos M, Storm G, Nijsen JF, Hennink WE. Polymeric micelles in anticancer therapy: targeting, imaging and triggered release. *Pharm Res.* 2010;27(12):2569–2589.
55. Kim DW, Kim SY, Kim HK, Kim SW, Shin SW, Kim JS, Park K, Lee MY, Heo DS. Multicenter phase II trial of Genexol-PM, a novel Cremophor-free, polymeric micelle formulation of paclitaxel, with cisplatin in patients with advanced non-small-cell lung cancer. *Ann Oncol.* 2007 Dec;18(12):2009–2014.
56. Boddu SHS, Bhagav P, Karla PK, Jacob S, Adatiya MD, Dhameliya TM, Ranch KM, Tiwari AK. Polyamide/poly (Amino Acid) polymers for drug delivery. *J Funct Biomater.* 2021 Oct 8;12(4):58.
57. Mittal P, Saharan A, Verma RF, Altalbawy MA, Alfaidi MA, Batiha GE-S, Akter W, Gautam RK, Uddin S, Rahman S. Dendrimers: a new race of pharmaceutical nanocarriers. *Biomed Res Int.* 2021;2021:8844030.
58. Majoros I, Thomas T, Mehta C, Baker J. Poly (amidoamine) dendrimer-based multifunctional engineered nanodevice for cancer therapy. *J Med Chem.* 2005;48: 5892–5899.
59. Zuckerman JE, Gritli I, Tolcher A, Heidel JD, Lim D, Morgan R, Chmielowski B, Ribas A, Davis ME, Yen Y. Correlating animal and human phase Ia/Ib clinical data with CALAA-01, a targeted, polymer-based nanoparticle containing siRNA. *Proc Natl Acad Sci U S A.* 2014 Aug 5;111(31):11449–11454.
60. Wong CK, Stenzel MH, Thordarson P. Non-spherical polymersomes: formation and characterization. *Chem Soc Rev.* 2019;48:4019e4035.
61. Scheerstra JF, Wauters AC, Tel J, Abdelmohsen LK, Van Hest JC. Polymersomes as a potential platform for cancer immunotherapy. *Mater Today Advan.* 2022 Mar 1;13:100203.

62. Hammer DA, Robbins GP, Haun JB, Lin JJ, Qi W, Smith LA, Ghoroghchian PP, Therien MJ, Bates FS. Leuko-polymersomes. *Faraday Discuss*. 2008;139:129–41; discussion 213–28, 419–20.
63. Miao Y, Yang T, Yang S, Yang M, Mao C. Protein nanoparticles directed cancer imaging and therapy. *Nano Convergence*. 2022 Jan 8;9(1):2.
64. Moreno-Aspitia A, Perez EA. Nanoparticle albumin-bound paclitaxel (ABI-007): a newer taxane alternative in breast cancer. *Fut Oncol*. 2005;1:755–762.
65. Ma P, Mumper RJ. Paclitaxel nano-delivery systems: a comprehensive review. *J Nanomed Nanotechnol*. 2013 Feb 18;4(2):1000164.
66. Gonzalez-Angulo AM, Meric-Bernstam F, Chawla S, Falchook G, Hong D, Akcakanat A, Chen H, Naing A, Fu S, Wheler J, Moulder S, Helgason T, Li S, Elias I, Desai N, Kurzrock R. Weekly nab-Rapamycin in patients with advanced nonhematologic malignancies: final results of a phase I trial. *Clin Cancer Res*. 2013 Oct 1;19(19):5474–5484.
67. Tubbs A, Nussenzweig A. Endogenous DNA damage as a source of genomic instability in cancer. *Cell*. 2017 Feb 9;168(4):644–656
68. Kaminski RW, Wu M, Turbyfill KR, Clarkson K, Tai B, Bourgeois AL, Van De Verg LL, Walker RI, Oaks EV. Development and preclinical evaluation of a trivalent, formalin-inactivated Shigella whole-cell vaccine. *Clin Vaccine Immunol*. 2014 Mar;21(3):366–82.
69. Degli Esposti L, Carella F, Iafisco M. Inorganic nanoparticles for theranostic use. in Vincenzo Guarino, Luigi Ambrosio (Eds.), *Electrofluidodynamic technologies (EFDTs) for biomaterials and medical devices*. 2018 Jan 1 (pp. 351–376). Woodhead Publishing, United Kingdom.
70. Uhljar LÉ, Ambrus R. Electrospinning of potential medical devices (wound dressings, tissue engineering scaffolds, face masks) and their regulatory approach. Pharmaceutics. 2023;15:417. https://doi.org/10.3390/pharmaceutics15020417.
71. Wolinsky JB, Colson YL, Grinstaff MW. Local drug delivery strategies for cancer treatment: gels, nanoparticles, polymeric films, rods, and wafers. *J Control Release*. 2012 Apr 10;159(1):14–26.
72. Salimi M, Mosca S, Gardner B, Palombo F, Matousek P, Stone N. Nanoparticle-mediated photothermal therapy limitation in clinical applications regarding pain management. *Nanomaterials (Basel)*. 2022 Mar 10;12(6):922.
73. Strenge P, Lange B, Draxinger W, Grill C, Danicke V, Theisen-Kunde D, Hagel C, Spahr-Hess S, Bonsanto MM, Handels H, Huber R, Brinkmann R. Differentiation of different stages of brain tumor infiltration using optical coherence tomography: comparison of two systems and histology. *Front Oncol*. 2022 Aug 30;12:896060.
74. Libutti SK, Paciotti GF, Byrnes AA, Alexander HR Jr, Gannon WE, Walker M, Seidel GD, Yuldasheva N, Tamarkin L. Phase I and pharmacokinetic studies of CYT-6091, a novel PEGylated colloidal gold-rhTNF nanomedicine. *Clin Cancer Res*. 2010 Dec 15;16(24):6139–49.
75. Zeng L, Li W, Chen CS. Breast cancer animal models and applications. *Zool Res*. 2020 Sep 18;41(5):477–494.
76. Yetisgin AA, Cetinel S, Zuvin M, Kosar A, Kutlu O. Therapeutic nanoparticles and their targeted delivery applications. *Molecules*. 2020 May 8;25(9):2193.
77. Morgan T, Muddana H, Altinoğlu E, Rouse S, Tabaković A, Tabouillot T, Russin T, Shanmugavelandy SS, Butler P, Eklund P, Yun J, Kester M, Adair, J. Encapsulation of organic molecules in calcium phosphate nanocomposite particles for intracellular imaging and drug delivery. *Nano Lett*. 2009; 8:4108–4115.
78. Zhang DX, Zou AP, Li PL. Ceramide reduces endothelium-dependent vasodilation by increasing superoxide production in small bovine coronary arteries. *Circ Res*. 2001 Apr 27;88(8):824–831.
79. Weng Y, Huang Q, Li C, Yang Y, Wang X, Yu J, Huang Y, Liang XJ. Improved nucleic acid therapy with advanced nanoscale biotechnology. *Mol Ther Nucl Acids*. 2020 Mar 6;19:581–601.
80. Nsairat H, Khater D, Sayed U, Odeh F, Al Bawab A, Alshaer W. Liposomes: structure, composition, types, and clinical applications. *Heliyon*. 2022 May 13;8(5):e09394.
81. Sengupta S, Eavarone D, Capila I, Zhao G, Watson N, Kiziltepe T, Sasisekharan R. Temporal targeting of tumour cells and neovasculature with a nanoscale delivery system. *Nature*. 2005;436:568–572.
82. Sivadasan D, Sultan MH, Madkhali O, Almoshari Y, Thangavel N. Polymeric lipid hybrid nanoparticles (PLNs) as emerging drug delivery platform-a comprehensive review of their properties. *Preparation Methods Ther Appl Pharm*. 2021 Aug 18;13(8):1291.

83. Karatoprak GŞ, Küpeli Akkol E, Genç Y, Bardakci H, Yücel Ç, Sobarzo-Sánchez E. Combretastatins: an overview of structure, probable mechanisms of action and potential applications. *Molecules*. 2020 May 31;25(11):2560.
84. Thevenot J, Troutier AL, David L, Delair T, Ladavière C. Steric stabilization of lipid/polymer particle assemblies by poly(ethylene glycol)-lipids. *Biomacromolecules*. 2007 Nov;8(11):3651–60.
85. Zhang L, Chan JM, Radovic-Moreno A, Shaikh MR, Farokhzad OC Biofunctionalized targeted nanoparticles for therapeutic applications. *Expert Opin Biol Ther*. 2008;8: 1063–1070.
86. Bromma K, Chithrani DB. Advances in gold nanoparticle-based combined cancer therapy. *Nanomaterials (Basel)*. 2020 Aug 26;10(9):1671.
87. Seyfried TN, Huysentruyt LC. On the origin of cancer metastasis. *Crit Rev Oncogenesis*. 2013;18(1–2).
88. Seyfried TN. *Cancer as a Metabolic Disease: On the Origin, Management, and Prevention of Cancer*. John Wiley & Sons; Hoboken: 2012. p. 432.
89. Lopes LF, Bacchi CE. Imatinib treatment for gastrointestinal stromal tumour (GIST). *J Cell Mol Med*. 2010 Jan;14(1–2):42–50
90. Bayat Mokhtari R, Homayouni TS, Baluch N, Morgatskaya E, Kumar S, Das B, Yeger H. Combination therapy in combating cancer. *Oncotarget*. 2017 Jun 6;8(23):38022–38043.
91. Farjadian F, Ghasemi A, Gohari O, Roointan A, Karimi M, Hamblin MR. Nanopharmaceuticals and nanomedicines currently on the market: challenges and opportunities. *Nanomedicine (Lond)*. 2019 Jan;14(1):93–126.
92. Tiwari H, Rai N, Singh S, Gupta P, Verma A, Singh AK, Kajal, Salvi P, Singh SK, Gautam V. Recent advances in nanomaterials-based targeted drug delivery for preclinical cancer diagnosis and therapeutics. *Bioengineering (Basel)*. 2023 Jun 25;10(7):760. doi: 10.3390/bioengineering10070760.
93. Chinen AB, Guan CM, Ferrer JR, Barnaby SN, Merkel TJ, Mirkin CA. Nanoparticle probes for the detection of cancer biomarkers, cells, and tissues by fluorescence. *Chem Rev*. 2015 Oct 14;115(19):10530–10574.
94. Anselmo AC, Mitragotri S. Nanoparticles in the clinic: an update. *Bioeng Transl Med*. 2019 Sep 5;4(3):e10143.
95. Venditto VJ, Simanek EE. Cancer therapies utilizing the camptothecins: a review of the in vivo literature. *Mol Pharm*. 2010 Apr 5;7(2):307–49.
96. Ying V, Haverstick K, Page RL, Saltzman WM. Efficacy of camptothecin and polymer-conjugated camptothecin in tumor spheroids and solid tumors. *J Biomater Sci Polym Ed*. 2007;18(10):1283–1299.
97. Ma P, Mumper RJ. Paclitaxel nano-delivery systems: a comprehensive review. *J Nanomed Nanotechnol*. 2013 Feb 18;4(2):1000164.
98. Meerum Terwogt JM, ten Bokkel Huinink WW, Schellens JH, Schot M, Mandjes IA, Zurlo MG, Rocchetti M, Rosing H, Koopman FJ, Beijnen JH. Phase I clinical and pharmacokinetic study of PNU166945, a novel water-soluble polymer-conjugated prodrug of paclitaxel. *Anticancer Drugs*. 2001 Apr;12(4):315–323.
99. Numbenjapon T, Wang J, Colcher D, Schluep T, Davis ME, Duringer J, Kretzner L, Yen Y, Forman SJ, Raubitschek A. Preclinical results of camptothecin-polymer conjugate (IT-101) in multiple human lymphoma xenograft models. *Clin Cancer Res*. 2009 Jul 1;15(13):4365–4373.
100. Ernsting MJ, Murakami M, Roy A, Li SD. Factors controlling the pharmacokinetics, biodistribution and intratumoral penetration of nanoparticles. *J Control Release*. 2013 Dec 28;172(3):782–794.
101. Barua S, Mitragotri S. Challenges associated with penetration of nanoparticles across cell and tissue barriers: a review of current status and future prospects. Nano Today. 2014 Apr 1;9(2):223–243.
102. Lundqvist M, Stigler J, Elia G, Lynch I, Cedervall T, Dawson KA. Nanoparticle size and surface properties determine the protein corona with possible implications for biological impacts. *Proc Natl Acad Sci USA* 2008;105:14265–14270.
103. Brewer A, Dror I, Berkowitz B. The mobility of plastic nanoparticles in aqueous and soil environments: a critical review. *ACS ES&T Water*. 2020 Oct 12;1(1):48–57.
104. Amreddy, N, Muralidharan, R, Babu, A, Mehta, M, Johnson, EV, Zhao, YD, et al. Tumor-targeted and pH-controlled delivery of doxorubicin using gold nanorods for lung cancer therapy. *Int J Nanomed*. 2015;10: 6773–6788.
105. Friedman AD, Claypool SE, Liu R. The smart targeting of nanoparticles. *Curr Pharm Des*. 2013;19(35):6315–6329.

106. Goulet DR, Atkins WM. Considerations for the design of antibody-based therapeutics. *J Pharm Sci.* 2020 Jan;109(1):74–103.
107. Wu PH, Opadele AE, Onodera Y, Nam JM. Targeting integrins in cancer nanomedicine: applications in cancer diagnosis and therapy. *Cancers (Basel).* 2019 Nov 13;11(11):1783.
108. Nimjee SM, White RR, Becker RC, Sullenger BA. Aptamers as therapeutics. *Annu Rev Pharmacol Toxicol.* 2017 Jan 6;57:61–79.
109. Bethge, WA, Sandmaier, BM. Targeted cancer therapy using radiolabeled monoclonal antibodies. *TCRT* 2005;4:393–406.
110. Lesniak, MS. Novel advances in drug delivery to brain cancer. *TCRT* 2005;4:417–428.
111. Dorbeck-Jung BR, Chowdhury N. Is the European medical products authorisation regulation equipped to cope with the challenges of nanomedicines? *Law Policy* 2011;33:276e303.
112. WangR, Billone PS, Mullett WM. Nanomedicine in action: an overview of cancer nanomedicine on the market and in clinical trials. *J Nanomater.* 2013;2013:12.
113. Wagner V, Dullaart A, Bock AK, Zweck A. The emerging nanomedicine landscape. *Nat Biotechnol* 2006;24:1211e1217.
114. RS Gaspar. Therapeutic products: regulating drugs and medical devices. in GA Hodge, DM Bowman, AD Maynard (Eds.), *International Handbook on Regulating Nanotechnologies.* Edward Elgar Publishing Limited, Northampton, MA, USA: 2010. pp. 291e320.
115. Gaspar R, Florindo H, Silva L, Videira M, Corvo ML, Martins B, Silva-Lima B. Regulatory aspects of oncologicals: nanosystems main challenges. in MJ Alonso, M Garcia-Fuentes (Eds.), *Nano-oncologicals.* Springer International Publishing, Singapore: 2014. pp. 425e452.
116. Dobrovolskaia MA, McNeil SE. Understanding the correlation between in vitro and in vivo immunotoxicity tests for nanomedicines. *J Control Release.* 2013;172:456e466.
117. Ehmann F, Sakai-Kato K, Duncan R, Hernan Perez de la Ossa D, Pita R, Vidal JM, Kohli A, Tothfalusi L, Sanh A, Tinton S, Robert JL, Silva Lima B, Amati MP. Next-generation nanomedicines and nanosimilars: EU regulators' initiatives relating to the development and evaluation of nanomedicines. *Nanomedicine (Lond).* 2013;8:849e856.
118. Gaspar R, Duncan R. Polymeric carriers: preclinical safety and the regulatory implications for design and development of polymer therapeutics. Adv *Drug Deliv Rev.* 2009;61:1220e1231.
119. Bawa R, Audette GF, Reece B. *Handbook of Clinical Nanomedicine: Law, Business, Regulation, Safety, and Risk, Pan Stamford Series on Nanomedicine.* CRC Press, Taylor and Francis, Boca Raton, Florida, USA: 2016: vol. 2.
120. Sharifi S, Reuel N, Kallmyer N, Sun E, Landry MP, Mahmoudi M. The issue of reliability and repeatability of analytical measurement in industrial and academic nanomedicine. *ACS Nano.* 2022 Dec 27;17(1):4–11.
121. Kroll A, Pillukat MH, Hahn D, Schnekenburger J. Interference of engineered nanoparticles with in vitro toxicity assays. *Arch Toxicol.* 2012 Jul;86:1123–1136.
122. Edmondson R, Broglie JJ, Adcock AF, Yang L. Three-dimensional cell culture systems and their applications in drug discovery and cell-based biosensors. assay and drug development technologies. *Assay Drug Dev Technol.* 2014 May 1;12(4):207–18.
123. Dickinson AM, Godden JM, Lanovyk K, Ahmed SS. Assessing the safety of nanomedicines: a mini review. *Appl In Vitro Toxicol.* 2019 Sep 1;5(3):114–122.
124. Hoskins C, Wang L, Cheng WP, Cuschieri A. Dilemmas in the reliable estimation of the in-vitro cell viability in magnetic nanoparticle engineering: which tests and what protocols? *Nanoscale Res Lett.* 2012 Dec;7:1–2.
125. Foulkes R, Man E, Thind J, Yeung S, Joy A, Hoskins C. The regulation of nanomaterials and nanomedicines for clinical application: current and future perspectives. *Biomater Sci.* 2020;8(17):4653–4664.

3 Targeted Therapy for Cancer with Nanomedicine

3.1 INTRODUCTION

Cancer and its surrounding environs have been treated using a variety of treatment techniques. In the year 1942, Louis Goodman along with his colleagues studied the use of nitrogen mustard in the treating non-lymphoma, Hodgkin's the first use of chemotherapy. When chemotherapy was first developed, it was able to halt cancer progression. A wide variety of chemotherapeutic drugs are now being tried in clinical trials to treat a variety of malignancies, including doxorubicin, paclitaxel, gemcitabine, and cisplatin, among others [1]. Advanced cancer diagnosis often causes multidrug resistance despite therapeutic progress. Because oxygen supply and angiogenesis are essential to cancer cell survival and dissemination, tumor microenvironment treatments have been studied. The complicated interaction between cancer cells, stromal cells, and blood arteries affects tumor growth [2]. Cancer cells have higher vulnerablility to damage from radiation than healthy cells; hence radiotherapy is an example of a strategy for eliminating them [3]. The utilization of gene therapy and immunotherapy in the treatment of cancer is also documented [4, 5]. The majority of them, however, are linked to adverse effects, resistance, or recurrence after first therapy [6].

As a result, chemotherapy failure in the clinical context directly contributed to the death of approximately 90% of patients with cancer [7]. As a result of tumor cells becoming resistant to chemotherapeutic drugs that are not in the same chemical family or function, MDR might emerge, posing a problem for the therapy [8]. According to one theory, the molecular mechanisms of MDR improve drug targeting by enhancing the DNA repair mechanism, detoxification by reducing drug activation as well as potentiating drug metabolism, detoxification by increasing efflux of membrane transport proteins, blocking cell death, and altering regulation of cell cycle (Figure 3.1) [9]. Because of its complex interaction, multidrug resistance (MDR) in cancer poses a serious barrier to traditional therapy. Changing membrane transport proteins, especially ATP-binding cassette (ABC) proteins and transmembrane transporters, is an effective method of combating MDR. ABC proteins and transmembrane transporters inhibit cancer cell cytotoxic drug accumulation via drug efflux mechanisms. Overexpression or changed activity may greatly affect anticancer therapies [10]. Modulating these proteins might improve traditional anticancer medicines and enable individualized cancer therapy. The most prevalent ABC protein, P-glycoprotein (P-gp, MDR1, or ABCB1), known to be the cause of MDR, is overexpressed.

A nucleotide-binding domain (NBD) and six transmembrane domains (TMD) are found in either half of P-gp [10]. Figure 3.1 depicts anticancer drug-resistant tumors have distinct molecular pathways.

Epipodophyllotoxins, Vinca alkaloids, taxanes, and anthracyclines are all frequent substrates for the P-gp transporter in chemotherapy regimens [11]. For example, natural compounds that block P-gp activity or MDR-1 gene downregulation have been tested to circumvent the efflux pump [12, 13]. They then reverse MDR and block P-gp activity, increasing the therapeutic effectiveness [14]. These MDR systems cannot stand a chance against the NP scan [15, 16].

DOI: 10.1201/9781003451020-3

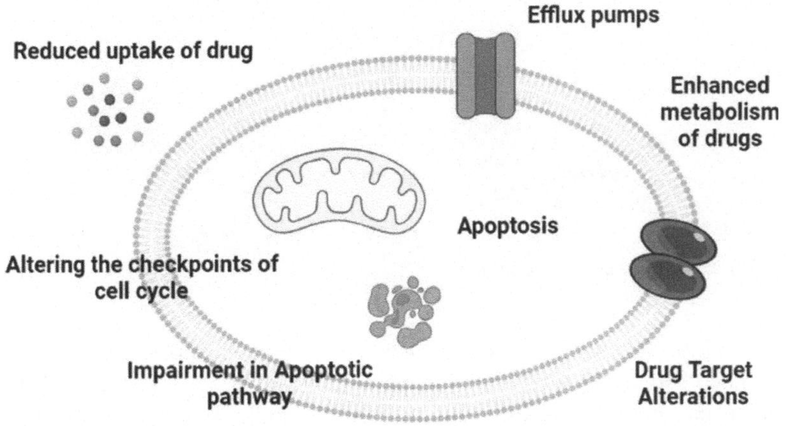

FIGURE 3.1 Illustration to show that tumors that are resistant to anticancer drugs follow specific biological pathways.

In order to increase treatment effectiveness and combat cancer medication resistance, it makes sense to look for a combination therapy that uses a more accurate method. A number of studies have shown encouraging results when utilizing NPs in combination with chemotherapeutic medicines or employing NPs during radiation to treat cancer [17]. Chemotherapeutic drugs in nanoparticle form provide a number of benefits over normal chemotherapy dosages. When a low-molecular-weight medicine is packaged in a nanoparticle, its bioavailability is improved and its removal by the liver and kidneys is minimized [18]. In comparison to conventional chemotherapy, chemotherapeutic nanoparticles provide a notable benefit in the form of reduced systemic toxicity and increased drug concentrations within tumor tissues. This is accomplished by nanoparticles' specific features, such as enhanced permeability and targeted accumulation in malignancies. Due to their reduced size and optimized surface characteristics, they are able to more effectively penetrate tumors with leaky vasculature and limit their exposure to healthy tissues. Chemotherapeutic nanoparticles provide a more focused and efficient drug delivery mechanism, potentially improving therapeutic effectiveness with fewer adverse effects [19].

3.2 CANCER TREATMENT USING CONJUGATED NANOPARTICLES

For focused and effective cancer therapy, conjugated nanoparticles are a potential new technique. These nanoparticles, which are often made up of materials such as carbon nanotubes (CNTs) [20] are functionalized or conjugated with certain ligands, antibodies, or medicines in order to increase their selectivity for cancer cells [21]. Drug delivery techniques benefit from CNTs' large surface area, mechanical strength, and cell membrane penetration [22]. These nanoparticles have the ability to preferentially detect and attach to cancer cells while sparing healthy tissues when they are coupled with targeting moieties, such as antibodies that recognize cancer-specific antigens [23]. Conjugating therapeutic compounds onto nanoparticles permits regulated and prolonged drug release, decreasing off-target effects and improving treatment effectiveness [24]. Due of non-specific medication distribution, traditional chemotherapy typically causes systemic toxicity. This tailored drug delivery strategy may solve this problem. Conjugated nanoparticles may transport drugs and be used for imaging and diagnosis. The utilization of imaging agents for functionalization purposes allows for the continuous observation of the nanoparticles' intracellular distribution and their interactions with cancer cells [25]. Conjugated nanoparticles are useful in the field of theragnostic because of their ability to serve as both a diagnostic tool and a therapeutic agent. However, problems such as biocompatibility, toxicity, and scalability must be carefully addressed to enable conjugated nanoparticles'

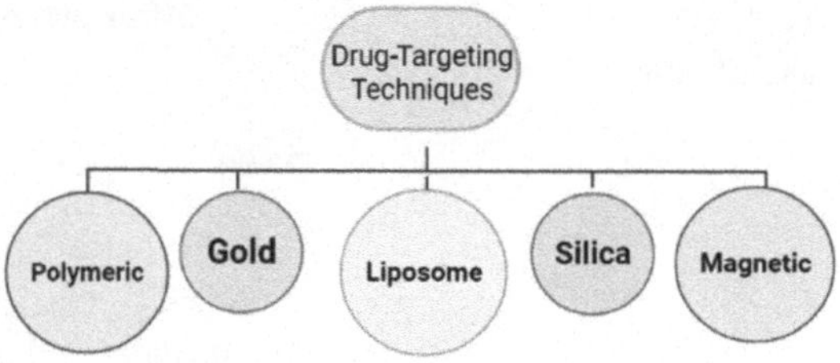

FIGURE 3.2 Typical drug-targeting techniques.

clinical translation [26]. Regulatory issues are also important in establishing the viability and safety of these novel nanotherapeutic methods. Nanoparticle conjugation, especially CNTs, for cancer therapy is a promising multidimensional approach. These conjugated nanoparticles show promise for improved and individualized cancer treatments in the future by integrating diagnostic capabilities with targeted drug delivery, a development that contributes to precision medicine. To counter MDR systems, the activity is thought to be an important benefit for NPs. An extensive discussion on the many forms of NPs including lipid and nanocapsule (Figure 3.2) [27–29], polymeric (NPs), metal and dendrimer (NPs), as well as dendrimers and liposomes.

3.3 OBSTACLES IN THE TREATMENT OF TUMORS ARE SURMOUNTED BY NANOPARTICLES

When cellular resistance to the medication is discovered, it is viewed as a cellular hindrance to the anticancer therapy's effectiveness. Chemotherapy penetration into the solid tumor is challenging because of the clinical characteristics of solid tumors, including aberrant blood artery architecture and function, interstitial hypertension, lack of lymphatics, and dilated angiogenesis [30].

A significant obstacle to conventional chemotherapy is its lack of selectivity, which may result in systemic toxicity and off-target consequences. Nanoparticles provide cancer-targeted drugs without harming healthy tissues. Functionalizing nanoparticles with tumor marker ligands or antibodies improve their capacity to identify and bind cancer cells, enhancing medication delivery [31]. There is still a big problem with chemotherapy: multidrug resistance once it has reached tumors. When treating common cancers, MDR remains the biggest obstacle to standard chemotherapy.

Liposome was the first discovery in the pharmaceutical history of nanoparticles [32]. The physicochemical features of nanoparticles help to overcome medication resistance, which is a key barrier in cancer therapy. Nanoparticles can potentially encapsulate several therapeutic compounds or circumvent efflux systems, which may improve treatment effectiveness and decrease the chances of resistance development [33]. Because nanoparticles (NPs) are small, they may be safely supplied intravenously and are a preferred therapy option because they boost therapeutic drug selectivity and overcome tumor resistance.

Improving the potential of regularly used medications by boosting their effectiveness and minimizing their toxicity and maintaining stable concentrations over a long length of time, with the help of NP therapeutic index is key [34]. As a result, half-life of the NPs coated with drug has to be long enough to maximize their effectiveness. Nanoparticles may passively accumulate in tumor tissues due to the increased permeability and retention (EPR) effect, which is a feature of tumor vasculature. This event enables the transportation of therapeutic substances to the location of the tumor, effectively addressing the difficulties associated with the infiltration of drugs into solid tumors [35]. The development of novel, more potent pharmaceuticals is made possible by the solubility and stability of the chemical being improved by nanoparticles. NPs are perfect for the intended purpose as their surface chemistry permits conjugation of ligands targeting transporter/receptor active sites. As discussed by Haley et al. [36] various sartigies have been used for the delivery of NP (Figure 3.3).

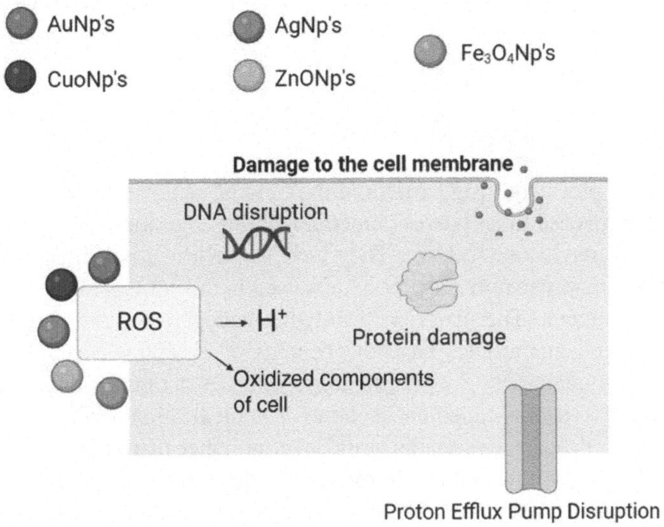

FIGURE 3.3 Application of nanoparticulate systems to combat medication resistance cancer cells.

Drug delivery to solid tumors is still a challenge, the body's principal defensive mechanism for swiftly removing NPs from the circulation is the reticuloendothelial system (RES), also referred as "mononuclear phagocytes" [37].

3.4 VARIOUS NPS USED FOR CANCER THERAPY

3.4.1 Liposomes

Liposomes, a subtype of nanoparticles, have emerged as flexible and efficient carriers in the field of cancer treatment, demonstrating their capacity to overcome significant obstacles related to drug administration. Phospholipid-based liposomes are colloidal drug delivery devices. It is made up of concentric bilayer vesicles surrounded by layers of aqueous medium. Their particle size ranges from around 20 to 80 nm, and they are made up of an outer layer that is made up of fats, and an inner core that is water. These lipid bilayer structures, which are spherical, can include several types of medicinal substances, such as chemotherapeutic medicines, nucleic acids, and imaging agents [38–40]. Liposomes may include medications that are either hydrophobic or hydrophilic. Hydrophobic drugs dissolve within the lipid layers as opposed to hydrophilic pharmaceuticals, which are disseminated in the aqueous core. Visudyne®, AmBisome® (amphotericin B), and Doxil® (doxorubicin hydrochloride) are just some of the liposomal medications now on the market (verteporfin). P-gp efflux is inhibited or bypassed via an endocytosis route by these preparations [41, 42]. There are two types of liposomes: those that include chemotherapy and those that do not. Head and tail are hydrophilic and hydrophobic in phospholipids. For cancer therapy, liposome is one of the most often used NPs [43–45]. Due to liposomes' ability to decrease chemotherapeutic drug clearance, boost targeting, and lessen harmful side effects, liposomes are often administered as a possible targeting and delivery strategy for chemotherapy [46]. Liposomes aid in addressing the pharmacokinetic challenges associated with certain medications. Manipulating the lipid content and size of liposomes allows for prolonged circulation durations and regulated release patterns, resulting in continuous drug exposure to cancer cells [47]. Liposomes have a wide range of applications beyond drug administration, since they may also function as vehicles for imaging agents, facilitating the concurrent detection and treatment of cancer. The capacity to perform theranostics is especially beneficial for assessing the effectiveness of therapy and improving therapeutic plans [48]. Pharmaceutically, using a liposome boosts cancer patient survival because of its ability to improve pharmacokinetic and pharmacodynamic features of the medicine utilized.

3.4.2 Polymer Nanoparticles

Polymers are the most prevalent drug carriers in the field of nanomedicine. The polymers used for medication-controlled release must possess biocompatibility and non-toxicity, with no presence of any contaminants that may cause leakage. They have to possess a half-life that is adequate and a physiologically appropriate structure. The polymers used in the composition of polymer NPs might be either natural or synthetic. The majority of polymer nanoparticles are chosen because they are biodegradable. Polymer nanoparticles have the benefits of exceptional stability and the capacity to be produced in large quantities. Polymer nanoparticles consist of vesicular structures known as nanocapsules and matrix systems called nanospheres. The medication is contained in a polymer container in nanocapsules. Nanospheres scatter drugs over polymer matrix [49–51]. Abraxane was the first polymer nanodrug to be successfully introduced to the market for pharmaceuticals in the year 2005. The substance consists of nanoparticles containing the medication paclitaxel, which are linked to albumin. There is no chromophore-electroluminescent (EL) component in this formulation. Paclitaxel becomes more soluble when it is treated with chromophore-EL. According to Weissig, Pettinger, and Murdock [52], it may have a deadly impact on certain individuals by causing severe allergic reactions and symptoms. According to McNeil [53], it has been established that nanotechnology has the potential to overcome the restrictions that are associated with the science of formulation.

3.4.3 Polymer Micelles and Polymersomes

Polymer micelles are formed by the self-assembly of macromolecules composed of block copolymers possessed together by non-covalent interactions. The structure of block copolymer micelles is characterized by a core–shell configuration. Critical micelle concentration (CMC), cumulative number, size, and morphology of the final structure are distinctive characteristics of micelles. These features depend on the polymer chains in the copolymer blocks. Polymer micelles exhibiting a lower critical micelle concentration (CMC) provide enhanced solubility for the encapsulated medication and increased stability of the micelle structure [54]. Micelles have exceptional efficacy in drug delivery systems (DDSs) due to their exceptional capacity, adjustable drug loading, strong durability under physiological conditions, reduced dissolution rate, enhanced drug accumulation at the desired site, and the opportunity for surface changes. Two polymer micelles, known as NK911 and NK105, have been commercially launched as drug carriers. NK911 contains doxorubicin, while NK105 contains paclitaxel [55, 56]. Polymersomes are composed of bilayer-structured amphiphilic copolymers in water. Additionally, a three-layer structure will be present if they are a three-block copolymer type. The cellular permeation of these structures is comparatively lesser than that of liposomes, which possess a visceral phospholipid structure. The characteristic will be enhanced in copolymers with longer hydrophobic segments. Additionally, it is a beneficial characteristic for regulating the release of medication. Copolymers have superior mechanical and biological stability compared to liposomes due to less interaction with visceral and macrophage structures. Drug protection will thus be quite strong [57, 58].

3.4.4 Polymer–Drug Interactions

Polymer–drug interactions are essential in the creation of effective and specific drug delivery systems, especially in the context of resolving multidrug resistance (MDR) issues in cancer therapy. Poly(N-(2-hydroxypropyl) methacrylamide) (polyHPMA) and its copolymers are potential non-immunogenic synthetic polymers since they can be dissolved in water and combat MDR. The water-soluble polymer polyhydroxypropylmethylacrylate (PolyHPMA) is a great vehicle for the conjugation and delivery of drugs. Due to its biocompatibility and absence of immunogenicity, it is a very appealing option for biomedical applications [59]. Researchers can enhance the effectiveness of chemotherapeutic medications in treating multidrug resistance (MDR) by conjugating them to polyHPMA, resulting in polymer–drug conjugates that have various benefits [60]. The medicine is released through the polymer–drug conjugate via endocytosis after being broken down by an enzymatic mechanism in the cells' lysosomes. HPMA conjugates reduced MDR1 expression and hence the resistance of resistant cells to Taxol [60, 61]. Apoptosis signaling pathways are activated as well as DNA repair is slowed down by the suppression of detoxification genes producing glutathione and UDP. Paclitaxel (nab-paclitaxel; Abraxane) is the most widely used albumin-based NP. Using albumin-based nanomedicine, hydrophobic chemotherapy may be created in injections with broad-spectrum dosages and rapidly achieves plasma maximum concentrations with better bioavailability [62, 63]. Nab-paclitaxel (IV) is converted to paclitaxel and albumin with few alterations to pharmacokinetics or tissue distribution [64]. Patients' chances of responding to nab-paclitaxel and slowing their cancer's development were greatly improved when the drug was given for longer periods (up to several weeks) [65].

3.4.5 Pluronic Micelles

Amphiphilic block copolymers, or phosphoonic micelles, play a crucial role as carriers in facilitating the internalization of water-insoluble lipids and micronutrients. They are able to self-assemble into layers and cores that are hydrophobic because they include both hydrophobic and hydrophilic components [66]. The hydrophobic core of these micelles contains compounds that are insoluble in water, which makes it easier for the individual to absorb them into the body. Additionally, they perform the function of carriers by building complexes with bile salts, which are referred to as mixed micelles. These micelles help with the emulsification of dietary lipids, as well as the effective digestion and absorption of these lipids. The amphiphilic nature of these entities enhances the overall efficacy of lipid digestion [67]. Adjuvant solubilizing agents, such as ethanol, are often used to help water-insoluble medicines dissolve intravenously [68, 69]. To prevent the use of the hazardous adjuvant, these hydrophobic medicines are frequently formulated in micelle nanoparticles. Conjugated poly (foliate) (ethylene glycol) FA receptor-mediated endocytosis enhances the cytotoxicity of doxorubicin in -b-copolycarbonates as well as methoxy poly(ethylene glycol)-b-polycarbonates [70]. In clinical investigations, pluronic L61 and F127 SP1049C-doxorubicin micelles were used for treating metastatic GIT adenocarcinoma. Tumors have higher doxorubicin concentrations than normal tissues with normal polymer dispersion [71]. For micelles to work, they alter the membrane shape, reduce membrane fluidity, and block efflux transporters, like P-gp as well as MRPs, from working and expressing [72–74]. These then increase the susceptibility of cancer cells to chemotherapy treatments, The mitochondrial respiratory chain is inhibited [75], glutathione (GSH) as well as glutathione-S-transferase (GST) activity is decreased [75], oxygen consumption is decreased, both mitochondrial membrane potentials are decreased [76], reactive oxygen species are produced, and cytochrome C is released in MDR cells [77].

3.5 NANOPARTICLES IN CHEMOTHERAPEUTIC CANCER TREATMENT

Chemotherapeutic cancer therapy has been improved by nanoparticles because they provide novel ways to optimize drug distribution, increase therapeutic effectiveness, and reduce systemic adverse effects. A variety of engineered nanoparticles, including micelles, polymeric nanoparticles, and liposomes, transport chemotherapeutic drugs to the location of a tumor in a regulated and targeted manner [78]. Nanoparticles use the increased permeability and retention (EPR) effect to preferentially accumulate in tumor tissues while sparing normal cells due to their tiny size and unique physicochemical features [79]. Moreover, surface modifications have the potential to enhance the specificity of drug delivery to cancer cells by facilitating active targeting [80]. By minimizing off-target effects, lowering dose needs, and reducing systemic toxicity, this focused method effectively addresses significant problems associated with conventional chemotherapy [78]. Additionally, nanoparticles play a role in surmounting multidrug resistance (MDR) through the implementation of sustained drug release and the bypassing of efflux mechanisms [81]. Nanoparticle design, surface engineering, and combination therapy studies might improve cancer treatment results. Several cancer therapy techniques use conjugated NPs. The following methods have been combined with nanoparticles to combat multidrug resistance and/or increase treatment sensitivity.

3.5.1 Topoisomerase Inhibitor Drug-Conjugated NPs

Topoisomerase inhibitor drug-conjugated nanoparticles are a potential way to treat cancer because they target topoisomerase enzymes, which are very important for DNA replication and repair. These drugs improve the accuracy and efficacy of cancer treatment when administered via nanoparticles; they accomplish this by interfering with the enzyme's regular operation, thereby inducing DNA damage that cells are unable to restore. Cell cycle arrest follows, enabling cells to repair the damage before continuing with the cell cycle [81]. If the damage is beyond repair, cells undergo apoptosis. By combining topoisomerase inhibitors with nanoparticles, their solubility, stability, and circulation time are enhanced, effectively resolving the difficulties related to restricted bioavailability and systemic toxicity [82, 83]. Nanoparticles enhance therapy effectiveness by releasing the medicine in a regulated and sustained manner, which prolongs the therapeutic benefits [84]. Doxorubicin has long been recognized by the Food and Drug Administration (FDA) as a powerful chemotherapeutic agent. It causes DNA and RNA polymerase to halt their activities [85]. It is also possible that doxorubicin might cause apoptosis by the activation of AMPK, which in turn activates downstream targets including p53, JNK, and mTORC [86–88] via the activation of AMPK. Doxorubicin has anticancer properties, although resistance has been found in certain cancers. Irinotecan is another chemotherapeutic medication that works by inhibiting isomerase. Semisynthetic camptothecin is derived from Camptotheca acuminata, a tree native to Central and South America. To induce cell death, the medication targets topoisomerase I. The FDA has authorized Doxil, a liposomal doxorubicin conjugate, for the therapy of Kaposi sarcoma, ovarian cancer, as well as multiple myeloma; The European and Canadian governments have approved Myocet, a liposomal doxorubicin conjugation, for treating metastatic breast cancer. M-302 is being examined in clinical trials for the treating human epidermal growth factor receptor 2 (HER2) breast cancer, while ThermoDox, a liposome combined with doxorubicin, is being investigated in clinical trial III for the treatment of hepatocellular carcinoma [36]. The combined use of doxorubicin, as well as verapamil in liposome preparation, demonstrated a stronger cytotoxic impact over a single drug in both *in vitro* as well as *in vivo* resistant animals [89]. Human transferrin (Tf) was added to liposomes to improve them and enhance their affinity towards Tf receptors. In resistant leukemia K562 cells (overexpressed Tf receptor+), Tf-conjugated coloaded liposomes proved more cytotoxic compared to non-targeted coloaded liposomes as well as Tf-conjugated doxorubicin liposomes. Treatment resistance was abolished by TfR-targeted liposomes that were loaded with doxorubicin as well as verapamil and specifically targeted cancer cells. In a preclinical investigation, it was discovered that liposome doxorubicin (SpHL-DOX) which is pH-sensitive significantly reduced the cardiotoxic effects of DOX [90, 91].

3.5.2 NPs Conjugated with DNA Replication-Targeting Drugs

Nanoparticles that have been conjugated with medications that target DNA replication provide a complex and focused approach to the treatment of cancer. This is accomplished by blocking processes that are essential for the growth of tumor cells. DNA replication is an essential stage in the cell cycle, and interfering with this process is a crucial approach to impede the proliferation of cancer cells. The conjugation of DNA replication-targeting medicines with nanoparticles improves their distribution, effectiveness, and overall treatment outcome [92, 93]. These medications are preserved in a nanoparticle environment, which ensures their delivery to specific cancer cells and prevents their breakdown. The regulated release of medications from nanoparticles allows for the pharmaceuticals to remain in circulation for a longer period, which maximizes the length of therapy. Drugs that target DNA replication generally disturb the precise duplication of genetic material by interfering with enzymes such as DNA polymerase or topoisomerase. By conjugating these medications with nanoparticles, it becomes possible to deliver them specifically to cancer cells while reducing their exposure to healthy tissues. By employing this targeted strategy, the adverse effects and maximized therapeutic efficacy that are characteristic of conventional chemotherapy are reduced [94]. The precise and directed administration of these medications amplifies their capacity to trigger apoptosis in cancerous cells while preserving normal cells. Numerous chemotherapeutic drugs target DNA replication. For instance, the chemotherapy drug cisplatin has significantly changed how cancer is treated. By interfering with the replication of DNA through the purine nucleotides in DNA, protein crosslinks of DNA are created. When Cisplatin disrupts DNA, several cellular processes are brought to life. Through the activation of cell cycle checkpoints as well as subsequent inhibition of Cdc2-cyclin A, which results in G2 arrest, it initiates the S phase [95, 96]. Additionally activated is P16INK4A, a type of inhibitor of cyclin-dependent kinase 4, which arrests the G1 cell cycle [97].

Drug resistance as well as systemic side effects in cancer patients are the main factors limiting cisplatin's therapeutic effectiveness. GSH levels inside cells have been shown to rise in response to cisplatin. Recently, NPs having a high disulfide density composed of poly (disulfide amide) polymers and cisplatin prodrugs have been developed to overcome cisplatin resistance in cancer cells [98]. The GSH scavenging mechanism of the nanoparticle platform is proposed to involve a polymer disulfide group. Aldehyde and the amino group were combined to create TAT-ASA-MNPs@CDDP nanoparticles, which were subsequently coordinated to cisplatin, which had stronger cytotoxic as well as apoptotic effects compared to the prodrug [99]. There may only be a few more cases of cisplatin combined with NPs. Cisplatin and a polymeric micelle have been combined using the anticancer medication NK-105. Phase III research on the chemical is focused on non-small-cell lung cancer.

3.5.3 NPs in Nonchemotherapeutic Cancer Treatment Methods

Nanoparticles have surfaced as multifunctional instruments in the realm of non-chemotherapeutic cancer treatment, presenting novel strategies that expand conventional chemotherapy. Within the field of immunotherapy, nanoparticles may be used as carriers for antigens, adjuvants, or immunomodulatory drugs, therefore augmenting the stimulation of the immune system in its fight against cancer cells [100, 101]. NPs may also target cancer cell receptors to deliver therapeutic chemicals like siRNA or gene-editing tools to inhibit cancer cell growth or cause apoptosis [102]. Hyperthermia therapy is a non-chemotherapeutic technique that involves the conversion of energy from external sources by nanoparticles into heat. The process of targeted heating may be used to specifically target and eliminate cancer cells while limiting harm to nearby healthy tissues [103]. Furthermore, NPs have the potential to improve diagnostic methodologies such as imaging and early cancer detection through their utilization as contrast agents or imaging agent carriers [104]. NPs' multifunctionality in non-chemotherapeutic techniques shows their potential to transform cancer therapy by giving more focused and less intrusive options. It is not only chemotherapy that has been utilized in the past to treat cancer patients. For example, radiotherapy, which has been used in cancer treatment for many decades, has demonstrated a positive effect on specific cancer types and cancer patient survival. Radiation therapy is the treatment of choice for tumors in their latter stages

[104]. It activates several signaling pathways, notably the p53 pathway, which are required for cell death. Upstream DNA damage signaling proteins such as ATM and ATR have been demonstrated to increase radiation sensitivity [105, 106]. Photodynamic cancer treatment was enhanced by the use of NPs like chlorin e6-loaded chitosan. Radiation activates Nanobiotix (NBTXR3) hafnium oxide, which after being administered consistently and targeting cancer cells, causing energy release and the death of cancer cells [107]. NPs have previously been studied in radiotherapy for cancer treatment. Soft tissue sarcoma therapy is now in phase III [107]. The use of chitosan nanoparticles loaded with chlorin e6 and highly biocompatible has been found to enhance photodynamic treatment for cancer.

In addition to chemotherapy, immunotherapy has also been employed in the treatment of cancers. A technique known as "immune surveillance" may be used by immune cells to destroy cancerous cells in premalignant tumors that have already undergone some change. Malignancy may occur if the system is impaired [108, 109]. As the immune system has the ability to eradicate tumor cells at its earliest stages, researchers have attempted to treat cancer by boosting immunity. For example, sipuleucel-T (prostate cancer treatment) and CTLA-4 antibody (melanoma treatment) have been licenced by the FDA for use in immunotherapy. Antigen vaccination and dendritic cell treatment are tw examples of immunotherapy that may be used to stimulate the immune system [110, 111]. For treating cancer, gene therapy and nanoparticles have been tried together. A transmembrane glycoprotein Mucin 1 (MUC1) antigen coupled to liposome, for example, is used in clinical trial III for non-small-lung cancer therapy. dHER2+As15, an antigen made from human HER2 and AS15 and used to treat metastatic breast cancer, is currently undergoing trial II [112].

Gene therapy is a technique for altering, replacing, or removing mutated genes from host cells. Gene therapy has become more popular in cancer research because cancer cells have mutated genes that lead to uncontrolled development [4]. Thus, the ability to insert whole genes into cancerous cells or even dormant stem cells could be used to regulate the development of malignancies. Liposomes and nanoparticles are examples of non-viral vectors that can be employed to introduce genetic material to host cells. Genetic nanoparticles for cancer gene therapy have been shown. Phase II studies have demonstrated the efficacy of two liposome nanoparticles, for instance, SGT53 and PNT2258, in the treatment of pancreatic cancer, non-Hodgkin lymphoma, and diffuse B-cell lymphoma [113] and are now in clinical trials. An antirecurrent B cell malignancy therapy using polyethyleniminenps coupled with an EIF5A vector has been described [114]. To treat pancreatic cancer in phase I/II, Atu027 is a liposome particle containing small interfering RNA (siRNA) N3 kinase. Phase I/II clinical trials using PLK1 siRNA-conjugated lipid nanoparticles TKM-080301 for the therapy of hepatocellular carcinoma as well as neuroendocrine tumors have been conducted.

To improve the specific delivery of doxorubicin (Dox) as well as curcumin (Cur) into the human breast cancer cell line MCF-7 with a better cardiotoxicity profile on an *in vivo* zebrafish model, new pH-sensitive prodrug nanoparticles were made using self-assemblage of a synthetic amphiphilic macromolecular prodrug. New disulfide-crosslinked nanoparticles of sodium alginate comprising doxorubicin were created and tested for cardiotoxicity as well as cytotoxicity only to tumor cells (Hep-G2 and HeLa), as well as in normal human liver cells (L-O2) to increase the effectiveness of the drug [115].

3.6 CONCLUSION

Cancer treatment resistance is being addressed due to advances in pharmaceutical delivery methods and nanotechnology. Nanoparticles might target cancer cells by reducing their acidity, offering a new cancer therapy. Acidic conditions allow stomach epithelial cells to proliferate, whereas high-specificity NPs like MM-398 hinder malignant cell DNA replication. However, manufacturing quality remains an issue, and quality control must be performed at each step of NP production. Nanomedicine laws may also be affected by drug development legislation. In order to make safe and successful plans for using NPs in cancer care, researchers, government bodies, and drug companies need to work together. The FDA has authorized chemotherapy-loaded nanoparticle compositions, although they cannot improve therapeutic efficacy. NPs may be activated by pH fluctuations, redox potentials, enzyme activity, temperature gradients, magnetic fields, light, or numerous stimuli, making them promise safe and effective cancer treatments.

REFERENCES

1. Goodman LS, Wintrobe MM, Dameshek W, Goodman MJ, Gilman A, McLennan MT. Landmark article Sept. 21, 1946: nitrogen mustard therapy. Use of methyl-bis (beta-chloroethyl) amine hydrochloride and tris (beta-chloroethyl) amine hydrochloride for Hodgkin's disease, lymphosarcoma, leukemia and certain allied and miscellaneous disorders. *JAMA*. 1984;251(17):2255–61.
2. Muriithi W, Macharia LW, Heming CP, Echevarria JL, Nyachieo A, Filho PN, et al. ABC transporters and the hallmarks of cancer: roles in cancer aggressiveness beyond multidrug resistance. *Cancer Biol Med*. 2020 May 5;17(2):253–69.
3. Baskar R, Dai J, Wenlong N, Yeo R, Yeoh KW. Biological response of cancer cells to radiation treatment. *Front Mol Biosci*. 2014;1:24.
4. Amer MH. Gene therapy for cancer: present status and future perspective. *Mol Cell Ther*. 2014;2(1):27.
5. Topalian SL, Weiner GJ, Pardoll DM. Cancer immunotherapy comes of age. *J Clin Oncol*. 2011;29(36):4828–36.
6. Frank KM, Hogarth DK, Miller JL, Mandal S, Mease PJ, Samulski RJ, et al. Investigation of the cause of death in a gene-therapy trial. *N Engl J Med*. 2009;361(2):161–9.
7. Xue X, Liang XJ. Overcoming drug efflux-based multidrug resistance in cancer with nanotechnology. *Chin J Cancer*. 2012;31(2):100–9.
8. Moitra K. Overcoming multidrug resistance in cancer stem cells. *BioMed Res Int*. 2015;2015:Article ID 635745, 8.
9. Gottesman MM. Mechanisms of cancer drug resistance. *Annu Rev Med*. 2002;53(1):615–27.
10. Mohammad IS, He W, Yin L. Understanding of human ATP binding cassette superfamily and novel multidrug resistance modulators to overcome MDR. *Biomed Pharmacother*. 2018 Apr 1;100:335–48.
11. Wink M, Ashour ML, El-Readi MZ. Secondary metabolites from plants inhibiting ABC transporters and reversing resistance of cancer cells and microbes to cytotoxic and antimicrobial agents. *Front Microbiol*. 2012;3:130.
12. Eid SY, El-Readi MZ, Wink M. Carotenoids reverse multidrug resistance in cancer cells by interfering with ABC-transporters. *Phytomedicine*. 2012;19(11):977–87.
13. El-Readi MZ, Eid S, Ashour ML, Tahrani A, Wink M. Modulation of multidrug resistance in cancer cells by chelidonine and *Chelidonium majus* alkaloids. *Phytomedicine*. 2013;20(3–4):282–94.
14. Shabbits JA, Krishna R, Mayer LD. Molecular and pharmacological strategies to overcome multidrug resistance. *Expert Rev Anticancer Ther*. 2001;1(4):585–94.
15. Wang Y, Dou L, He H, Zhang Y, Shen Q. Multifunctional nanoparticles as nanocarrier for vincristine sulfate delivery to overcome tumor multidrug resistance. *Mol Pharm*. 2014;11(3):885–94.
16. Ganassin R, Horst FH, Camargo NS, Chaves SB, Morais PC, Mosiniewicz-Szablewska E, et al. Selolnanocapsules with a poly(methylvinyl ether-co-maleic anhydride) shell conjugated to doxorubicin for combinatorial chemotherapy against murine breast adenocarcinoma *in vivo*. *Artif Cells Nanomed Biotechnol*. 2018;46(sup2):1046–52.
17. Gurunathan S, Kang MH, Qasim M, Kim JH. Nanoparticle-mediated combination therapy: two-in-one approach for cancer. *Int J Mol Sci*. 2018 Oct 20;19(10):3264.
18. Matsumura Y. Poly (amino acid) micelle nanocarriers in preclinical and clinical studies. *Adv Drug Deliv Rev*. 2008;60(8):899–914.
19. Qi SS, Sun JH, Yu HH, Yu SQ. Co-delivery nanoparticles of anti-cancer drugs for improving chemotherapy efficacy. *Drug Deliv*. 2017 Jan 1;24(1):1909–26.
20. Bianco A, Kostarelos K, Prato M. Applications of carbon nanotubes in drug delivery. *Curr Opin Chem Biol*. 2005;9(6):674–9.
21. Peer D, Karp JM, Hong S, FaroKhzad OC, Margalit R, Langer R. Nanocarriers as an emerging platform for cancer therapy. *Nat Nanotechnol*. 2007;2(12):751–60.

22. Liu Z, Chen K, Davis C, Sherlock S, Cao Q, Chen X, et al. Drug delivery with carbon nanotubes for in vivo cancer treatment. *Cancer Res*. 2008;68(16):6652–60.
23. Shi K, Long Y, Xu C. QD-loaded nanoparticles for molecular imaging and cancer therapy. *Sci World J*. 2014;2014:531609.
24. Kamaly N, Yameen B, Wu J, Farokhzad OC. Degradable controlled-release polymers and polymeric nanoparticles: mechanisms of controlling drug release. *Chem Rev*. 2016;116(4):2602–63.
25. Liu Z, Fan AC, Rakhra K, Sherlock S, Goodwin A, Chen X, et al. Supramolecular stacking of doxorubicin on carbon nanotubes for in vivo cancer therapy. *Angew Chem Int Ed Engl*. 2009;48(41):7668–72.
26. Nel AE, Mädler L, Velegol D, Xia T, Hoek EM, Somasundaran P, et al. Understanding biophysicochemical interactions at the nano-bio interface. *Nat Mater*. 2009;8(7):543–57.
27. Bi Y, Hao F, Yan G, Teng L, Lee RJ, Xie J. Actively targeted nanoparticles for drug delivery to tumor. *Curr Drug Metab*. 2016;17(8):763–82.
28. Schroeder A, Heller DA, Winslow MM, Dahlman JE, Pratt GW, Langer R, et al. Treating metastatic cancer with nanotechnology. *Nat Rev Cancer*. 2011;12(1):39–50.
29. Dong X, Mumper RJ. Nanomedicinal strategies to treat multidrug-resistant tumors: current progress. *Nanomedicine (Lond)*. 2010;5(4):597–615.
30. Campbell RB. Tumor physiology and delivery of nanopharmaceuticals. *Anti Cancer Agents Med Chem*. 2006;6(6):503–12.
31. Bangham AD, Standish MM, Watkins JC. Diffusion of univalent ions across the lamellae of swollen phospholipids. *J Mol Biol*. 1965;13(1):238–52.
32. Peer D, Karp JM, Hong S, Farokhzad OC, Margalit R, Langer R. Nanocarriers as an emerging platform for cancer therapy. *Nat Nanotechnol*. 2007;2(12):751–60.
33. Farokhzad OC, Langer R. Impact of nanotechnology on drug delivery. *ACS Nano*. 2009;3(1):16–20.
34. Tummala S, Kuppusamy G, Satish Kumar MNS, Praveen TK, Wadhwani A. 5-fluorouracil enteric-coated nanoparticles for improved apoptotic activity and therapeutic index in treating colorectal cancer. *Drug Deliv*. 2016;23(8):2902–10.
35. Maeda H, Nakamura H, Fang J. The EPR effect for macromolecular drug delivery to solid tumors: improvement of tumor uptake, lowering of systemic toxicity, and distinct tumor imaging in vivo. *Adv Drug Deliv Rev*. 2013;65(1):71–9.
36. Haley B, Frenkel E. Nanoparticles for drug delivery in cancer treatment. *Urol Oncol*. 2008;26(1):57–64.
37. Li SD, Huang L. Nanoparticles evading the reticuloendothelial system: role of the supported bilayer. *Biochim Biophys Acta*. 2009;1788(10):2259–66.
38. Torchilin VP. Recent advances with liposomes as pharmaceutical carriers. *Nat Rev Drug Discov*. 2005;4(2):145–60.
39. US National Library of Medicine; 2016. ClinicalTrials.gov. Available from: https://clinicaltrials.gov/ct2/show/NCT02314052?term.
40. US National Library of Medicine; 2011. ClinicalTrials.gov. Available from: https://clinicaltrials.gov/ct2/show/NCT00882180?term.
41. Capek I. Polymer decorated gold nanoparticles in nanomedicine conjugates. *Adv Colloid Interface Sci*. 2017;249:386–99.
42. Motomura M, Ichihara H, Matsumoto Y. Nano-chemotherapy using cationic liposome that strategically targets the cell membrane potential of pancreatic cancer cells with negative charge. *Bioorg Med Chem Lett*. 2018;28(7):1161–5.
43. Bhowmik S, Bhowmick S, Maiti K, Chakra A, Shahi P, Jain D, et al. Two multicenter Phase I randomized trials to compare the bioequivalence and safety of a generic doxorubicin hydrochloride liposome injection with Doxil® or Caelyx® in advanced ovarian cancer. *Cancer Chemother Pharmacol*. 2018;82(3):521–32.
44. Qu MH, Zeng RF, Fang S, Dai QS, Li HP, Long JT. Liposome-based co-delivery of siRNA and docetaxel for the synergistic treatment of lung cancer. *Int J Pharm*. 2014;474(1–2):112–22.
45. Nsairat H, Khater D, Sayed U, Odeh F, Al Bawab A, Alshaer W. Liposomes: structure, composition, types, and clinical applications. *Heliyon*. 2022;8(5):e09394.
46. Park JW. Liposome-based drug delivery in breast cancer treatment. *Breast Cancer Res*. 2002;4(3):95–9.
47. Gabizon A, Catane R. Prolonged circulation time and enhanced accumulation in malignant exudates of doxorubicin encapsulated in polyethylene-glycol coated liposomes. *Cancer Res*. 1991;51(16):3941–7.

48. Lammers T, Aime S, Hennink WE, Storm G, Kiessling F. Theranostic nanomedicine. *Acc Chem Res.* 2011;44(10):1029–38.
49. Elmowafy M, Samy A, Abdelaziz AE, Shalaby K, Salama A, Raslan MA, et al. Polymeric nanoparticles based topical gel of poorly soluble drug: formulation, ex-vivo and in vivo evaluation. *Beni Suef Univ J Basic Appl Sci.* 2017;6(2):184–91.
50. Guterres SS, Alves MP, Pohlmann AR. Polymeric nanoparticles, nanospheres and nanocapsules, for cutaneous applications. *Drug Target Insights.* 2007;2:147–57.
51. Hickey JW, Santos JL, Williford JM, Mao HQ. Control of polymeric nanoparticle size to improve therapeutic delivery. *J Control Release.* 2015;219:536–47.
52. Weissig V, Pettinger TK, Murdock N. Nanopharmaceuticals (part 1): products on the market. *Int J Nanomed.* 2014;9:4357–73.
53. McNeil SE. Unique benefits of nanotechnology to drug delivery and diagnostics. *Methods Mol Biol.* 2011;697:3–8.
54. Zhang Y, Huang Y, Li S. Polymeric micelles: nanocarriers for cancer-targeted drug delivery. *AAPS Pharm Sci Tech.* 2014;15(4):862–71.
55. Hong RL, Tseng YL. Phase I and pharmacokinetic study of a stable, polyethylene-glycolated liposomal doxorubicin in patients with solid tumors: the relation between pharmacokinetic property and toxicity. *Cancer.* 2001;91(9):1826–33.
56. Matsumura Y, Hamaguchi T, Ura T, Muro K, Yamada Y, Shimada Y, et al. Phase I clinical trial and pharmacokinetic evaluation of NK911, a micelle-encapsulated doxorubicin. *Br J Cancer.* 2004;91(10):1775–81.
57. Zhao Y, Li X, Zhao X, Yang Y, Li H, Zhou X, et al. Asymmetrical polymer vesicles for drug delivery and other applications. *Front Pharmacol.* 2017;8(374):374.
58. Petit J, Polenz I, Baret JC, Herminghaus S, Bäumchen O. Vesicles-on-a-chip: a universal microfluidic platform for the assembly of liposomes and polymersomes. *Eur Phys J E Soft Matter.* 2016;39(6):59.
59. Kopeček J, Kopečková P. HPMA copolymers: origins, early developments, present, and future. *Adv Drug Deliv Rev.* 2010;62(2):122–49.
60. Kopecek J, Kopecková P, Minko T, Lu Z. HPMA copolymer-anticancer drug conjugates: design, activity, and mechanism of action. *Eur J Pharm Biopharm.* 2000;50(1):61–81.
61. Minko T, Kopečková P, Kopeček J. Comparison of the anticancer effect of free and HPMA copolymer-bound adriamycin in human ovarian carcinoma cells. *Pharm Res.* 1999;16(7):986–96.
62. Minko T, Kopečková P, Kopeček J. Chronic exposure to HPMA copolymer-bound adriamycin does not induce multidrug resistance in a human ovarian carcinoma cell line. *J Control Release.* 1999;59(2):133–48.
63. Dranitsaris G, Yu B, Wang L, Sun W, Zhou Y, King J, et al. Abraxane® versus Taxol® for patients with advanced breast cancer: a prospective time and motion analysis from a Chinese health care perspective. *J Oncol Pharm Pract.* 2016;22(2):205–11.
64. Park J, Park JE, Hedrick VE, Wood KV, Bonham C, Lee W, et al. A comparative in vivo study of albumin-coated paclitaxel nanocrystals and Abraxane. *Small.* 2018;14(16):article 1703670.
65. Bhattacharyya J, Bellucci JJ, Weitzhandler I, McDaniel JR, Spasojevic I, Li X, et al. A paclitaxel-loaded recombinant polypeptide nanoparticle outperforms Abraxane in multiple murine cancer models. *Nat Commun.* 2015;6(1):article 7939.
66. Gradishar WJ, Tjulandin S, Davidson N, Shaw H, Desai N, Bhar P, et al. Phase III trial of nanoparticle albumin-bound paclitaxel compared with polyethylated castor oil-based paclitaxel in women with breast cancer. *J Clin Oncol.* 2005;23(31):7794–803.
67. Amidon GL, Lennernäs H, Shah VP, Crison JR. A theoretical basis for a biopharmaceutic drug classification: the correlation of in vitro drug product dissolution and in vivo bioavailability. *Pharm Res.* 1995;12(3):413–20.
68. Sugahara T, Takamatsu Y, Bhadani A, Akamatsu M, Sakai K, Abe M, et al. Characterization of the micelle structure of oleic acid-based gemini surfactants: effect of stereochemistry. *Phys Chem Chem Phys.* 2018;20(13):8874–80.
69. Kloover JS, den Bakker MA, Gelderblom H, van Meerbeeck JP. Fatal outcome of a hypersensitivity reaction to paclitaxel: a critical review of premedication regimens. *Br J Cancer.* 2004;90(2):304–5.

70. Rijcken CJF, Soga O, Hennink WE, van Nostrum CF. Triggered destabilisation of polymeric micelles and vesicles by changing polymers polarity: an attractive tool for drug delivery. *J Control Release.* 2007;120(3):131–48.
71. Lv Y, Yang B, Li YM, He F, Zhuo RX. Folate-conjugated amphiphilic block copolymer micelle for targeted and redox-responsive delivery of doxorubicin. *J Biomater Sci Polym Ed.* 2018;29(1):92–106.
72. Sakai-Kato K, Nanjo K, Kusuhara H, Nishiyama N, Kataoka K, Kawanishi T, et al. Effect of knockout of *Mdr1a* and *Mdr1b* ABCB1 genes on the systemic exposure of a doxorubicin-conjugated block copolymer in mice. *Mol Pharm.* 2015;12(9):3175–83.
73. Batrakova EV, Li S, Vinogradov SV, Alakhov VY, Miller DW, Kabanov AV. Mechanism of pluronic effect on P-glycoprotein efflux system in blood-brain barrier: contributions of energy depletion and membrane fluidization. *J Pharmacol Exp Ther.* 2001;299(2):483–93.
74. Pawar A, Singh S, Rajalakshmi S, Shaikh K, Bothiraja C. Development of fisetin-loaded folate functionalized pluronic micelles for breast cancer targeting. *Artif Cells Nanomed Biotechnol.* 2018;46(sup1):347–61.
75. Qin L, Wu L, Jiang S, Yang D, He H, Zhang F, et al. Multifunctional micelle delivery system for overcoming multidrug resistance of doxorubicin. *J Drug Target.* 2018;26(4):289–95.
76. Bao Y, Yin M, Hu X, Zhuang X, Sun Y, Guo Y, et al. A safe, simple and efficient doxorubicin prodrug hybrid micelle for overcoming tumor multidrug resistance and targeting delivery. *J Control Release.* 2016;235:182–94.
77. Qi Y, Qin X, Yang C, Wu T, Qiao Q, Song Q, et al. Micelle system based on molecular economy principle for overcoming multidrug resistance and inhibiting metastasis. *Mol Pharm.* 2018;15(3):1005–16.
78. Peer D, Karp JM, Hong S, Farokhzad OC, Margalit R, Langer R. Nanocarriers as an emerging platform for cancer therapy. *Nat Nanotechnol.* 2007;2(12):751–60.
79. Maeda H, Nakamura H, Fang J. The EPR effect for macromolecular drug delivery to solid tumors: improvement of tumor uptake, lowering of systemic toxicity, and distinct tumor imaging in vivo. *Adv Drug Deliv Rev.* 2013;65(1):71–9.
80. Alexis F, Pridgen E, Molnar LK, Farokhzad OC. Factors affecting the clearance and biodistribution of polymeric nanoparticles. *Mol Pharm.* 2008;5(4):505–15.
81. Wilhelm S, Tavares AJ, Dai Q, Ohta S, Audet J, Dvorak HF, et al. Analysis of nanoparticle delivery to tumors. *Nat Rev Mater.* 2016;1(5):16014.
82. Peer D, Karp JM, Hong S, Farokhzad OC, Margalit R, Langer R. Nanocarriers as an emerging platform for cancer therapy. *Nat Nanotechnol.* 2007;2(12):751–60.
83. Pommier Y, Leo E, Zhang H, Marchand C. DNA topoisomerases and their poisoning by anticancer and antibacterial drugs. *Chem Biol.* 2010;17(5):421–33.
84. Zhang L, Gu FX, Chan JM, Wang AZ, Langer RS, Farokhzad OC. Nanoparticles in medicine: therapeutic applications and developments. *Clin Pharmacol Ther.* 2008;83(5):761–9.
85. Buchholz TA, Stivers DN, Stec J, Ayers M, Clark E, Bolt A, et al. Global gene expression changes during neoadjuvant chemotherapy for human breast cancer. *Cancer J.* 2002;8(6):461–8.
86. Carvalho C, Santos RX, Cardoso S, Correia S, Oliveira PJ, Santos MS, et al. Doxorubicin: the good, the bad and the ugly effect. *Curr Med Chem.* 2009;16(25):3267–85.
87. Jones RG, Plas DR, Kubek S, Buzzai M, Mu J, Xu Y, et al. AMP-activated protein kinase induces a p53-dependent metabolic checkpoint. *Mol Cell.* 2005;18(3):283–93.
88. Gwinn DM, Shackelford DB, Egan DF, Mihaylova MM, Mery A, Vasquez DS, et al. AMPK phosphorylation of raptor mediates a metabolic checkpoint. *Mol Cell.* 2008;30(2):214–26.
89. Liu LF, Duann P, Lin CT, D'Arpa P, Wu J. Mechanism of action of camptothecin. *Ann N Y Acad Sci.* 1996;803(1):44–9.
90. Wang J, Goh B, Lu W, Zhang Q, Chang A, Liu XY, et al. *In vitro* cytotoxicity of Stealth liposomes co-encapsulating doxorubicin and verapamil on doxorubicin-resistant tumor cells. *Biol Pharm Bull.* 2005;28(5):822–8.
91. Wu J, Lu Y, Lee A, Pan X, Yang X, Zhao X, et al. Reversal of multidrug resistance by transferrin-conjugated liposomes co-encapsulating doxorubicin and verapamil. *J Pharm Pharm Sci.* 2007;10(3):350–7.
92. Peer D, Karp JM, Hong S, Farokhzad OC, Margalit R, Langer R. Nanocarriers as an emerging platform for cancer therapy. *Nat Nanotechnol.* 2007;2(12):751–60.

93. Zhang L, Gu FX, Chan JM, Wang AZ, Langer RS, Farokhzad OC. Nanoparticles in medicine: therapeutic applications and developments. *Clin Pharmacol Ther*. 2008;83(5):761–9.
94. Pommier Y, Leo E, Zhang H, Marchand C. DNA topoisomerases and their poisoning by anticancer and antibacterial drugs. *Chem Biol*. 2010;17(5):421–33.
95. Prestayko AW, D'Aoust JC, Issell BF, Crooke ST. Cisplatin (*cis*-diamminedichloroplatinum II). *Cancer Treat Rev*. 1979;6(1):17–39.
96. Shi L, Nishioka WK, JTh'ng. DW Litchfield, Greenberg AH. Premature p34cdc2 activation required for apoptosis. *Science*. 1994;263(5150):1143–5.
97. Shapiro GI, Harper JW. Anticancer drug targets: cell cycle and checkpoint control. *J Clin Invest*. 1999;104(12):1645–53.
98. Shapiro GI, Edwards CD, Ewen ME, Rollins BJ. $p16^{INK4A}$ participates in a G_1 arrest checkpoint in response to DNA damage. *Mol Cell Biol*. 1998;18(1):378–87.
99. Ling X, Chen X, Riddell IA, Tao W, Wang J, Hollett G, et al. Glutathione-scavenging poly(disulfide amide) nanoparticles for the effective delivery of Pt(IV) prodrugs and reversal of cisplatin resistance. *Nano Lett*. 2018;18(7):4618–25.
100. Shi J, Kantoff PW, Wooster R, Farokhzad OC. Cancer nanomedicine: progress, challenges, and opportunities. *Nat Rev Cancer*. 2017;17(1):20–37.
101. Blanco E, Shen H, Ferrari M. Principles of nanoparticle design for overcoming biological barriers to drug delivery. *Nat Biotechnol*. 2015;33(9):941–51.
102. Rastinehad AR, Anastos H, Wajswol E, Winoker JS, Sfakianos JP, Doppalapudi SK, et al. Gold nanoshell-localized photothermal ablation of prostate tumors in a clinical pilot device study. *Proc Natl Acad Sci U S A*. 2019;116(37):18590–6.
103. Jokerst, Lobovkina JV, T, Zare RN, Gambhir SS. Nanoparticle pegylation for imaging and therapy. *Nanomedicine (Lond)*. 2011;6(4):715–28.
104. Quan LM, Zhong Y, Weng HH. Synthesis of cell penetrating peptide decorated magnetic nanoparticles loading cisplatin for nasopharyngeal cancer therapy. *Lin Chuang Er Bi Yan Hou Tou Jing Wai Ke Za Zhi*. 2018;32(13):963–8.
105. Barcellos-Hoff MH, Park C, Wright EG. Radiation and the microenvironment – tumorigenesis and therapy. *Nat Rev Cancer*. 2005;5(11):867–75.
106. Rainey MD, Charlton ME, Stanton RV, Kastan MB. Transient inhibition of ATM kinase is sufficient to enhance cellular sensitivity to ionizing radiation. *Cancer Res*. 2008;68(18):7466–74.
107. Hickson I, Zhao Y, Richardson CJ, Green SJ, Martin NM, Orr AI, et al. Identification and characterization of a novel and specific inhibitor of the Ataxia-telangiectasia mutated kinase ATM. *Cancer Res*. 2004;64(24):9152–9.
108. Ding YF, Li S, Liang L, Huang Q, Yuwen L, Yang W, et al. Highly biocompatible chlorin e6-loaded chitosan nanoparticles for improved photodynamic cancer therapy. *ACS Appl Mater Interfaces*. 2018;10(12):9980–7.
109. Sharma P, Wagner K, Wolchok JD, Allison JP. Novel cancer immunotherapy agents with survival benefit: recent successes and next steps. *Nat Rev Cancer*. 2011;11(11):805–12.
110. Sharma P, Allison JP. Immune checkpoint targeting in cancer therapy: toward combination strategies with curative potential. *Cell*. 2015;161(2):205–14.
111. Schreibelt G, Tel J, Sliepen KH, Benitez-Ribas D, Figdor CG, Adema GJ, de Vries IJ. Toll-like receptor expression and function in human dendritic cell subsets: implications for dendritic cell-based anti-cancer immunotherapy. *Cancer Immunol Immunother*. 2010;59(10):1573–82.
112. Lasaro MO, Ertl HCJ. Targeting inhibitory pathways in cancer immunotherapy. *Curr Opin Immunol*. 2010;22(3):385–90.
113. Sharma B, Crist RM, Adiseshaiah PP. Nanotechnology as a delivery tool for precision cancer therapies. *AAPS J*. 2017 Nov;19(6):1632–42..
114. Hirsch LR, Stafford RJ, Bankson JA, Sershen SR, Rivera B, Price RE, et al. Nanoshell-mediated near-infrared thermal therapy of tumors under magnetic resonance guidance. *Proc Natl Acad Sci U S A*. 2003;100(23):13549–54.
115. Gao C, Tang F, Gong G, Zhang J, Hoi MPM, Lee SMY, et al. pH-responsive prodrug nanoparticles based on a sodium alginate derivative for selective co-release of doxorubicin and curcumin into tumor cells. *Nanoscale*. 2017;9(34):12533–42.

4 Effective Nanomedicine for Cancer Therapy

4.1 INTRODUCTION

Since the 1971 National Cancer Act, the campaign against cancer has lasted for 4 decades. Despite significant advancements in the cataloging of environmental factors and the cellular and molecular structure of this dreaded ailment, the distinctions between a cancer cell and a healthy cell remain imprecise. Anticancer treatment may be improved with the use of nanomedicine [1]. As an outcome, nanomedicines have historically been used to modify the biodistribution as well as target site accumulation of chemotherapeutic drugs to increase their effectiveness and decrease their toxicities. Nanomedicines, in preclinical settings usually increase tumor growth inhibition and lengthen life compared to non-formulated medications, but in clinical settings, patients often only benefit from nanomedicines because of decreased or altered side effects [2].

Nanomedicine anticancer medications Onivyde and Vyxeos (liposomal daunorubicin with cytarabine) have recently been approved, however clinical translation success remains poor despite that, the apparent mismatch between the increasing number of preclinical studies describing the development of more complex nanomedicines and the small number of nanomedicine products with clinical licenses has received a lot of attention [3, 4].

The imbalance is caused by a variety of biological, pharmacological, and translational barriers [5]. Biological barriers include correct intracellular processing and trafficking, perfusion, penetration and distribution from and in the target cells (in addition to endo/lysosomal escape), and distribution to and into target cells. Aspects of nanoformulation and manufacture are both included in pharmaceutical barriers. To ensure optimal stability in blood circulation, advantageous biodistribution of the medication in the body, an acceptable toxicity profile as well as logical mechanisms for drug release and biodegradation/elimination are just a few of the concerns that need to be addressed. In terms of clinical translation, selecting the correct medicine and the proper combination regimen, as well as applying them to the right illness indication and the suitable patient group, is the most important hurdle.

Defining important strategic directions to guide the design of nanomedicine clinical trials and provide demonstrable therapeutic benefits for patients is critical to tackling the correct translational problems. "Smart" cancer nanomedicine, is an umbrella term encompassing plausible and practical "Strategies and Materials to Advance and Refine Treatments," there are four strategies to increase the use and efficacy of nanomedicine. Nanomaterials have numerous benefits for society, including nanomedicine, solar cell production, and battery efficiency. Nanotechnology simplifies food and agriculture processes, improving control and offering the potential for pharmaceutical chemistry to produce nanomedicines for disease treatment. These are the classification of smart patient, smart pharmaceutical choice, smart combination therapies, and smart immunomodulation (Figure 4.1).

DOI: 10.1201/9781003451020-4

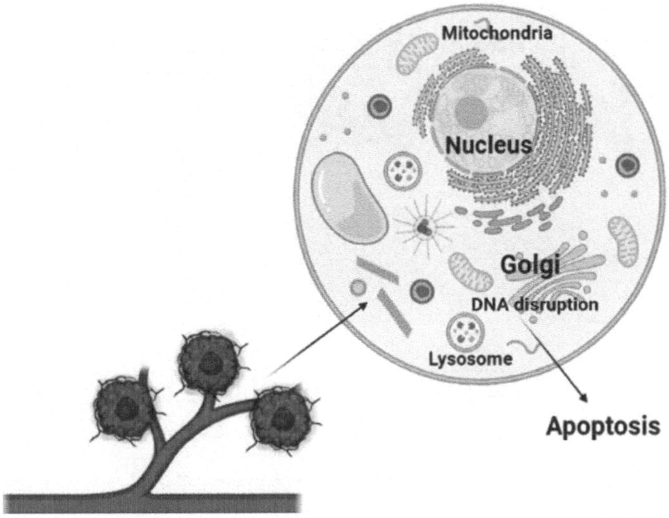

FIGURE 4.1 Targeted cellular therapy site of cancer using nanomedicine.

4.2 PATIENT STRATIFICATION

Nanomedicine is transforming cancer therapy by providing individualized and precise medical treatment. This process entails classifying people into subgroups according to different molecular, genetic, or clinical attributes, hence enabling the implementation of more efficient and personalized treatment approaches. Nanoparticles may be designed to selectively bind to these indicators, facilitating accurate administration of medication to cancerous cells while limiting harm to healthy tissues [6]. Companion diagnostics, which can determine which patients will benefit from a given nanotherapeutic intervention, may also be more easily developed using this method. Diagnostic nanoparticles, often used as imaging agents, could assist in the non-invasive surveillance of disease advancement, evaluation of therapy effectiveness, and identification of possible drug resistance. Incorporating patient stratification into nanomedicine improves treatment results by maximizing therapeutic effectiveness and decreasing negative side effects [7]. However, before being widely used, issues including regulatory concerns, ethical considerations, and uniformity of diagnostic criteria must be resolved. To confirm the effectiveness and safety of these customized treatments and provide strong recommendations for clinical use, continuous research, and clinical studies are necessary. Biomarkers and companion diagnostics are used widely in modern cancer medication development for patient stratification. Molecularly focused therapies like antibodies that block growth factor receptors or tyrosine kinase inhibitors have been successfully translated into the clinic with the aid of the companion diagnostics, which addresses the significant heterogeneity, which is characteristic of tumor. Patients with high HER2 expression levels were preselected for the Herceptin, Perjeta, and Kadcyla trials using pathological stains and/or fluorescence *in situ* hybridization, ensuring enrichment of patients likely to respond and exclusion of anticipated non-responders in these studies [8]. The initial "general biomarker" in the field of immuno- to be discovered that is connected to a particular genetic signature rather than an organ or cancer genesis. A more extensively applicable biomarker, MSI-H (MSI-H), or dMMR, is used to stratify patients for immune checkpoint inhibitor therapy [9].

4.3 BIOMARKERS INVOLVED IN CANCER NANOMEDICINE

Biomarkers play a pivotal role as essential indicators within the domain of cancer nanomedicine, thereby enabling the advancement of therapeutic interventions that are both targeted and

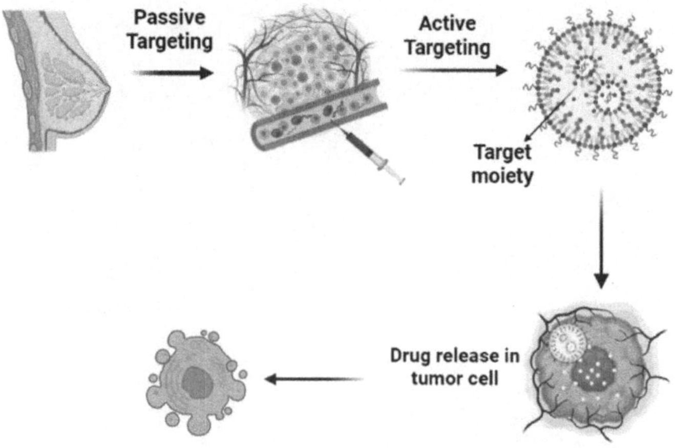

FIGURE 4.2 Clinical approaches for the selective treatment of cancer cells.

individualized. The molecular signatures, which include genetic, protein, microRNA, metabolic, and circulating biomarkers, are crucial in developing novel methods for cancer diagnosis, therapy, and monitoring. Genetic biomarkers, including mutations and amplifications, provide valuable insights into the distinctive genetic characteristics of malignancies. Cancer nanomedicine nanoparticles may target genetic changes to deliver drugs to cancer cells while protecting healthy tissues [10]. Biomarkers and companion diagnosis are presently not being utilized to modify nanomedicine therapy in patients, which is surprising (Figure 4.2). Antibody-drug conjugates are a significant exception to the norm, as they are frequently omitted from lists of nanomedicines because of their more biotechnological compared to nanotechnological character (although they should be included by the generally recognized definition). Kadcyla (ado-trastuzumab emtansine, anti-HER2); Besponsa (inotuzumab ozogamicin, anti-CD22); Adcetris (brentuximab vedotin, anti-CD30) as well as Mylotarg (ado-trastuzumab emtansine, anti-HER2) have just gained regulatory clearance (gemtuzumabozogamicin, anti-CD33). For each of these drugs, their clinical development has been aided by the inherent availability of biomarkers for patient classification.

Nanomedicines based on liposomes, micelles as well as polymeric nanoparticles may have recently failed in the clinic because to a lack of biomarker integration. Nanoparticles that target the prostate-specific membrane antigen, like BIND-014 (docetaxel-loaded polyethylene glycol-polylactic acid nanoparticles), CRLX101 (campthotecin-loaded polyethylene glycol-cyclodextr0in micelles), and NK105 (paclitaxel-loaded polyethylene glycol-polyaspartate-based micelles), have not been able to demonstrate convincing response rates in patient populations with predetermined stratification [10–12]. A retrospective question is whether or not the expectation that these nanodrugs might produce large reaction rates in a mixed (as well as highly pretreated) patient population without stratification was reasonable. Even while nanomedicines like Abraxane, which have been authorized by the FDA, have improved the quality of life and reduced toxicity in thousands of patients. Due to the fact that they are employed with non-segregated patient populations, their potential for therapy may not yet be completely realized [13]. As a result, we should start developing biomarkers to facilitate patient stratification and starting to incorporate nanomedicines into early clinical development phases, especially in combination regimens. Biomarkers of microRNAs, which play a role in controlling gene expression, add complexity to cancer nanomedicine. Nanoparticles may be designed to deliver microRNA-based therapies by regulating particular microRNAs linked to cancer development and metastasis

The EPR effect is often used to explain nanomedicine accumulage in solid tumors. The number of those opposed to the approach has, nevertheless, grown during the past few years.

The EPR effect, according to some nanomedicine researchers, is only present in mice, and not in human beings. Passive accumulation of nanocarriers in tumors does occur in patients, regardless of whether the word "EPR" is the most appropriate pathophysiological phrase to characterize the mechanisms underpinning nanocarrier localization in tumors. Nanomedicine accumulation and effectiveness need to be monitored and predicted, and methodologies and materials to do so are needed [14]. Nanomedicines that target ligands, like BIND-014, use both EPR as well as active recognition of receptors excessively expressed at diseased locations, making it possible to classify patients reasonably readily, for example, by detecting immunohistochemically the expression of PSMA in tumor biopsies [15]. Another option is positron emission tomography (PET) or single-photon emission computed tomography (SPECT) to assess PSMA receptor expression on cancerous cells and/or angiogenic endothelium in metastatic patients, allowing for patient stratification [16]. Retrospective CTC analysis in a BIND-014 phase II clinical study showed that effective therapy associated with fewer PSMA-positive CTC10, which is another option. PSMA-positive (and other) CTCs should be investigated further since they may be used as biomarkers for stratifying patients as well as indicators of therapy responses. Figure 4.2 illustrates clinically sound approaches to cancer nanomedicine patient stratification.Activated targeting depends heavily on passive targeting, which needs a considerable period to be circulated. The mononuclear phagocytic system (MPS) is a key player in the clearance of nanomedicines from the bloodstream, and the introduction of targeted ligands may help [17]. Before attaching to target cells, actively targeted nanomedicines should extravasate from the blood vessels of tumors and metastases, travel through the interstitium, and cross numerous cell layers. The designated binding-site barrier, that may prevent nanomedicines from entering cells, could be a challenge for the future [18]. Active targeting's usefulness depends heavily on the size of the nanocarrier. For instance, it has been shown that nanocarriers with a diameter of fewer than 7 nm significantly increase tumor formation when actively targeted because of their higher retention [19]. There was no difference in tumor accumulation between both passive and active targeting for nanocarriers having a diameter of under 14 nm [20]. However, active targeting altered the nanocarriers' intratumoural compartmentalization, enhancing their absorption by cancer cells. Although they did not reach higher tumor concentrations, HER2-targeted gold nanoparticles as well as 100-nm-sized HER2-targeted liposomes22 appeared to cluster in tumor cells to a greater extent than in macrophages [21]. These two potential results may be used to critically assess the extra benefit of active targeting in tumor nanomedicine applications [22]. When it comes to treating hematological cancers (which have a high concentration of cancer cells in the blood and/or MPS organs) plus other conditions requiring intracellular delivery of the therapeutic payload. We think active targeted nanomedicines are likely to be especially helpful, such as when RNA medications are used to control gene expression.

4.4 NANOTECHNOLOGIES FOR BIOIMAGING AND DETECTION

Molecular imaging of living cells and complete animals is a valuable resource for researching the biology of cancer and evaluating the effectiveness of tumor treatments. The development of fluorescent probes known as quantum dots [23–25] has greatly improved this form of imaging. Semiconductor quantum dots (QDs) are very small crystals or particles, typically measuring between 1 and 10 nm, that possess distinct photochemical and photophysical characteristics that are not seen in typical organic dyes and fluorescent proteins [26]. QDs produce distinct hues of light when stimulated at certain wavelengths, depending on their size. Typically, a shorter wavelength of light is emitted by a smaller particle in comparison to the subsequent larger dimension. QDs are ideal for *in vivo* imaging at molecular, cellular, organ, and animal levels due to their stability, enhanced fluorescence capacity, and multicolor fluorescence emission. While there are various nanoparticles that can serve this function [27–29], QDs currently seem to provide the most flexibility for cancer investigations conducted *in vivo*. Altered quantum dots may serve as durable immunofluorescent tools for identifying cancer indicators like Her2 and other biological targets on potential tumor cells [30]. Modified quantum dots may be attached to immunoglobulins to provide fluorescent imaging tests that can detect particular antigens on both fixed and living cells. This method has several benefits: the signal is stronger, there is more signal to noise, and the QDs are more photostable than other fluorescent molecules [30, 31]. Furthermore, QDs have the potential to be employed in the long-term labeling of living cells [32–34]. The quantum dots may be targeted to specific cell surface markers using conjugated antibodies, or they can be taken up by the cells by endocytic uptake [32]. Using amphipathic peptides, particles may be transported from the endosome to the cytosol or nucleus after internalization. The cells may be monitored for weeks and fluorescence data captured at various time periods since the particles are stable. QDs are excellent for biotical coding of live cells in drug compound screens, multiplexed experiments, and tracking individual cells in mixed cell populations [35, 36]. Various-sized QDs or various amounts of the particles are transfected into cells to analyze mixed cell populations.

The wavelength length(s) of the light that the cell types produce may then be used to differentiate them. A procedure that may be used in the construction of several multiplex assays is the ability to generate more than 100 different codes. The capability to observe complete organs or tumor masses in living creatures *in situ* is an essential component for research in the fields of cancer biology and therapies [36–38]. This capability is used in combination with single-cell analysis techniques. In a preliminary investigation [39], quantum dots were covered with a peptide that specifically targets the lungs. This was done to illustrate the precise localization and buildup of the probes in the lungs after intravenous administration. Additionally, two distinct peptides were used to guide the probes towards blood veins or lymphatic vessels that are linked to malignancies. The practicality of employing QDs for *in vivo* targeting of particular organs or tissues was illustrated in this study. Such capabilities may prove advantageous in the identification of specific diseases and the administration of drugs. B16F10 tumor cells tagged with QDs were utilized to follow cellular extravasation into lung tissue in mice injected with these cells as part of a metastasis study [40].

Investigators found QDs useful for analyzing the metastatic behavior and potential of different cell types *in vivo*. Their study demonstrated that the biological characteristics of the labeled cells were identical to those of the unlabeled cells. Furthermore, by attaching a distinct quantum dot to each cell, they were able to monitor up to five distinct groups of cells. The assessment of lymph node involvement plays an essential part in diagnosing and predicting the progression of many types of malignancies. The sentinel lymph node, the first node in the lymphatic basin where the main tumor drains, is commonly targeted for surgical excision by oncologists but may be difficult to locate or observe. A new nanoparticle, the near-infrared fluorescent type II quantum dot, labels sentinel nodes for mapping and imaging [41]. Near-infrared quantum dots have similarities with the aforementioned QDs, with the exception that their emission spectrum falls just outside the range of colors detectable by the human eye, namely in the infrared region. These particles have the advantage that infrared may enter live tissue far deeper than visible light, allowing near-infrared QDs to photograph and identify items that visible-wavelength QDs are unable to detect. This QD technology enables surgeons to see the lymph node in real-time during surgery and certify completion by watching the disappearance of intense fluorescence in the region. Nanoparticles (QDs) may detect and diagnose cancer *in vivo*. Multifunctional nanoparticle probes may target cancer targets and enable *in vivo* tumor imaging, according to preliminary mouse tests. A copolymer covering protected these probes from degradation, several polyethylene glycol molecules increased biocompatibility, and monoclonal antibodies recognized prostate tumor antigens. Drug delivery is another potential application of the multifunctional QDs described in this study, thereby providing a versatile platform for both diagnosis and therapy. Early tumor diagnosis improves survival chances because *in situ* cancers are simpler to remove than metastasized ones.

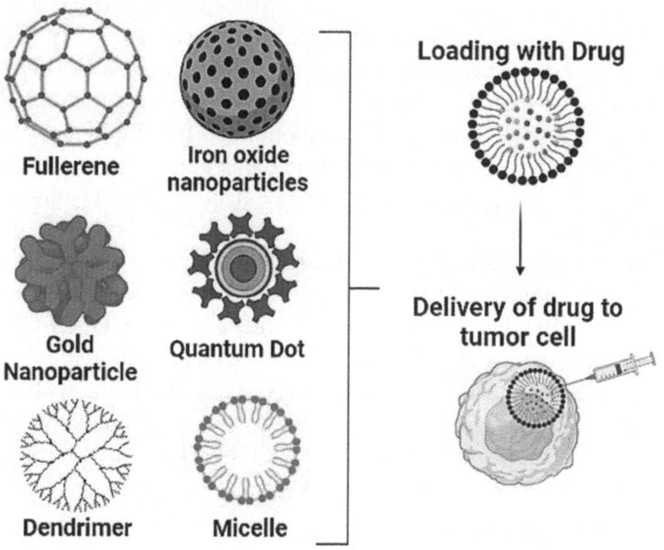

FIGURE 4.3 Smart medication selection in nanotechnology for cancer treatment.

4.5 DRUG SELECTION

For cancer nanomedicines to be a clinical and economic success, rational medication selection is essential. Except for antibody-drug conjugates, all clinically approved cancer nanomedicines to date have been based on conventional cytostatics like doxorubicin, paclitaxel, daunorubicin, vincristine, as well as irinotecan [42]. While nanomedicine reformulation increases the therapeutic index for all of these drugs, the majority of the time it does so by reducing side effects rather than by enhancing therapeutic responses considerably. We must be aware of specific adverse effects, like complement-mediated infusion reactions, in order to fully utilize the therapeutic effectiveness of nanomedicines [43]. As it requires a greater mechanistic understanding of these effects, as well as identifying effective strategies of dealing with them. Future research in the field of cancer nanomedicine medication development should concentrate on nanocarriers for the administration of non-standard pharmaceuticals such biologics. Also recommended are clever techniques like drug derivatization, library screening, and modular nanocarrier design (Figure 4.3).

4.6 DRUG CLASSES

Doxorubicin and paclitaxel, two common chemotherapy medications, have adverse effects, although they are generally well tolerated by patients, otherwise they would not have made it to the market. Auristatins, for example, are too poisonous to be given to patients in their pure form. Several antibody–drug conjugates, such as brentuximab vedotin (Adcetris), have been created to allow the use of auristatins *in vivo*. In contrast, the payloads of antibody–drug conjugates are often rather small. Thousands of auristatin molecules were packed into polymeric nanoparticles as a means of exploring formulations with greater auristatin concentrations [44]. That was the first study to show that nanoparticles may effectively limit tumor development and extend longevity in an animal model without substantial systemic toxicities. Similarly, reformulation in PEG-PLA-based nanoparticles improved effectiveness and decreased toxicity in numerous preclinical models of a strong Aurora B kinase inhibitor that generated unacceptable side effects in a phase II clinical trial in free form [45].

DNA and RNA-based therapeutics benefit greatly from the use of nanocarrier technology. Agents containing nucleic acids need intracellular delivery and must be protected against breakdown in the bloodstream. The nanotechnology used in Onpattro's drug (patisiran, liver-targeted siRNA-containing lipid nanoparticles for combating transthyretin-related hereditary amyloidosis) may aid in the development of RNA-based vaccinations for treating infections and cancer [46]. Therapeutic proteins may be produced in the liver using RNA encoded for therapeutic proteins in vaccines that target hepatocytes [47, 48]. In the same way, antitumor effects may be induced by delivering RNA-encoded cancer antigens to antigen-presenting cells in the liver and spleen [49–52]. Recently, some of these cases have started employing nucleic acid-based nanovaccines in clinical investigations for cancer immunotherapy [53].

Proteins are another type of therapy that may benefit from the delivery of nanocarriers due to the systemic toxicity of immunostimulatory medicines, including interleukin-2 (IL2) for immuno-oncology applications [54]. Biochemically, the biologic medication NKTR-214 (bempegaldesleukin) suppressed tumor development in an aldehyde-treated melonoma mice model substantially more than unmodified aldehyde-treated aldehyde, and it worked in conjunction with checkpoint inhibitor therapy [55]. Patients suffering from advanced or metastatic solid tumors56 and non-human primates55 were both reported to respond favorably to NKTR-214 treatment [56].

4.7 MODULAR STRUCTURE

For each innovative nanodrug, the carrier material as well as formulation process must be customized to the payload's physicochemical properties. Nanomedicine design has traditionally been formulation-driven. Therapeutics with comparable properties may be used, despite its inherent inflexibility [57]. Drugs like doxorubicin, which are both amphiphilic and ionizable, have been encapsulated in liposomes via pH gradient-based remote loading. As an alternative, molecules of drugs can be (re) engineered to make them more compatible with nanocarriers. Doxorubicin's hydrophobicity and miscibility with PLGA nanoparticles were improved via rational chemical derivatization, which was done to increase drug–nanocarrier compatibility and effectiveness [58]. On the other hand, a docetaxel-conjugated hydrolysable ester linker ensured stable inclusion in polymeric micelles with a core crosslink while also authorizing for regulated release of drug. In a breast cancer cell line model, single intravenous injection of polymeric micelles carrying docetaxel derivatives completely regressed the tumor [59]. In a phase II trial, the technique is currently being used to treat patients with ovarian cancer [60]. Utilizing an identical ester linker technique, fatty acids connected to cabazitaxel drove prodrugs plus PEG-lipids to assemble themselves into nanoparticles. While free cabazitaxel was more toxic and less effective in mice with breast cancer, the PEGylated version of the medicine was less toxic and more effective [61].

Derivatization methods are increasingly being employed to construct modular nanomedicine platforms. The physical disparities between drug molecules may be reduced by synthesizing prodrugs that are stable in nanocarriers, enhancing the encapsulation prediction of drugs having various features. It is also possible to limit systemic exposure and negative effects by using modular prodrug nanomedicines. In fibrosarcoma-bearing mice, for instance, a clever prodrug-based nanomedicine platform allowed for the stable co-encapsulation of doxorubicin as well as monomethyl auristatin E, two drugs with very different physicochemical properties, as well as improved selectivity and therapeutic efficacy [62].

4.8 SCREENING NANOMEDICINE LIBRARIES

The creation of nanomedicine libraries for the identification of potential therapeutic candidates during preclinical nanodrug development has been made easier by the combination of drug derivatization and modular ideas with quick and scalable manufacturing techniques. As a result, effective screening procedures for both *in vitro* as well as *in vivo* evaluation must be developed. If a novel nanomedicine has different qualities, such as its size and surface charge, traditional methodologies simply alter these two factors while investigating its pharmacological performance and medicinal properties. As a result of novel manufacturing technologies like microfluidics, it is now possible to generate vast nanomedical libraries that can be used for multiple parameter screenings. When developing BIND-014 (PSMA-targeted polymeric nanoparticles with docetaxel), these microfluidic manufacturing procedures were used. To improve BIND-014, a combinatorial polymeric nanoparticle library was developed and assessed for nanoparticle size, density of the ligand, encapsulation of the drug, as well as release kinetics. The most suitable formulation was assessed in people following pharmacokinetic, distribution in the body, pharmacotolerability, and therapeutic efficacy studies in animal models [63].

A library of lipoprotein-like nanoparticles was tested for biodistribution and immune cell selectivity using PET imaging and flow cytometry in search of novel nanoimmunotherapeutics. Ovalbumin52-specific CD8+ T cells were found in lipid nanoparticle libraries 7 days after subcutaneous injection of mRNA encoding for the model protein, and the information was used to further cancer vaccine research. For mice with B16-F10 melanoma tumors, increased survival was seen when mRNA for tumor-associated antigens was fed into the formulation that generated the most specific CD8+ T cells after two rounds of library selection. Barcoding methods are advantageous for library screenings. A formulation of nanoparticles capable of delivering functional siRNA as well as sgRNA to the bone marrow endothelial cells was found after intravenous administration of 30 nucleic acid barcoded lipid nanoparticles [64]. Tumors were extracted 48 hours after mice were given PEGylated liposomes with DNA barcodes and chemotherapeutics. In accordance with PCR barcode identification plus cell viability assessment in isolated tumor cells, the most effective chemotherapeutic treatment in a mouse model of breast cancer is predicted.

4.9 COMBINATION THERAPIES

Nanomedicine is a comprehensive and strategic methodology that attempts to optimize treatment effectiveness while minimizing potential obstacles, including systemic toxicity and drug resistance. Nanoparticle-facilitated synergistic integration of several therapeutic modalities offers significant potential for cancer treatment. Nanoparticles are adaptable carriers, enabling for the simultaneous administration of many therapeutic drugs with diverse modes of action. Encapsulating chemotherapeutic, immunotherapeutic, or nucleic acid-based medicines in nanoparticles allows targeted delivery to cancer cells [65]. This method minimizes harm to healthy tissues while optimizing the therapeutic effect on malignant cells. Moreover, combination treatment has the ability to target many cancer hallmarks at the same time, including tumor cell growth inhibition, apoptosis induction, and tumor microenvironment modification. Nanoparticles may be customized to release therapeutic drugs in a regulated and coordinated way, hence enhancing treatment timing and spatial coordination [66].

Surgery, radiation, chemotherapy, and/or immunotherapy may be used to treat various types of cancer, depending on their location, stage as well as grade. Surprisingly, clinical studies incorporating nanomedicines are almost always conducted as single-agent treatments in order to evaluate their effectiveness. Nanomedicine formulations cannot be compared with standard of care in terms of effectiveness since it does not take use of some of the inherent characteristics of nanomedicines. Because they can co-encapsulate various pharmaceuticals, nanomedicines may be used in combination with normal chemotherapy treatments, and they are more effective than free-form drugs when it comes to interacting with environmental stimuli. (1) Small molecule drugs are more dependent on blood flow as well as permeability compared to nanomedicines are, and these characteristics benefit from employing pharmacological as well as physical combination therapies. (2) Nanomedicines deliver greater amounts of drugs to pathological sites, and they stay there for longer periods of time. (3) Nanomedicines are often designed to respond in particular to pharmacological or physical combination treatments, which can be more effective at treating localized conditions. These features

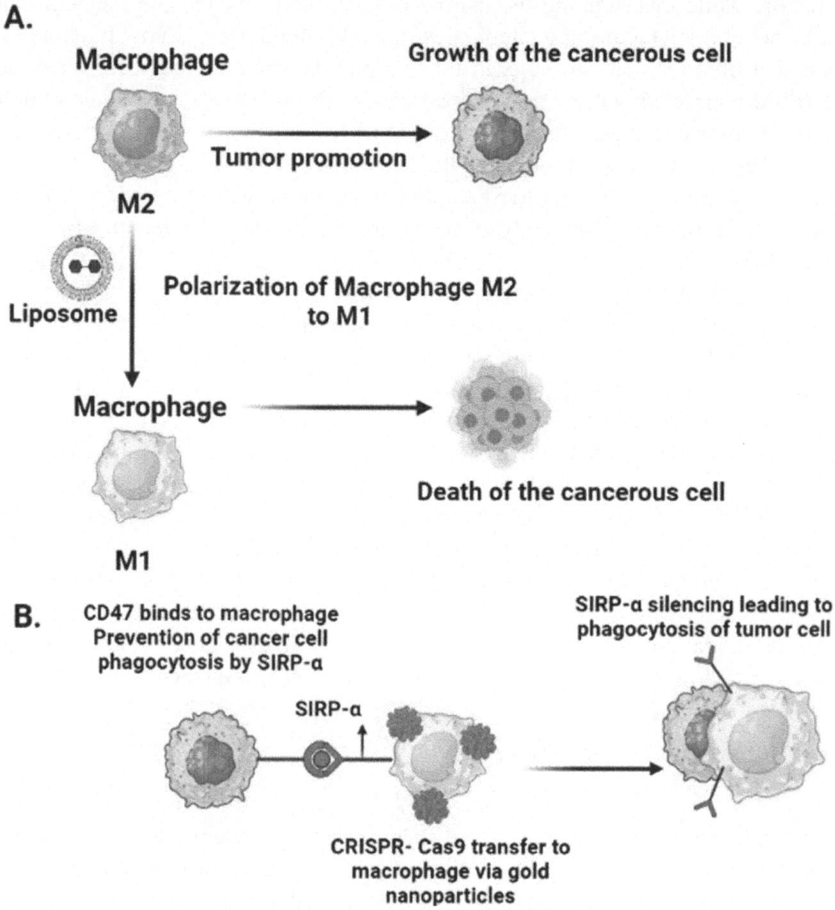

FIGURE 4.4 Combination therapy based on cancer nanomedicine.

should be used to their full potential in order to develop more potent anticancer combo treatments (Figure 4.4).

4.9.1 Systemic Combination Therapies

Liposomal irinotecan (Onivyde), newly licenced in conjunction with 5-fluorouracil (5-FU) plus leucovorin (LV) for treating pancreatic cancer, demonstrates the efficacy of nanomedicines in systemic combination therapy [67]. A powerful anticancer medicine like Irinotecan is difficult to administer in free form because of its significant adverse effects. Compared to 5-FU/LV, liposomal irinotecan by itself did not increase overall survival in patients suffering from pancreatic cancer, but when combined with 5-FU/LV, overall survival was dramatically improved while the safety profiles were highly acceptable [68]. Therapy of triple-negative breast cancer with atezolizumab (Abraxane) and nanoparticle albumin-bound paclitaxel has also demonstrated promising outcomes [69].

Tumor-targeted medication delivery is increasingly being paired with systemically delivered cancer nanomedicines. Increasing the clinical effect and efficacy of cancer nanomedicine requires overcoming several biological, immunological, and translational barriers. Tumor metabolism, interstitial fluid pressure, and extracellular matrix density all function as biological barriers. Inhibiting TGF-signaling and lowering collagen formation by cancer-associated fibroblasts, Both conventional nanomedicines as well as 100-nm-sized oncolytic viruses may benefit from the use of losartan to increase their dispersion and efficacy [70, 71]. Losartan has been shown to dramatically increase the percentage of R0 resections following neoadjuvant chemotherapy using FOLFIRINOX in pancreatic cancer, according to recent studies [72, 73]. Because of their higher cellular metabolism, tumors have low extracellular pH (pH 6.5–7), which can be improved by increasing extracellular pH (pH 6.5–7). When sodium bicarbonate-loaded liposomes were tested, they were shown to be able to raise the intratumoral pH to 7.4 and so enhance uptake of doxorubicin by inhibiting protonation and hydrophilization [74].

Systemic combination treatment may also benefit from nanomedicines. For instance, Vyxeos is a liposomal nanomedicine preparation that can be used to "ratiometrically" kill cancer cells. It contains both daunorubicin and cytarabine at a synergistic drug proportion of 5:1. Vyxeos received fast-track FDA clearance after a phase III study found that it extended median survival time in patients suffering from acute myeloid leukaemia from 6 to 10 months as compared to the standard of treatment [75].

4.9.2 Local Combination Therapies

Radiotherapy, ultrasound, and heat are all effective treatments that may be used in conjunction with cancer nanomedicines. In the same way that pretreatment with radiation improves radiochemotherapy results by increasing nanomedicine accumulation and penetration, nanocarrier materials also enhance those outcomes [76, 77]. Liposomal irinotecan, when administered in conjunction with radiotherapy and cyclophosphamide, has been shown to be more effective and to be delivered to tumors with more efficiency [78]. The abscopal effect, which is enhanced by nanomedicines, may improve immunotherapy results by capturing and delivering antigens produced by radiation to antigen-presenting cells [79].

For tumor-targeted drug administration by sonopermeation, ultrasound may be used in conjunction with microbubbles to open interendothelial junctions, promote endocytosis and transfer of the medication into cells, and improve blood flow to the tissues, especially in highly stromal tumors [80]. Gemcitabine, ultrasound, and microbubbles were shown to increase median survival in pancreatic cancer patients from 9 months to 18 months in the first clinical proof of concept study using sonopermeation [81]. When combined with intravenous microbubbles, SonoCloud, an ultrasonic device that can be implanted into the skull, may help glioblastoma patients with their BBB [82]. In individuals who have primary brain tumors, it is feasible and safe to use targeted external ultrasound that is guided by magnetic resonance [83].

Temperature-sensitive doxorubicin-loaded liposomes are currently the most sophisticated method of integrating nanomedicines with locally applied physical therapy. In a phase III study for treating hepatocellular carcinoma (HCC), Thermodox was unable to achieve its primary objective for a number of reasons, including the use of radiofrequency ablation. However, it demonstrated an improvement in progression-free as well as overall survival in a sample of patients [84]. We eagerly anticipate the findings of a recently finished follow-up phase III trial in HCC along with painstakingly adjusted RFA parameters [85]. Thermodox is also being tested in conjunction with targeted ultrasound-based hyperthermia for a variety of cancers in children and adults, including several types of breast cancer [80, 86].

4.9.3 Immunomodulation

Recent clinical breakthroughs in immunotherapy as well as chimeric antigen receptor (CAR) T-cell treatments have caused a paradigm change in cancer treatment [87, 88]. By boosting the body's immune system, patients with cancer types and phases that were previously believed to be challenging or impossible to treat have shown long-lasting antitumor responses. A tiny percentage of

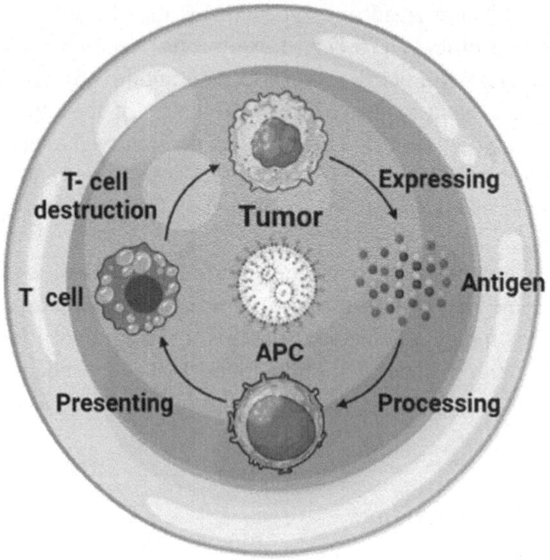

FIGURE 4.5 Nanomedicine-based immunomodulation.

people have experienced full recovery for up to 10 years, per extensive studies. Unfortunately, for a great deal of cancer patients, immunotherapy is ineffective. To maximize the effects of immunotherapy, the understanding of both local and systemic tumor immune microenvironment (TIME) must be increased [89]. The development of more effective immuno-oncological treatments will benefit from the insight.

In the late 1990s, while cancer nanomedicine was initially explored, the idea was to find ways to circumvent the immune system while still delivering therapeutic payloads to tumor cells. As we have just found, the true promise of nanomedicines may lie in their ability to stimulate the immune system. For one to employ nanotherapeutics in induced immune (Figure 4.5), it is required to use them to regulate the adaptive and/or innate immune systems [90–92]. With the help of nanomedicines that boost the immune system's ability to fight cancer, a new generation of immunotherapies with less adverse reactions is soon to be available [93, 94].

4.10 ADAPTIVE IMMUNE SYSTEM TARGETING

The majority of immunomodulating nanomedicines address the adaptive immune system in line with already-approved immunotherapeutics for cancer. These formulations frequently aim to induce or increase CD4+ and CD8+ T-cell responses, induction or enhancement of antigen presentation (signal 1), regulation of co-stimulatory signals (signal 2), and/or production of cytokines (signal 3) to produce antitumor effects. To increase a patient's receptivity to immunotherapy, researchers may also design nanomedicines that alter the immune system's TIME.

By administering chemotherapeutics like doxorubicin and oxaliplatin to tumors, immunogenic cell death (ICD) may increase the effectiveness of checkpoint blockade immuno therapeutics [95]. ICD-inducing nanomedicines outperform free pharmaceuticals, which induce ICD in terms of immunotherapy because the former have less systemic drug exposure and less systemic immunodepression, that is one of the main causes. Indoleamine 2,3-dioxygenase, a soluble immuno-inhibitor, may also be inhibited by nanomedicines (IDO) [96]. IDO encourages tryptophan's conversion to kynurenine, which suppresses the immune system in cancer cells. A metabolic pathway that suppresses the immune system is rendered inactive by nanomedicines containing IDO inhibitors. Following both local and systemic treatment of nanoparticles that included the anticancer oxaliplatin and an IDO inhibitor, pancreatic ductal tumors in mice were reduced in size [97]. In addition, a co-formulation of doxorubicin with an IDO inhibitor enhanced anti-PD-1 therapy in a mice model with metastatic breast cancer [98].

The most cutting-edge use of genetic medicine in oncology is the creation of customized cancer vaccines, as detailed in Sec. 4.5. These vaccines contain patient-specific tumor antigens encoded by mRNA in a lipid-based carrier system that is ionizable. As a result of subcutaneous or intravenous injection of a nanocarrier formulation to preserve the payload, it is a successful method in triggering T-cell responses against tumors by delivering antigen to cells that present antigen. Interchangeable RNA payloads can be built to encode either patient-specific neoepitopes or tumor-associated self-antigens that are shared by patients with a particular type of tumor to generate entirely customized cancer vaccines.

As indicated in Sec. 4.9, radiation therapy may work in conjunction with immune checkpoint blockade treatment in some circumstances. Additionally, the abscopal effect, which occurs when local radiation therapy at the initial tumor site causes distant metastatic lesions to retreat, may improve immunotherapy, particularly when combined with intelligent nanomedicine formulations [99, 100].

4.11 INNATE IMMUNE SYSTEM TARGETING

The bulk of nanoimmunotherapies today concentrate on affecting the adaptive immune system, but the innate immune system's components have received less attention [101]. The innate immune system acts as an immediate and mostly non-specific first line of defense against infections through the complement system along with cells like phagocytes as well as natural killer cells. These cells' pattern-recognizing receptors (PRRs) (DAMPs) are capable of detecting both PAMPs plus damage-associated molecular patterns (DAMPs). Innate immunological responses may be triggered by PAMPs and DAMPs, which in turn can activate the adaptive immune system. A basic form of innate immunological memory known as "trained immunity," that remains intact in the bone marrow by hematopoietic cell stem and progenitor cells, is orchestrated by metabolic and epigenetic changes that underpin these reactions [102, 103]. Because bone marrow-targeted nanomedicines may produce trained immunity, they may assist in reducing both local and metastatic tumor development.

A different strategy involves using nanomedicine to activate innate antitumor immune responses on dendritic cells (DCs) by activating PRRs such as TLRs, RLRs and activators of interferon genes on the PRRs, such as RLRs, on DCs in the TIME (STING) [104]. Transcriptional activation of type I interferons is one of many signalling pathways triggered by PRR activation (IFN-1). By utilizing IFN-1 to activate DCs and produce antitumor T-cell immunity, it is conceivable to reprogramme immunologically "cool" tumors into "hot" tumors that are responsive to checkpoint inhibitor therapy. Cyclodextrin nanoparticles carrying the TLR7/8 agonist R848 that encourage TAM polarization concerning an M1-like phenotype, like an example, may improve cancer immunotherapy. Monotherapy with nanoparticles inhibited tumor development via modulating immunosuppressive TIME. Additional checkpoint inhibitor treatment was increased by the R848-containing formulation in an insensitive tumor model. RLRs are cytosolic double-stranded RNA sensor proteins. RNA that has been 5'-triphosphorylated as well as short double-stranded RNA is specifically recognised by RIG-1. As a result, 5'-triphosphate-end bispecific siRNAs may be engineered to silence an oncogene while simultaneously activating RIG-1. Anti-Bcl2 siRNA-treated lipid-coated calcium phosphate nanoparticles decreased tumor formation and prolonged life in mice with orthotopic pancreatic cancer using two-pronged strategy. STING, an essential regulatory protein (dsDNA), detects cytosolic double-stranded DNA and initiates the activation of IFN-1. The STING-binding molecule cyclic guanosine monophosphate-adenosine monophosphate (cGAMP) is produced as a result of the type I interferon response to DsDNA, which is recognized by cyclic GMP-AMP synthase (cGAS). Nanomedicines are a good tool for inducing immunological response since cGAMP as well as STING agonists are cyclic dinucleotides therefore must be present within the cell in order to be recognized by cGAS. Examples include polymersomes that improve cytosolic transport of cGAMP, which suppressed tumor development and extended life in mice with a murine melanoma model [105].

4.12 CONCLUSION

Cancer nanomedicines may be improved by using a combination of logical reasoning and sound judgement. Four strategic paths for cancer nanomedicine performance, translation, and exploitation are presented. Much like other oncology medication research sectors, clinical trials for cancer nanomedicine crucially need probes and methodologies for patient classification. In order to guarantee that preclinical formulations developed and evaluated in the lab will function properly in patients when they are put into use, library screening and modular drug as well as nanocarrier design may be helpful. Rationally designed pharmacological as well as physical combination regimens will increase the pharmacokinetics and/or pharmacodynamic benefits provided by entrapping drugs in nanomedicine formulations. The development of immunomodulatory nanomedicines as a reaction to the pathophysiological aspects identified as limiting the effectiveness of present cancer immune therapies may improve the results of immune oncological interventions and increase the proportion of long-term survival.

Additionally, there are a number of other avenues that may be taken to enhance the effectiveness of cancer nanomedicine. Standardizing preclinical nanomedicine research and enhancing repeatability, quantitative comparisons, meta-analysis, and modeling may be accomplished by establishing minimal information reporting guidelines. Different than intravenous application, it may be beneficial to look at other methods of delivery for nanomedicines. In contrast to clinical intravenous administration, at-home self-administration of antibody-based medicines like Humira (adalimumab; anti-TNF) reduces the requirement for hospitalization by working effectively with subcutaneous self-injection. Nanomedicines may benefit from alternate methods of administration that have received little attention so far, but these benefits might be considerable.

The subject of cancer nanomedicine has grown rapidly in the last several years. Even while various novel materials and articles are being developed, only a small number of anticancer nanomedicines (including antibody–drug conjugates) have reached the market. We need to rethink that approach to translational cancer nanomedicine research and abandon the practise of creating ever-more complicated nanomedicine materials in order to make a difference. We need to devise a strategy that will help as many people as possible benefit from nanomedicines. In order to make the shift, a conglomeration of academics, pharmaceutical companies, regulatory authorities, and clinicians must work together in an integrated and concerted way. The strategic directions presented in the publication, which intends to streamline translational cancer nanomedicine research, will improve the clinical impact and patient performance of nanomedicine anticancer medications.

REFERENCES

1. Peer D, et al. Nanocarriers as an emerging platform for cancer therapy. *Nat Nanotechnol.* 2007;2:751–760.
2. Shi, J, Kantof PW, Wooster R, Farokhzad OC. Cancer nanomedicine: progress, challenges and opportunities. *Nat Rev Cancer.* 2017;17:20–37.
3. Tinkle S, McNeil SE, Mühlebach S, Bawa R, Borchard G, Barenholz Y, Tamarkin L, Desai N. Nanomedicines: addressing the scientific and regulatory gap. *Ann N Y Acad Sci.* 2014 Apr;1313(1):35–56.
4. Van der Meel R, Lammers T, Hennink WE. Cancer nanomedicines: oversold or underappreciated? *Expert Opin Drug Deliv.* 2017;14:1–5.

5. Anchordoquy TJ, et al. Mechanisms and barriers in cancer nanomedicine: addressing challenges, looking for solutions. *ACS Nano.* 2017;11:12–18.
6. McGranahan N, Swanton C. Biological and therapeutic impact of intratumor heterogeneity in cancer evolution. *Cancer Cell.* 2015;27(1):15–26.
7. Wicki A, Witzigmann D, Balasubramanian V. Nanomedicine in cancer therapy: challenges, opportunities, and clinical applications. *J Control Release.* 2015;200:138–157.
8. Verma S, et al. Trastuzumab emtansine for HER2-positive advanced breast cancer. *N Engl J Med.* 2012;367:1783–1791.
9. van der Meel R, Sulheim E, Shi Y, Kiessling F, Mulder WJ, Lammers T. Smart cancer nanomedicine. *Nat Nanotechnol.* 2019 Nov;14(11):1007–1017.
10. Bobo D, Robinson KJ, Islam J, Thurecht KJ, Corrie SR. Nanoparticle-based medicines: a review of FDA-approved materials and clinical trials to date. *Pharmaceut Res.* 2016;33(10):2373–2387.
11. Voss MH, et al. A randomized phase II trial of CRLX101 in combination with bevacizumab versus standard of care in patients with advanced renal cell carcinoma. *Ann Oncol.* 2017;28:2754–2760.
12. Fujiwara Y, et al. A multi-national, randomised, open-label, parallel, phase III non-inferiority study comparing NK105 and paclitaxel in metastatic or recurrent breast cancer patients. *Br J Cancer.* 2019;120:475–480.
13. Petersen GH, Alzghari SK, Chee W, Sankari SS, La-Beck NM. Meta-analysis of clinical and preclinical studies comparing the anticancer efcacy of liposomal versus conventional non-liposomal doxorubicin. *J Control Release.* 2016;232:255–264.
14. Lammers T, Rizzo LY, Storm G, Kiessling F. Personalized nanomedicine. *Clin Cancer Res.* 2012;18:4889–4894.
15. Bravaccini, S. et al. PSMA expression: a potential ally for the pathologist in prostate cancer diagnosis. *Sci Rep.* 2018;8:1–8.
16. Han S, Woo S, Kim YJ, Suh CH. Impact of 68Ga-PSMA PET on the management of patients with prostate cancer: a systematic review and meta-analysis. *Eur Urol.* 2018;74:179–190.
17. Lu J, Gao X, Wang S, He Y, Ma X, Zhang T, Liu X. Advanced strategies to evade the mononuclear phagocyte system clearance of nanomaterials. *Exploration.* 2023 Feb;3(1):20220045.
18. Juweid M, et al. Micropharmacology of monoclonal antibodies in solid tumors: direct experimental evidence for a binding site barrier. *Cancer Res.* 1992;52:5144–5153.
19. Danhier F, Feron O, Préat V. To exploit the tumor microenvironment: passive and active tumor targeting of nanocarriers for anti-cancer drug delivery. *J Control Release.* 2010 Dec 1;148(2):135–146.
20. Tsvetkova Y, et al. Balancing passive and active targeting to diferent tumor compartments using ribofavin-functionalized polymeric nanocarriers. *Nano Lett.* 2017;17:4665–4674.
21. Choi CHJ, Alabi CA, Webster P, Davis ME. Mechanism of active targeting in solid tumors with transferrin-containing gold nanoparticles. *Proc Natl Acad Sci USA.* 2010;107:1235–40.
22. Kirpotin DB, et al. Antibody targeting of long-circulating lipidic nanoparticles does not increase tumor localization but does increase internalization in animal models. *Cancer Res.* 2006;66:6732–6740.
23. Alivisatos AP. Semiconductor clustors, nanocrystals, and quantum dots. *Science.* 1996; 271:933–937.
24. Alivisatos P. The use of nanocrystals in biological detection. *Nat Biotechnol.* 2004; 22:47–52.
25. Bruchez Jr M, Moronne M, Gin P, Weiss S, Alivisatos AP. Semiconductor nanocrystals as fluorescent biological labels. *Science* 1998; 281:2013–2016.
26. Smith AM, Gao X, Nie S. Quantum dot nanocrystals for in vivo molecular and cellular imaging. *Photochem Photobiol.* 2004;80: 377–385.
27. Anderson SA, Glod J, Arbab AS, Noel M, Ashari P, Fine HA, et al. Noninvasive MR imaging of magnetically labeled stem cells to directly identify neovasculature in a glioma model. *Blood.* 2005; 105:420–425.
28. Hutten A, Sudfeld D, Ennen I, Reiss G, Hachmann W, Heinzmann U, et al. New magnetic nanoparticles for biotechnology. *J Biotechnol.* 2004;112:47–63.
29. Lian W, Litherland SA, Badrane H, Tan W, Wu D, Baker HV, et al. Ultrasensitive detection of biomolecules with fluorescent dye-doped nanoparticles. *Anal Biochem.* 2004; 334:135–144.
30. Wu X, Liu H, Liu J, Haley KN, Treadway JA, Larson JP, et al. Immunofluorescent labeling of cancer marker Her2 and other cellular targets with semiconductor quantum dots. *Nat Biotechnol.* 2003; 21:41–46.

31. Smith AM, Nie S. Chemical analysis and cellular imaging with quantum dots. *Analyst.* 2004;129:672–677.
32. Jaiswal JK, Goldman ER, Mattoussi H, Simon SM. Use of quantum dots for live cell imaging. *Nat Methods*. 2004;1:73–78.
33. Jaiswal JK, Mattoussi H, Mauro JM, Simon SM. Long-term multiple color imaging of live cells using quantum dot bioconjugates. *Nat Biotechnol*. 2003;21:47–51.
34. Michalet X, Pinaud FF, Bentolila LA, Tsay JM, Doose S, Li JJ, et al. Quantum dots for live cells, in vivo imaging, and diagnostics. *Science*. 2005;307:538–544.
35. Han M, Gao X, Su JZ, Nie S. Quantum-dot-tagged microbeads for multiplexed optical coding of biomolecules. *Nat Biotechnol.* 2001;19: 631–635.
35. Mattheakis LC, Dias JM, Choi YJ, Gong J, Bruchez MP, Liu J, et al. Optical coding of mammalian cells using semiconductor quantum dots. *Anal Biochem.* 2004;327:200–208.
36. Jain RK, Stroh M. Zooming in and out with quantum dots. *Nat Biotechnol*. 2004;22:959–960.
37. Jiang W, Papa E, Fischer H, Mardyani S, Chan WC. Semiconductor quantum dots as contrast agents for whole animal imaging. *Trends Biotechnol*. 2004;22:607–609.
38. Larson DR, Zipfel WR, Williams RM, Clark SW, Bruchez MP, Wise FW, et al. Water-soluble quantum dots for multiphoton fluorescence imaging in vivo. *Science*. 2003;300:1434–1436.
39. Akerman ME, Chan WC, Laakkonen P, Bhatia SN, Ruoslahti E. Nanocrystal targeting in vivo. *Proc Natl Acad Sci U S A*. 2002;99: 12617–12621.
40. Kim S, Lim YT, Soltesz EG, De Grand AM, Lee J, Nakayama A, et al. Near-infrared fluorescent type II quantum dots for sentinel lymph node mapping. *Nat Biotechnol*. 2004;22:93–97.
41. Ji H, Hu C, Yang X, et al. Lymph node metastasis in cancer progression: molecular mechanisms, clinical significance and therapeutic interventions. *Sig Transduct Target Ther*. 2023;8:367. https://doi.org/10.1038/s41392-023-01576-4.
42. Hare JI, et al. Challenges and strategies in anti-cancer nanomedicine development: an industry perspective. *Adv Drug Deliv Rev*. 2017;108:25–38.
43. Szebeni J, Simberg D, González-Fernández Á, Barenholz Y, Dobrovolskaia MA. Roadmap and strategy for overcoming infusion reactions to nanomedicines. *Nat Nanotechnol*. 2018;13:1100–1108.
44. Qi R, et al. Nanoparticle conjugates of a highly potent toxin enhance safety and circumvent platinum resistance in ovarian cancer. *Nat Commun*. 2017;8:2166.
45. Ashton S, et al. Aurora kinase inhibitor nanoparticles target tumors with favorable therapeutic index in vivo. *Sci Transl Med*. 2016;8:325ra17.
46. Adams D, et al. Patisiran, an RNAi therapeutic, for hereditary transthyretin amyloidosis. *N Engl J Med*. 2018;379:11–21.
47. Sahin U, Türeci Ö. Personalized vaccines for cancer immunotherapy. *Science.* 2018;359:1355–1360.
48. Pardi N, Hogan MJ, Porter FW, Weissman D. mRNA vaccines – a new era in vaccinology. *Nat Rev Drug Discov*. 2018;17:261–279.
49. Pardi N, et al. Administration of nucleoside-modifed mRNA encoding broadly neutralizing antibody protects humanized mice from HIV-1 challenge. *Nat Commun*. 2017; 8:14630.
50. Kranz LM, et al. Systemic RNA delivery to dendritic cells exploits antiviral defence for cancer immunotherapy. *Nature*. 2016;534:396–401.
51. Kreiter S, et al. Mutant MHC class II epitopes drive therapeutic immune responses to cancer. *Nature.* 2015;520:692–696.
52. Oberli MA, et al. Lipid nanoparticle assisted mRNA delivery for potent cancer immunotherapy. *Nano Lett*. 2017;17:1326–1335.
53. Sahin U, et al. Personalized RNA mutanome vaccines mobilize poly-specifc therapeutic immunity against cancer. *Nature.* 2017;547:222–226.
54. Zhang Y, Li N, Suh H, Irvine DJ. Nanoparticle anchoring targets immune agonists to tumors enabling anti-cancer immunity without systemic toxicity. *Nat Commun*. 2018;9:6.
55. Doberstein SK. Bempegaldesleukin (NKTR-214): a CD-122-biased IL-2 receptor agonist for cancer immunotherapy. *Expert Opin Biol Ther*. 2019 Dec 2;19(12):1223–1228.
56. Bentebibel S-E, et al. A frst-in-human study and biomarker analysis of NKTR-214, a novel IL2Rβγ-biased cytokine, in patients with advanced or metastatic solid tumors. *Cancer Discov*. 2019; 9:711–721.

57. Cern A, Marcus D, Tropsha A, Barenholz Y, Goldblum A. New drug candidates for liposomal delivery identifed by computer modeling of liposomes' remote loading and leakage. *J Control Release.* 2017;252:18–27.
58. Zhao Y, et al. Augmenting drug–carrier compatibility improves tumournanotherapyefcacy. *Nat Commun.* 2016; 7:11221.
59. Hu Q, et al. Complete regression of breast tumour with a single dose of docetaxel-entrapped core-cross-linked polymeric micelles. *Biomaterials.* 2015;53:370–378.
60. Cristal Terapeutics. Efcacy study of CPC634 (CriPec® docetaxel) in platinum resistant ovarian cancer (CINOVA). ClinicalTrials.gov. 2018. https://clinicaltrials.gov/ct2/show/NCT03742713.
61. Wang H, et al. New generation nanomedicines constructed from self-assembling small-molecule prodrugs alleviate cancer drug toxicity. *Cancer Res.* 2017;77:6963–6974.
62. Miller MA, et al. Modular nanoparticulate prodrug design enables efcient treatment of solid tumors using bioorthogonal activation. *ACS Nano.* 2018;12:12814–12826.
63. Hrkach J, et al. Preclinical development and clinical translation of a PSMA-targeted docetaxel nanoparticle with a diferentiated pharmacological profle. *Sci Transl Med.* 2012;4:128ra39.
64. Wang ET, et al. Barcoded nanoparticles for high throughput in vivo discovery of targeted therapeutics. *Proc Natl Acad Sci USA.* 2017;114:2060–2065.
65. Peer D, Karp JM, Hong S, Farokhzad OC, Margalit R, Langer R. Nanocarriers as an emerging platform for cancer therapy. *Nat Nanotechnol.* 2007;2(12):751–760.
66. Dreaden EC, Alkilany AM, Huang X, Murphy CJ, El-Sayed MA. The golden age: gold nanoparticles for biomedicine. *Chem Soc Rev.* 2012;41(7):2740–2779.
67. Greene MK, Johnston MC, Scott CJ. Nanomedicine in pancreatic cancer: current status and future opportunities for overcoming therapy resistance. *Cancers.* 2021 Dec 7;13(24):6175.
68. Chen LT, et al. Final results of NAPOLI-1: a phase 3 study of nal-IRI (MM-398) ± 5-fuorouracil and leucovorin (5-FU/LV) vs 5-FU/LV in metastatic pancreatic cancer (mPAC) previously treated with gemcitabinebased therapy. *Ann Oncol.* 2016;27:622PD–622PD.
69. Schmid, P. et al. Atezolizumab and nab-paclitaxel in advanced triplenegative breast cancer. *N Engl J Med.* 2018;379:2108–2121.
70. Chauhan VP, et al. Angiotensin inhibition enhances drug delivery and potentiates chemotherapy by decompressing tumour blood vessels. *Nat Commun.* 2013;4:2516.
71. Diop-Frimpong B, Chauhan VP, Krane S, Boucher Y. Jain RK. Losartan inhibits collagen I synthesis and improves the distribution and efcacy of nanotherapeutics in tumors. *Proc. Natl Acad. Sci. USA* . 2011;108:2909–2914.
72. Murphy JE, et al. Potentially curative combination of TGF-b1 inhibitor losartan and FOLFIRINOX (FFX) for locally advanced pancreatic cancer (LAPC): R0 resection rates nd preliminary survival data from a prospective phase II study. *J Clin Oncol.* 2018;36:4116.
73. Murphy JE, et al. Total neoadjuvant therapy with FOLFIRINOX in combination with losartan followed by chemoradiotherapy for locally advanced pancreatic cancer. *JAMA Oncol.* 2019;5:1020.
74. Abumanhal-Masarweh H, et al. Sodium bicarbonate nanoparticles modulate the tumor pH and enhance the cellular uptake of doxorubicin. *J Control Release.* 2019;296:1–13.
75. Lancet JE, et al. CPX-351 (cytarabine and daunorubicin) liposome for injection versus conventional cytarabine plus daunorubicin in older patients with newly diagnosed secondary acute myeloid leukemia. *J Clin Oncol.* 2018;36:2684–2692.
76. Davies CDL, et al. Radiation improves the distribution and uptake of liposomal doxorubicin (Caelyx) in human osteosarcoma xenografs. *Cancer Res.* 2004;64:547–553.
77. Lammers T, et al. Image-guided and passively tumour-targeted polymeric nanomedicines for radiochemotherapy. *Br J Cancer.* 2008;99:900–910.
78. Miller MA, et al. Radiation therapy primes tumors for nanotherapeutic delivery via macrophage-mediated vascular bursts. *Sci Transl Med.* 2017;9:eaal0225.
79. Min Y, et al. Antigen-capturing nanoparticles improve the abscopal efect and cancer immunotherapy. *Nat Nanotechnol.* 2017;12:877–882.
80. Snipstad S, et al. Sonopermeation to improve drug delivery to tumors: from fundamental understanding to clinical translation. *Expert Opin Drug Deliv.* 2018;15:1249–1261.
81. Dimcevski G, et al. A human clinical trial using ultrasound and microbubbles to enhance gemcitabine treatment of inoperable pancreatic cancer. *J Control Release.* 2016;243:172–181.

82. Carpentier A, et al. Clinical trial of blood-brain barrier disruption by pulsed ultrasound. *Sci Transl Med.* 2016;8:343re2.
83. Mainprize T, et al. Blood-brain barrier opening in primary brain tumors with non-invasive MR-guided focused ultrasound: a clinical safety and feasibility study. *Sci Rep.* 2019;9:321.
84. Tak WY, et al. Phase III HEAT study adding lyso-thermosensitive liposomal doxorubicin to radiofrequency ablation in patients with unresectable hepatocellular carcinoma lesions. *Clin Cancer Res.* 2018;24:73–83.
85. Celsion. Study of TermoDox with standardized radiofrequency ablation (RFA) for treatment of hepatocellular carcinoma (HCC) (OPTIMA). *ClinicalTrial.gov.* 2014. https://clinicaltrials.gov/ct2/show/NCT02112656
86. Kim, A. A phase I study of lyso-thermosensitive liposomal doxorubicin and MR-HIFU for pediatric refractory solid tumors. *ClinicalTrial.gov.* 2015. https://clinicaltrials.gov/ct2/show/NCT02536183?term=thermodox&rank=10.
87. Ribas A, Wolchok, JD. Cancer immunotherapy using checkpoint blockade. *Science.* 2018;359:1350–1355.
88. June CH, et al. CAR T cell immunotherapy for human cancer. *Science.* 2018;359:1361–1365.
89. Jain RK, et al. Understanding the tumor immune microenvironment (TIME) for efective therapy. *Nat Med.* 2018;24:541–550.
90. Riley RS, June CH, Langer R, Mitchell MJ. Delivery technologies for cancer immunotherapy. *Nat Rev Drug Discov.* 2019;18:175–196.
91. Sun Q, et al. Nanomedicine and macroscale materials in immunooncology. *Chem Soc Rev.* 2019;48:351–381.
92. Mulder WJM, Ochando J, Joosten LAB, Fayad ZA, Netea MG. Terapeutic targeting of trained immunity. *Nat Rev Drug Discov.* 2019;18:553–566.
93. Jiang W, et al. Designing nanomedicine for immuno-oncology. *Nat Biomed Eng.* 2017;1:0029.
94. Friedman CF, Proverbs-Singh TA, Postow MA. Treatment of the immune-related adverse efects of immune checkpoint inhibitors: a review. *JAMA Oncol.* 2016;2:1346–1353.
95. Pfrschke C, et al. Immunogenic chemotherapy sensitizes tumors to checkpoint blockade therapy. *Immunity.* 2016;44:343–354.
96. Prendergast GC, Malachowski WP, DuHadaway JB, Muller AJ. Discovery of IDO1 inhibitors: from bench to bedside. *Cancer Res.* 2017;77:6795–6811.
97. Lu J, et al. Nano-enabled pancreas cancer immunotherapy using immunogenic cell death and reversing immunosuppression. *Nat Commun.* 2017;8:1811.
98. Lu J, et al. Breast cancer chemo-immunotherapy through liposomal delivery of an immunogenic cell death stimulus plus interference in the IDO-1 pathway. *ACS Nano.* 2018;12:11041–11061.
99. Hwang WL, Pike LRG, Royce TJ, Mahal BA, Loefer JS. Safety of combining radiotherapy with immune-checkpoint inhibition. *Nat Rev Clin Oncol.* 2018;15:477–494.
100. Ngwa W, et al. Using immunotherapy to boost the abscopal efect. *Nat Rev Cancer.* 2018;18:313–322.
101. Borden EC. Interferons α and β in cancer: therapeutic opportunities from new insights. *Nat Rev Drug Discov.* 2019;18:219–234.
102. Netea MG, Latz E, Mills KHG, O'Neill LAJ. Innate immune memory: a paradigm shif in understanding host defense. *Nat Immunol.* 2015;16:675–679.
103. Netea MG, et al. Trained immunity: a program of innate immune memory in health and disease. *Science.* 2016;352:aaf1098.
104. Marongiu L, Valache M, Facchini FA, Granucci F. How dendritic cells sense and respond to viral infections. *Clin Sci.* 2021 Oct;135(19):2217–42.
105. Shae D, et al. Endosomolyticpolymersomes increase the activity of cyclic dinucleotide STING agonists to enhance cancer immunotherapy. *Nat Nanotechnol.* 2019;14:269–278.

5 Enhancing Cancer Immunotherapy Using Nanoparticle-Based Smart Carriers

5.1 INTRODUCTION

Cancer immunotherapy has emerged as a groundbreaking approach in the treatment of various malignancies, leveraging the body's immune system to target and eliminate cancer cells. It is now well-accepted that immunotherapy may be used to treat a broad range of illnesses by manipulating the host's immune system [1]. Depending on whether a medication inhibits or enhances the immune response of the host, it can be classified as immunosuppressive or immunostimulatory. Several forms of autoimmune disorders may be treated with immunosuppressive medication such as diabetes type 1, rheumatoid arthritis, atherosclerosis, as well as obesity. Contrarily, immunostimulatory therapy refers to therapies that boost the immune system intending to treat cancer along with other infectious diseases [2].

Recently, immunomodulatory approaches to cancer treatment have become more popular owing to their lesser side effects compared to chemotherapy, radiation, and surgery [3]. There has been increased use of immunomodulatory medicines. Using tumor antigens, the immune system can tell the difference between cancerous and healthy cells [4]. The immune system can recognize two different types of TSAs: tumor-specific (TSAs), which are distinct molecules generated only by tumor cells, like PSA, or prostrate-specific antigens (highly selective for recognizing cancer and triggering host immune response), as well as tumor-associated (TAAs), which are distinct molecules produced by both healthy and cancerous cells. However, the immunosuppressive nature of the tumor microenvironment (TME) hinders the host's immune system from efficiently battling tumor cells [5]. However, the tumor microenvironment (TME) has an immunosuppressive character, which prevents the host immune system from working efficaciously against tumor cells [6]. Immune checkpoint blockers, cell-based therapies, monoclonal antibodies, and cancer vaccines can all be utilized for stimulating the immune system of the host, which is very efficacious in many patients [7]. Tumor immunotherapy not only kills cancer cells but also stops them from spreading and coming back, making it a significant advance over current cancer therapies. Existing cancer immunotherapy has significant drawbacks, including the production of damaging autoimmunity and the inability to transmit cancer antigens to immune cells effectively [8]. Additionally, the immunosuppressive TME inherently minimizes the effectiveness of immunotherapy for cancer.

Nanoparticles, due to their unique physical and chemical properties, offer an innovative platform for delivering therapeutic agents precisely to tumor sites. By incorporating advanced materials into these smart carriers, researchers can modulate the release kinetics of immunotherapeutic payloads, ensuring sustained and targeted delivery. This approach not only maximizes the therapeutic impact on cancer cells but also minimizes systemic side effects, a critical consideration for improving patient outcomes [9]. Small particle size, customizable form, high cell penetrating capacity, and

DOI: 10.1201/9781003451020-5

improved magnetic, electrical mechanical, and optical capabilities relative to its bulk structures are some of the distinctive attributes of nanoparticles (NPs) [10]. NPs are frequently employed in a variety of biological applications because of their extraordinary features. A wide range of disorders have been treated using NPs because of their immunomodulatory properties (immunoinhibitory or immunostimulatory) [11]. When it comes to the therapy of inflammation and autoimmune illnesses, immunosuppressants and immunostimulatory are utilized, respectively. Because of all of its benefits, including their multiple advantages, nanoparticles (NPs) are also frequently used as carriers and delivery systems in cancer immunotherapy: (1) antigen and adjuvants are delivered to identical antigen presentation cells (APCs) simultaneously; (2) preventing bioactive molecules carrying cargo from being destroyed by enzymes; (3) effective delivery with targeting ligands to particular cells or regions; (4) for elevating the release of cancer antigens and stimulate the immune system, nanoparticles may be made using photodynamic therapy (PDT), photothermal therapy (PTT), or radiosensitizers, which could eradicate tumors [12]. Anti-inflammatory and anti-immunosuppressive applications of nanoparticles have been shown in Figure 5.1.

Photo- and radio-based immunotherapy will be discussed in a future literature review, as the focus of the current chapter is on using nanoparticles as delivery systems for antigens and immunostimulants [13]. We would like to present some immunostimulatory NPs that have been broadly utilized in immunotherapy. For cancer immunotherapy, NPs may be used as clever transporters of antigens and adjuvants [14]. In the discussion that follows, we will examine the interactions that NPs, antigens, and adjuvants have with immune system cells and how various environmental factors affect these interactions. In addition, the effects of NPs in the TME on dendritic cells (DCs), T lymphocytes (T lymphocytes), as well as natural killer cells (NK cells), among others, will be thoroughly discussed

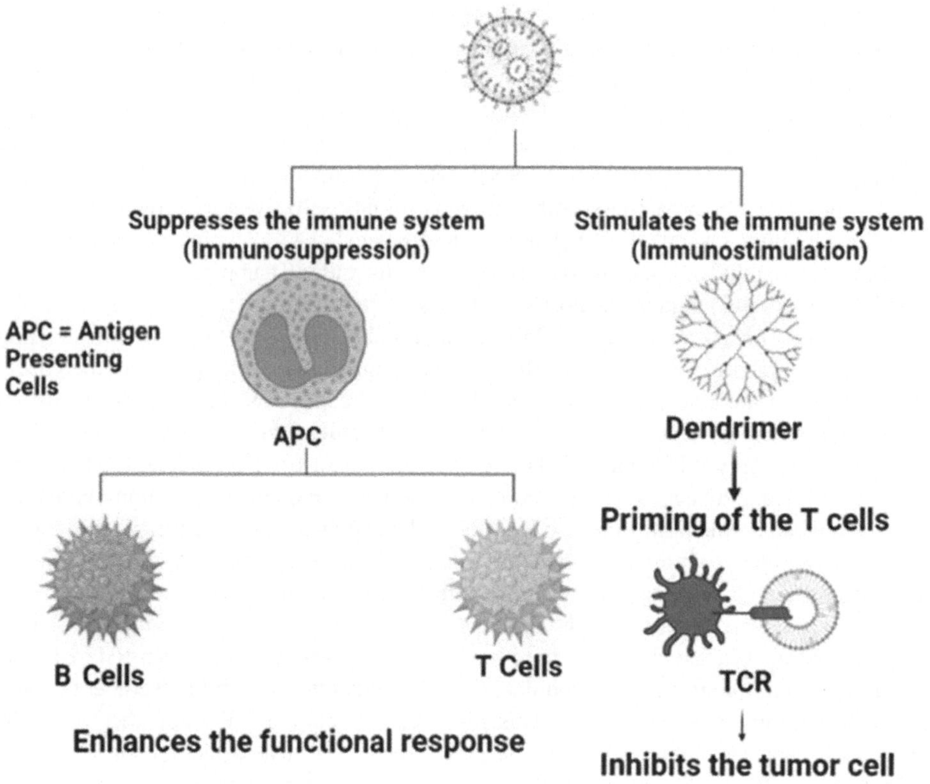

FIGURE 5.1 Utilization of nanoparticles to lower inflammatory levels and suppress immune responses.

[15]. This paper aims to provide a comprehensive overview of the current advancements, challenges, and prospects in harnessing the potential of nanoparticle-based smart carriers to augment the efficacy of cancer immunotherapy.

5.2 CLASSIFICATION OF IMMUNOSTIMULATORY NANOPARTICLES

Molecules that can normalize and/or alter the immune system are known as immunomodulators. Two types of immunosuppressants and immunostimulants may be found in these compounds (which stimulate the immune system) [16].

5.2.1 Nanoparticles Derived from Polymers

Polymer-derived nanoparticles offer a customizable platform for drug delivery, diagnostics, and imaging in the realm of healthcare. The tunable properties of these nanoparticles, such as size, shape, and surface chemistry, allow for precise control over their interactions with biological systems. This has led to significant advancements in targeted drug delivery, where therapeutic agents can be encapsulated within polymer nanoparticles to enhance their stability, solubility, and bioavailability. Polymeric NPs utilized most frequently as immunostimulatory NPs because of their excellent biocompatibility, water solubility, biodegradability, chemical stability, plus considerable capability of loading immune-related components [17]. In cancer immunotherapy, polymeric NPs such as PLGA, PGA, PGA-PLG, PEG, PEI, and chitosan NPs are the most widely employed. As an efficient adjuvant for immunization, these NPs have been widely used [18]. If, for instance, Kim *et al.* discovered that PLGA NPs encapsulating the TLR 7/8 agonist boosted the co-stimulatory compounds (CD40, CD80, and CD86), then the stimulation of dendritic cells derived from bone marrow (BMDCs) led to a rise in CD40, CD80, and CD86 expression [19]. Due to their capacity to stimulate DCs along with CD8+ T cells (cytotoxic T cells), PLGA NPs are also useful adjuvants for cancer immunotherapy. Following subcutaneous administration of the nanoformulation, anticancer responses in the bladder, melanoma, as well as renal carcinoma models were each increased [20]. In a recent study published in the journal *Immunotherapy Cancer*, Poly (I: C) and Resiquimod NPs were employed to co-deliver two TLR agonists (poly (I: C) and Resiquimod) together with a chemokine, MIP 3 (Macrophage Inflammatory Protein-3 alpha), which notably improved the therapeutic effectiveness of cancer vaccines in tumor-carrying mice [21]. It was demonstrated that the co-delivery of such immune modulators using PLGA NPs remarkably made alterations to the populations of lymphoid along with myeloid cells in the tumor as well as lymph node. Additionally, nanovaccines increased the long-term lifespan of tumor-carrying mice by 75–100% and nearly doubled the animals' length of progression-free life [22].

5.2.2 Liposomes (Lipid Bilayer)

Liposomes, lipid bilayer structures with a versatile range of applications, stand at the intersection of biology and nanotechnology, offering unique advantages in drug delivery, diagnostics, and fundamental biological research [23]. These microscopic vesicles, composed of phospholipids or other amphiphilic molecules, mimic cell membranes and provide an ingenious platform for encapsulating and delivering therapeutic agents. It has also emerged as a major NP in the delivery of medicines, DNA, and vaccinations through liposomes. By delivering antigens to APCs and boosting the number of vaccination adjuvants, a variety of liposomal antigen delivery systems, such as DOTAP, DC-Chol, and DDA, are utilized to improve the immune response to various antigens [23]. According to Yuba and colleagues, DCs took up lysosomes carrying dextran-modified dextran liposomes responsive to pH and delivered OVA into the cytosol [24]. Subcutaneous treatment of the nanoformulation also boosted antigen-specific immune responses and suppressed tumor development in E.G7-OVA tumor-carrying mice [25]. Using a complex of a TLR9 agonist (CpG-ODNs) and a 3,5-didodecyloxybenzamidine (adjuvant) in liposomes modified with pH-responsive polymer, Gulijk *et al.* found that the combination increased DC production of co-stimulatory molecules plus cytokine, resulting in improved antigen-specific immunity [26]. These investigations revealed a broad range of potential uses for liposomes as antigen transporters as well as adjuvants in cancer immunotherapy. Additional research has shown that synthetic long-peptides (SLPs) may be successfully delivered to dendritic cells (DC) and activated CD8+ cytotoxic T cells by using liposome cationic liposomes [27]. That means that peptide-based cancer vaccines may be effectively delivered using liposomes.

5.2.3 Gold Nanoparticles

Gold nanoparticles, with their unique physicochemical properties and versatile applications, have emerged as key players in the fields of nanotechnology, medicine, catalysis, and materials science. These nanoscale entities, typically ranging from 1 to 100 nm in size, owe their distinct properties to the intriguing interplay between their size, shape, and surface characteristics. They may be employed in immunotherapy because of their minimal immunotoxicity, changeable surface chemistry, as well as their ability to be readily controlled in terms of form and size. It is crucial to remember that GNPs are a particular class of NPs that activate macrophages and lead to their development into dendritic-like cells, which promotes the expansion of T cells as well as the generation of cytokines [28]. To boost antibody production in mice, GNPs were employed as an adjuvant with CpG-ODNs, another immunostimulant, which proved to be much more effective. By altering the thiolated CpG-ODNs on the outermost layers of hollow GNPs, tumor formation is prevented. Immune cells absorb the modified nanoconjugate considerably more easily than free CpG-ODNs and display greater immune stimulatory activity. CpG-hollow GNPs elevated the release of TNF via cells of RAW264.7 by a factor of 15 when compared to CpG-ODNs alone [29].

5.2.4 Nanoparticles with a Magnetic Core

Nanoparticles with a magnetic core represent a fascinating class of nanomaterials that has garnered significant attention in various scientific and technological domains. The integration of a magnetic core within nanoparticles introduces multifunctionality, enabling applications ranging from targeted drug delivery and imaging in medicine to data storage and environmental remediation. Due to their advantages in current magnetic resonance imaging (MRI) techniques, magnetic NPs are broadly utilized in theranostics. For cancer theranostic applications, researchers are particularly intrigued by SPIONs, which are superparamagnetic iron oxide nanoparticles [30]. The aggregation of these NPs may be minimized by coating them with a biocompatible substance. According to Martins *et al.*, dimercaptosuccinic acid-coated SPIONs have been demonstrated to transmit an anti-tumorigenic cytokine, IFN-, to the site of the tumor by utilizing an outer magnetic field [31]. The outcomes revealed enhanced macrophage infiltration, T-cell populations, antiangiogenic activity, as well as tumor growth suppression. Furthermore, it has been demonstrated that applying a magnetic field from outside enhances T-cell activation plus inhibits the advancement of cancer cells using magnetic NPs coated using dextran plus functionalized using proteins that activate T cells. Another study revealed a synergistic enhancement of the anticancer immune reaction plus direct death of tumor cells when two TLR agonists, poly (I: C) as well as imiquimod (R837), were loaded onto micellar zinc-doped iron oxide magnetic NPs [32]. Recently, Luo and coworkers described the usage of ultrasmall iron oxide nanocomposites loaded with OVA promoting the maturation of DC along with the activation of T cells [33]. These nanocomposites' stimulation of macrophages encouraged an adaptive immune reaction against tumors. These nanocomposites might inhibit and prevent the growth of B16-OVA tumors in both the subcutaneous as well as metastatic regions, according to the *in vivo* findings. According to Kim and colleagues, OVA-coated and silica-coated magnetic NPs that were ingested by DCs induced antigen-selective CD4+ T helper type 1 (Th1) cell reactions and antigen-selective CD8+ cytotoxic T-cell (Tc) immune reactions simultaneously [34]. Additionally, these types of nanoformulations notably inhibited the advancement of tumors in animals with EG7-OVA tumors.

5.2.5 Nanoparticles Derived from Proteins

Nanoparticles derived from proteins have emerged as a dynamic and versatile class of nanomaterials, capitalizing on the inherent properties of proteins to address challenges in drug delivery, diagnostics, and biomedical research. The utilization of proteins, with their diverse structures and functionalities, as building blocks for nanoparticle design offers a unique and biocompatible approach to overcome limitations associated with traditional materials. To stimulate a potent anticancer immune response, tumor antigens along with adjuvants can also be delivered with the help of protein NPs. According to a recent study by Molino and colleagues, biomimicking protein NPs may efficiently co-deliver CpG-ODN activator plus peptide epitopes, leading to enhanced as well as prolonged activation of CD8+ T cell and improved antigen cross-presentation in DCs [35]. A further study found that the gp100 epitope associated with melanoma, CpG-ODN, and viral mimetic protein NPs all enhanced the proliferation of CD8+ T cells as well as IFN-production simultaneously. On the other hand, these multifunctional NPs extended the time that mice survived after vaccination by 40% and postponed the start of tumor formation in mice by 5.5 days. Thakur *et al.* employed HLA-A2-restricted epitopes of MAGE-A3 as well as NY-ESO-1 (E2 nanoparticle) to deliver two human cancer-testis antigens concurrently via the E2 subunit assembling of pyruvate dehydrogenase in 2018 [36]. They discovered that giving HLA-A2 transgenic mice the NY-ESO-1 epitope along with CpG-ODN at the very same time via E2 protein NPs boosted IFN-secretion 25 times and cell destruction activity 15 times, respectively. Mice were immunized using E2 NPs containing the MAGE-A3 epitope with CpG-ODN, which increased IFN production by a factor of 6 and cell lysis activity by a factor of 9. When supplied jointly, NYESO1-CpG E2 as well as MAGEA3-CpG E2 nanoformulations increased IFN- production along with cell lysis activity [37].

5.2.6 Micelles

Micelles, dynamic and self-assembling nanostructures formed by amphiphilic molecules, have emerged as versatile and efficient carriers in drug delivery, nanomedicine, and various technological applications. The unique ability of micelles to spontaneously organize into well-defined structures in solution, driven by the amphiphilic nature of their building blocks, contributes to their widespread use in enhancing solubility, stability, and targeted delivery of hydrophobic compounds. Micelles are utilized as excellent nanocarriers of adjuvants and antigens to increase the efficacy of cancer vaccines. Examples include an investigation by Li *et al.* [38] that utilized polymeric hybrid micelles (PHMs) to carry TRP2 as well as TLR-9 agonists, respectively (CpG-ODN). They discovered the effectiveness of nanovaccine in targeting the proximal lymph node as well as increased the quantity of antigen/adjuvant that was taken up by DCs. Using the co-delivery method, a potent anticancer impact was identified in a lung metastatic melanoma model, which further evoked antigen-selective CD8+ T-cell immune reactions. Li and coworkers developed polymeric hybrid micelles (PHMs) for the simultaneous administration of the CpG-ODN adjuvant and the Trp2 peptide antigen in a different study [39]. To create PHMs, PCL-PEI and PCL-PEG were employed. Compared to mixes of unengaged Trp2 or CpG or Trp2/PHM0/CpG with no PCL-PEI, PHMs containing 10% PCL-PEI were more effective at trapping DCs and triggering antigen-selective CD8+ T-cell reactions along with anticancer effectiveness. After some time in 2018, Li and colleagues conducted an additional study using carboxylated polymeric mixed micelles to efficiently deliver an OVA plus TLR-7 agonist (CL264) to DCs in lymph nodes [40]. They discovered that these nanovaccines promoted the maturation of DC, and production of cytokine, along with elevated antigen cross-presentation, every one of them boosted the immune response to the target antigen. The nanovaccine also has the potential to significantly decrease the growth of cancer cells in C57BL/6 mice.

5.2.7 Particles that Resemble Viruses

Nanoparticles designed to resemble viruses represent an innovative and promising class of nanomaterials with diverse applications in medicine, vaccine development, and targeted therapies. Drawing inspiration from the intricate structures of viruses, researchers have engineered synthetic particles that mimic certain aspects of viral morphology and behavior. These virus-mimicking nanoparticles leverage the advantages of viruses, such as their ability to interact with specific cells and deliver payloads, while mitigating the inherent risks associated with live viral vectors. Significant interest has also been shown in the application of virus-like particles (VLPs) as a type of nanovaccine platform for the enhancement of the effectiveness of cancer immunotherapy. According to an investigation by Lizotte and colleagues [41], when cowpea mosaic virus (CPMV) self-assembled VLPs were breathed by C57BL/6J mice, they significantly reduced B16F10 lung melanomas as well as activated neutrophils in the tumor microenvironment (TME). Recently, Kerstetter-Fogle and coworkers [42] gave an account that intracranial glioma, a brain tumor, was successfully treated with CPMV VLPs by inducing a potent anticancer immune reaction. Immune responses against HER-2 in HER2+ mice cancer models were generated by CPMV VLPs coupled with the CH401 peptide from the HER-2-derived antigenic CH401 peptide [43]. Nanovaccines also prevented tumor development and metastasis in mice, according to the researchers. 2020 saw the incorporation of CpG-ODNs specifically delivered to TME's tumor-associated macrophages using VLPs made from Cowpea Chlorotic Mottle Virus (CCMV)-derived CpG-ODNs. Additionally, they demonstrated that TAMs in TME quickly absorbed VLPs loaded with CpG-ODNs, which boosted their phagocytic activity and caused more potent anticancer effects than free CpG-ODNs in both *in vitro* as well as *in vivo* [44].

5.2.8 Nanoemulsions

Nanoemulsions (NEs) are often employed in the form of adjuvants or delivery systems for antigen/adjuvant since they strongly stimulate the antitumor immune response [45]. Bose and colleagues created a lectin receptor of C-type (Clec9A) functionalized tailored nanoemulsions (Clec9A- TNE) for antigen-specific immunotherapy [46]. They could stimulate the growth of antigen-selective CD4+ along with CD8+ T cells and induce antibody and CD8+ T-cell immunological reactions in cross-presenting DCs by using Clec9A-TNE as a nanocarrier [47]. Oncogenic HPV16 antigen, E6/E7 was loaded into Clec9A-TNE, as well as the researchers discovered that it greatly reduced tumor growth, triggered powerful antigen-specific IFN-responses, and improved mouse survival [48–50]. According to recent research by Kim and colleagues, NEs loaded with TLR7/8 agonist, paired with cancer cell antigens successfully incorporated an anticancer immune reaction by activation of DCs, T cells, along with modulating immunosuppressive TME without causing systemic harm [51]. Additionally, they depicted that NE (TLR 7/8) therapy in conjunction with immune checkpoint blockade therapy (ICBT) incorporated a synergistic anticancer immune response in the B16F10-OVA melanoma plus TC-1 cervical cancer model [52].

5.2.9 Nanogels

Nanogels have proven to be an efficacious antigen or protein system of delivery in the domain of cancer immunotherapy. Cui and coworkers developed the self-administering antigen delivery system using amphiphilic galactosyl dextran-retinal nanogels sensitive to pH (GDR) [53]. These types of nanovaccines (GDR/OVA) have been demonstrated to significantly enhance the maturation of DC, uptake of antigen by DCs, as well as antigen releases in the cytosol. Additionally, GDR nanogels promoted lysosomal disruption in DCs and increased the formation of ROS, they both increased DCs' ability to cross-present antigens and resulted in a potent antitumor immune response [54]. According to Yang *et al.*, disulfide bonds were employed to connect OVA to dextran nanogels, enabling intracellular OVA releases in a reductive environment [55]. It has been demonstrated that these OVA nanogels are easily absorbed by DCs and help the cells mature. Additionally, when paired with the adjuvant poly (I: C), these OVA-nanogels significantly produced potent antitumor effects combating melanoma *in vivo*. Recently, Li and colleagues (2019) created pullulan self-assembly nanogels harboring carbazol group modifications to induce a powerful adaptive immune response when administered to DCs [56].

5.2.10 Dendrimers

Nanovaccines based on dendrimers are being applied to treat several malignancies. In a study (Feng *et al.*) [57], it was discovered that polyamidoamine dendrimers modified with DGBA function like an efficient nanocarrier for simultaneously delivering OVA as well as CpG-ODN. The combined use of the DGBA, OVA, and CpG nanovaccines promoted DC maturation and lysosomal escape following the effective uptake by DCs, enabling them to give antigen cross-presentation more successfully. It has been demonstrated that a potent nanovaccine against the B16-OVA melanoma significantly boosts CD8+ T-cell immune reactions. Nanovaccine therapy for B16-OVA melanoma exhibited synergistic CD8+ T-cell immune reactions with the use of ICBT. To deliver CpG-ODN to DCs, Debele *et al.* recently created dendrimer-encased GNPs that were decorated with methylated polyethylene glycol (PEG-Au DENPs). It has been demonstrated that PEG-Au DENPs loaded with CpG are easily absorbed by DCs, which encourages the maturation of DC and stimulates T-cell activation to start an adaptive cellular antitumor immune response [58].

5.3 STRATEGIES TO ENHANCE IMMUNOSTIMULATORY NANOPARTICLES

There are three ways in which the host immune system is activated by NPs: (1) providing antigens, (2) functioning as self-adjuvantors, or (3) being delivered or acting as adjuvantors to induce immunogenic cancer cell death [59]. Furthermore, the following qualities must be considered necessary for NPs to be a successful delivery method.

5.3.1 Interaction between Antigens and Adjuvants with Nanoparticles

The kind of relationship that exists between NPs, as well as antigens, is essential for the efficient transport of antigens because it prevents the cargo molecules from being broken down by enzymes and then prematurely liberated into the circulatory system [60]. Antigen and/or adjuvant molecules have been physically adsorbable, encapsulated, or chemically conjugated to the NPs. The various ways that NPs and adjuvants can interact are shown in Figure 5.2.

5.3.2 Physical Adsorption

NPs can bind to antigens as well as adjuvant molecules through hydrophobic or electrostatic interactions [61]. The antigens in the NPs are expelled from the cell and delivered into the environment more quickly because the link is weaker. By customizing the surface of the NP with the right coating materials or functionalization, these interactions may be managed. Garg with his colleagues investigated BSA adsorption on the functionalized FDU-12 mesoporous silica surface

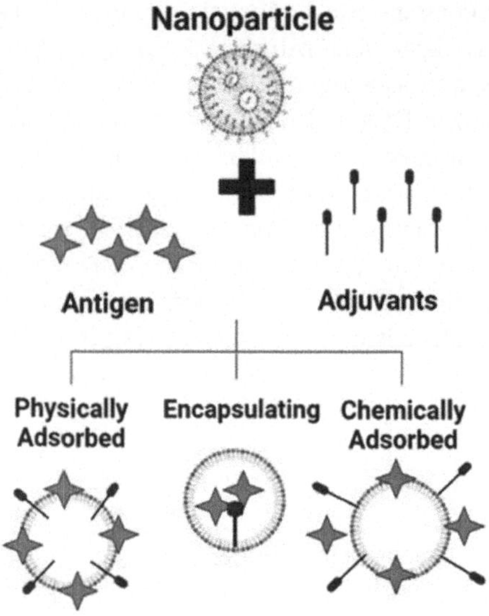

FIGURE 5.2 Nanoparticle interactions with adjuvants or antigens involve physical adsorption, encapsulation, and chemical conjugation.

[62]. They found out silica with vinyl functionalization adsorbed BSA with the help of hydrophobic interactivities, and silica with amino functionalization adsorbed BSA through electrostatic interactivities. Mahony and coworkers also discovered OVA adsorption on MSNs functionalized with amino groups with the help of electrostatic interactivities amongst positive charged amino groups located onto the NP surface with negatively charged protein [63]. In a different study, Perez-Potti and colleagues discovered noncovalent adsorption of TAA plus an adjuvant (CpG-ODN) onto the surface of MWCNTs, which are oxidized. OVA at the latest has been administered to DCs via physical adsorption onto the outermost layer of MWCNTs that have had their surface changed with mannose [64].

5.3.3 Encapsulation

Antigens and/or adjuvants may be encapsulated in polymeric NPs by combining them with the polymer, emulsifying them, and then evaporating the solvent. To encapsulate antigens and/or adjuvants, liposomal encapsulation methods such as dehydration-reabsorption procedures or freeze–thaw sonication may be used to accomplish these goals [65]. During encapsulation, the cargo molecules are more firmly attached to the NPs based on polymer or liposomes, plus the trapped molecules can be released inside the cytosol once the NPs have been ingested and broken down. Yuba *et al.* discovered that DCs could efficiently endocytose OVA while picking it up into their cells by using dextran-modified liposomes [24]. The antigens had been released in the cytosol when the liposomes ruptured in the somewhat acidic surrounding of the endosomes. Rosalia and colleagues used an improved PLGA nanoparticle vaccine formulation to deliver an OVA antigen plus two adjuvants, poly (I: C), a TLR3 ligand, as well as Pam3CSK4 (a TLR2 ligand), to DCs [66]. Das and colleagues also gave an account of the co-encapsulation of the antigen (OVA) along with adjuvant (poly (I: C)) in PLGA NPs for systematic delivery into DCs [67]. Following that research, Choo *et al.* observed that when they delivered a novel TLR7/8 agonist to DCs in PLGA nanoparticles, the antigen-specific immune response significantly increased [68].

5.3.4 Molecular Bonding (Chemical Conjugation)

Here, in such a type of interactivity, the antigen is bound chemically with the surface of NPs. For instance, Slütter and his colleagues (2010) covalently attached OVA with N-trimethyl chitosan (TMC) by utilizing a reducible disulfide link for enhancing the immune response of the antigens over OVA/TMC NPs [69]. Hu and his colleagues found a significant decrease in the growth of malignant melanomas when conventional and customized antigens (Trp2, M27, and M30) were coupled with an immunoadjuvant (CpG-ODN) in stacked double hydroxide nanoparticles [70]. Trp2, M27, and M30 peptides were initially chemically coupled to BSA via the creation of an amide bond before the BSA-antigens were placed on the surface of LDH NPs. Dykman *et al.* attached CpG-ODNs to GNPs and investigated their immunogenicity by creating a coordination link between GNPs and 5′-thiolated ODNs [71]. Another study used hollow gold nanospheres to attach CpG-ODNs altered with thiols to increase the immunostimulatory effect and effective delivery of CpG-ODNs.

5.4 PARAMETERS IMPACTING THE INTERACTION BETWEEN ANTIGEN-PRESENTING CELLS (APCS) AND NANOCARRIERS

The interaction between antigen-presenting cells (APCs) and nanocarriers is a critical aspect in the field of vaccine development and immunotherapy [72]. Nanocarriers, such as nanoparticles and liposomes, serve as delivery systems for antigens, enhancing their stability, targeting, and immunogenicity. The efficacy of these nanocarriers is intricately linked to their interactions with APCs, which include dendritic cells, macrophages, and B cells. Several parameters significantly impact the nature and effectiveness of this interaction, influencing the immune response and overall therapeutic outcomes. The strongest linkages are produced by NP-antigen chemical conjugation, which also enables an extended release of the payload's molecules [73]. Killer cells of the human body's immune system, such as natural killer (NK) cells/cytotoxic T cells, have a greater capacity to recognize antigens of a foreign or malignant origin [74,75]. Instead of getting rid of them, they provide them to the killer cells to incite an even stronger immune reaction. B cells, macrophages, dendritic cells (DC), as well as Langerhans cells—also referred to as antigen-presenting cells (APCs)—are a few of them. APCs also activate CD4+ helper T cells, which secrete cytokines to regulate immunological activity, or CD8+ cytotoxic T cells, which act as their APCs in addition to production of immune-regulating cytokines plus antibodies (especially in the case of B cells) [76]. Contrarily, it is important to emphasize that CD4+ helper T cells activate only if they recognize an antigenic peptide that is neither self nor cancerous and is expressed on MHC-II molecules only by the APCs [77,78]. To elicit an antitumor immune reaction, the tumor antigens, as well as adjuvants, should be delivered to the APCs through commendatory interactivity among the nanocarriers with APCs. The interactivity is influenced by the size, hydrophobicity, shape, surface functionalization, as well as charge on the surface of the NPs [79, 80]. In this complex interplay between nanocarriers and APCs, a nuanced understanding of these parameters is essential for the design of effective vaccines and immunotherapies [81]. Optimizing these factors can lead to enhanced antigen presentation, immune activation, and ultimately, improved therapeutic outcomes in various disease contexts [82].

5.5 CONCLUSION

Over the various previous decades, NP-based immunotherapy has experienced remarkable expansion in the domain of treating cancer as well as immunotherapy. The findings discussed the role of NPs in cancer immunotherapy through stimulating the APCs plus T cells as well as the targeting of selective cells accountable for immunosuppressive properties of the tumor microenvironment. The simultaneous administration of antigens, as well as adjuvant to APCs, may enhance tumor immunotherapy. NPs may function as self-adjuvants and increase the body's T and B cells' ability to absorb immunostimulatory chemicals. As a result, a greater challenge in the therapy of cancer is the clinical translation of NP immunostimulatory NPs. Immunostimulatory NPs must be secure since they communicate with the immune system. Therefore, a detailed investigation of immunotoxicity is required. When evaluating NPs' toxicity, it is also critical to take into account whether or not they have an impact on the intracellular signaling system. When NPs interact with serum proteins, the immune system may identify them as foreign substances, leading to autoimmunity against them. This is necessary because of the successful clinical application that relies on the NPs' ability to be tailored so that they do not trigger ROS, allergic sensitization, or hypersensitivity and can leave the body fast. Researchers involved in the domain of NPs that are immunostimulatory increasingly using NPs that are naturally obtained and are more secure as well as biologically compatible compared to the synthetic NPs. They even demand an in-depth study of how they interact with other biological elements, such as immunological cells inside the body. A fascinating new field of research that may result in new cancer treatments is immunostimulatory NPs for cancer therapy. Although its clinical use has several limits, greater study in the field and the development of safer nanocarriers for cancer patients may increase their therapeutic efficiency.

REFERENCES

1. Varadé J, Magadán S, González-Fernández Á. Human immunology andimmunotherapy: main achievements and challenges. *Cell Mol Immunol*. 2021 Apr;18(4):805–28.
2. Meng X, Lei Y, Zhang X, Sun K, Zhang L, Wang Z. Cancer immunotherapy: classification, therapeutic mechanisms, and nanomaterial-based synergistic therapy. *Appl Mater Today*. 2021 Sep 1; 24:101149.
3. Ventola CL. Cancer immunotherapy, Part 1: current strategies and agents. *PT*. 2017 Jun;42(6):375–83.
4. Papaioannou NE, Beniata OV, Vitsos P, Tsitsilonis O, Samara P. Harnessing the immune system to improve cancer therapy. *Ann Transl Med*. 2016 Jul;4(14):1–15.
5. Koury J, Lucero M, Cato C, Chang L, Geiger J, Henry D, Hernandez J, Hung F, Kaur P, Teskey G, Tran A. Immunotherapies: exploiting the immune system for cancer treatment. *J Immunol Res*. 2018 Mar 14; 2018:9585614.
6. Whiteside TL. The tumor microenvironment and its role in promoting tumor growth. *Oncogene*. 2008 Oct 6;27(45):5904–12.
7. Kubli SP, Berger T, Araujo DV, Siu LL, Mak TW. Beyond immune checkpoint blockade: emerging immunological strategies. *Nat Rev Drug Discov*. 2021 Dec;20(12):899–919.
8. Caspi RR. Immunotherapy of autoimmunity and cancer: the penalty for success. *Nat Rev Immunol*. 2008 Dec;8(12):970–6.
9. Shams F, Golchin A, Azari A, Mohammadi Amirabad L, Zarein F, Khosravi A, Ardeshirylajimi A. Nanotechnology-based products for cancer immunotherapy. *Mol Biol Rep*. 2022 Feb;49(2):1389–412.
10. Hasan A, Morshed M, Memic A, Hassan S, Webster TJ, Marei HE. Nanoparticles in tissue engineering: applications, challenges, and prospects. *Int J Nanomedicine*. 2018 Sep 24;13:5637–55.
11. Yuan C, Liu Y, Wang T, Sun M, Chen X. Nanomaterials as smart immunomodulator delivery system for enhanced cancer therapy. *ACS Biomater Sci Eng*. 2020 Jul 22;6(9):4774–98.
12. Pivetta TP, Botteon CEA, Ribeiro PA, Marcato PD, Raposo M. Nanoparticle systems for cancer phototherapy: an overview. *Nanomaterials (Basel)*. 2021 Nov 20;11(11):3132.
13. Wu YH, Chen RJ, Chiu HW, Yang LX, Wang YL, Chen YY, Yeh YL, Liao MY, Wang YJ. Nanoparticles augment the therapeutic window of RT and immunotherapy for treating cancers: pivotal role of autophagy. *Theranostics*. 2023 Jan 1;13(1):40–58.
14. Pati R, Shevtsov M, Sonawane A. Nanoparticle vaccines against infectious diseases. *Front Immunol*. 2018 Oct 4; 9:2224.
15. Han B, Song Y, Park J, Doh J. Nanomaterials to improve cancer immunotherapy based on ex vivo engineered T cells and NK cells. *J Control Release*. 2022 Mar 1;343:379–91.
16. Zdanowicz MM. The pharmacology of immunosuppression. *Am J Pharm Educ*. 2009 Dec 17;73(8):144.
17. Yu Z, Shen X, Yu H, Tu H, Chittasupho C, Zhao Y. Smart polymeric nanoparticles in cancer immunotherapy. *Pharmaceutics*. 2023 Feb 26;15(3):775.
18. Zhu M, Wang R, Nie G. Applications of nanomaterials as vaccine adjuvants. *Hum Vaccin Immunother*. 2014;10(9):2761–74.

19. Kim H, Niu L, Larson P, Kucaba TA, Murphy KA, James BR. Polymeric nanoparticles encapsulating novel TLR7/8 agonists as immunostimulatory adjuvants for enhanced cancer immunotherapy. *Biomaterials.* 2018;164: 38–53.
20. Gao L, Li J, Song T. Poly lactic-co-glycolic acid-based nanoparticles as delivery systems for enhanced cancer immunotherapy. *Front Chem.* 2022 Aug 15;10:973666.
21. Anfray C, Mainini F, Digifico E, Maeda A, Sironi M, Erreni M, Anselmo A, Ummarino A, Gandoy S, Expósito F, Redrado M, Serrano D, Calvo A, Martens M, Bravo S, Mantovani A, Allavena P, Andón FT. Intratumoral combination therapy with poly(I: C) and resiquimod synergistically triggers tumor-associated macrophages for effective systemic antitumoral immunity. *J Immunother Cancer.* 2021 Sep;9(9):e002408.
22. Fang X, Lan H, Jin K, Gong D, Qian J. Nanovaccines for cancer prevention and immunotherapy: an update review. *Cancers (Basel).* 2022 Aug 9;14(16):3842.
23. Khademi F, Taheri RA, Momtazi-Borojeni AA, Farnoosh G, Johnston TP, Sahebkar A. Potential of cationic liposomes as adjuvants/delivery systems for tuberculosis subunit vaccines. *Rev Physiol Biochem Pharmacol.* 2018;175:47–69.
24. Yuba E, Tajima N, Yoshizaki Y, Harada A, Hayashi H, Kono K. Dextran derivative-based pH-sensitive liposomes for cancer immunotherapy. *Biomaterials.* 2014 Mar;35(9):3091–101.
25. Mainini F, De Santis F, Fucà G, Di Nicola M, Rivoltini L, Eccles M. Nanobiotechnology and immunotherapy: two powerful and cooperative allies against cancer. *Cancers (Basel).* 2021 Jul 27;13(15):3765.
26. van Gulijk M, Dammeijer F, Aerts JGJV, Vroman H. Combination strategies to optimize efficacy of dendritic cell-based immunotherapy. *Front Immunol.* 2018 Dec 5;9:2759.
27. Kordalivand N, Tondini E, Lau CY, Vermonden T, Mastrobattista E, Hennink WE, Ossendorp F, van Nostrum CF. Cationic synthetic long peptides-loaded nanogels: an efficient therapeutic vaccine formulation for induction of T-cell responses. *J Control Release.* 2019 Dec 10;315:114–25.
28. Sallusto F, Lanzavecchia A. The instructive role of dendritic cells on T-cell responses. *Arthritis Res.* 2002;4 (Suppl 3):S127–32.
29. Cai H, Shukla S, Steinmetz NF. The antitumor efficacy of CpG oligonucleotides is improved by encapsulation in plant virus-like particles. *Adv Funct Mater.* 2020 Apr 14;30(15):1908743.
30. Wu M, Huang S. Magnetic nanoparticles in cancer diagnosis, drug delivery and treatment. *Mol Clin Oncol.* 2017 Nov;7(5):738–46.
31. Martins ES, Espindola A, Britos TN, Chagas C, Barbosa E, Castro CE, Fonseca FLA, Haddad PS. Potential use of DMSA-containing iron oxide nanoparticles as magnetic vehicles against the COVID-19 disease. *Chem Select.* 2021 Aug 20;6(31):7931–7935.
32. Huang L, Ge X, Liu Y, Li H, Zhang Z. The role of toll-like receptor agonists and their nanomedicines for tumor immunotherapy. *Pharmaceutics.* 2022 Jun 10;14(6):1228.
33. Luo Lijia, Iqbal Muhammad Zubair, Liu Chuang, Xing Jie, Akakuru Ozioma Udochukwu, Fang Qianlan, Li Zihou, Dai Yunlu, Li Aiguo, Guan Yong, Wu Aiguo. Engineered nano-immunopotentiators efficiently promote cancer immunotherapy for inhibiting and preventing lung metastasis of melanoma. *Biomaterials.* 2019;2232:119464.
34. Kim CG, Kye YC, Yun CH. The role of nanovaccine in cross-presentation of antigen-presenting cells for the activation of $CD8^+$ T cell responses. *Pharmaceutics.* 2019 Nov 15;11(11):612.
35. Molino NM, Anderson AK, Nelson EL, Wang SW. Biomimetic protein nanoparticles facilitate enhanced dendritic cell activation and cross-presentation. *ACS Nano.* 2013 Nov 26;7(11):9743–52.
36. Thakur N, Thakur S, Chatterjee S, Das J, Sil PC. Nanoparticles as smart carriers for enhanced cancer immunotherapy. *Front Chem.* 2020 Dec 21;8:597806.
37. Thakur N, Thakur S, Chatterjee S, Das J, Sil P. Nanoparticles as smart carriers for enhanced cancer immunotherapy. *Front Chem.* 2020;8:10.
38. Li H, Li Y, Wang X, Hou Y, Hong X, Gong T, Zhang Z, Sun X. Rational design of polymeric hybrid micelles to overcome lymphatic and intracellular delivery barriers in cancer immunotherapy. *Theranostics.* 2017 Sep 26;7(18):4383–98.
39. Li H, Li Y, Wang X, Hou Y, Hong X, Gong T. Rational design of polymeric hybrid micelles to overcome lymphatic and intracellular delivery barriers in cancer immunotherapy. *Theranostics.* 2017;7:4383.
40. Li C, Zhang X, Chen Q, Zhang J, Li W, Hu H. Synthetic polymeric mixed micelles targeting lymph nodes trigger enhanced cellular and humoral immune responses. *ACS Appl Mater Interfaces.* 2018;10:2874–89.

41. Lizotte PH, Wen AM, Sheen MR, Fields J, Rojanasopondist P, Steinmetz NF, Fiering S. In situ, vaccination with cowpea mosaic virus nanoparticles suppresses metastatic cancer. *Nat Nanotechnol.* 2016 Mar;11(3):295–303.
42. Kerstetter-Fogle A, Shukla S, Wang C, Beiss V, Harris PLR, Sloan AE, Steinmetz NF. Plant virus-like particle in situ vaccine for intracranial glioma immunotherapy. *Cancers (Basel).* 2019 Apr 10;11(4):515.
43. Hu H, Steinmetz NF. Development of a virus-like particle-based anti-HER2 breast cancer vaccine. *Cancers (Basel).* 2021 Jun 10;13(12):2909.
44. Kumari N, Choi SH. Tumor-associated macrophages in cancer: recent advancements in cancer nanoimmunotherapies. *J Exp Clin Cancer Res.* 2022;41: 68.
45. Dewangan HK, Tomar S. Nanovaccine for transdermal delivery system. *J Drug Deliv Sci Technol.* 2022 Jan 1;67:102988.
46. Bose RJC, Uday Kumar S, Zeng Y, Afjei R, Robinson E, Lau K. Tumor cell-derived extracellular vesicle-coated nanocarriers: an efficient theranostic platform for the cancer-specific delivery of anti-miR-21 and imaging agents. *ACS Nano.* 2018;12:10817–832.
47. Zeng B, Middelberg AP, Gemiarto A, MacDonald K, Baxter AG, Talekar M, Moi D, Tullett KM, Caminschi I, Lahoud MH, Mazzieri R, Dolcetti R, Thomas R. Self-adjuvanting nanoemulsion targeting dendritic cell receptor Clec9A enables antigen-specific immunotherapy. *J Clin Invest.* 2018 May 1;128(5):1971–84.
48. Wieking BG, Vermeer DW, Spanos WC, Lee KM, Vermeer P, Lee WT, Xu Y, Gabitzsch ES, Balcaitis S, Balint JP Jr, Jones FR, Lee JH. A non-oncogenic HPV 16 E6/E7 vaccine enhances the treatment of HPV-expressing tumors. *Cancer Gene Ther.* 2012 Oct;19(10):667–74.
49. Peng S, Ferrall L, Gaillard S, Wang C, Chi WY, Huang CH, Roden RBS, Wu TC, Chang YN, Hung CF. Development of DNA vaccine targeting E6 and E7 proteins of human papillomavirus 16 (HPV16) and HPV18 for immunotherapy in combination with recombinant vaccinia boost and PD-1 antibody. *mBio.* 2021 Jan 19;12(1):e03224–20.
50. Lee DW, Anderson ME, Wu S, Lee JH. Development of an adenoviral vaccine against E6 and E7 oncoproteins to prevent growth of human papillomavirus-positive cancer. *Arch Otolaryngol Head Neck Surg.* 2008 Dec;134(12):1316–23.
51. Kim SY, Kim S, Kim J-E, Lee SN, Shin IW, Shin HS. Lyophilizable and multifaceted toll-like receptor 7/8 agonist-loaded nanoemulsion for the reprogramming of tumor microenvironments and enhanced cancer immunotherapy. *ACS Nano.* 2019;13:12671–86.
52. Li Y, Ayala-Orozco C, Rauta PR, Krishnan S. The application of nanotechnology in enhancing immunotherapy for cancer treatment: current effects and perspective. *Nanoscale.* 2019 Oct 7;11(37):17157–78.
53. Cui Y, Li Y-Y, Li J, Zhang H-Y, Wang F, Bai X. STAT3 regulates hypoxia-induced epithelial-mesenchymal transition in oesophageal squamous cell cancer. *Oncol Rep.* 2016;36:108–16.
54. Chen W, Li C, Jiang X. Advanced biomaterials with intrinsic immunomodulation effects for cancer immunotherapy. *Small Methods.* 2023 Feb 21;7(5):2201404.
55. Yang Z, Ma Y, Zhao H, Yuan Y, Kim BYS. Nanotechnology platforms for cancer immunotherapy. *Wiley Interdiscip Rev Nanomed Nanobiotechnol.* 2020 Mar;12(2):e1590.
56. Li D, Sun F, Bourajjaj M, Chen Y, Pieters EH, Chen J. Strong *in vivo* antitumor responses induced by an antigen immobilized in nanogels via reducible bonds. *Nanoscale. 2016*;8:19592–604.
57. Feng X, Xu W, Li Z, Song W, Ding J, Chen X. Immunomodulatory nanosystems. *Adv Sci.* 2019;6:1900101.
58. Debele TA, Yeh CF, Su WP. Cancer immunotherapy and application of nanoparticles in cancer immunotherapy as the delivery of immunotherapeutic agents and as immunomodulators. *Cancers.* 2020 Dec 15;12(12):3773.
59. Ahmed A, Tait SWG. Targeting immunogenic cell death in cancer. *Mol Oncol.* 2020 Dec;14(12):2994–3006.
60. Vitulo M, Gnodi E, Meneveri R, Barisani D. Interactions between nanoparticles and intestine. *Int J Mol Sci.* 2022 Apr 14;23(8):4339.
61. al-Shakhshir RH, Regnier FE, White JL, Hem SL. Contribution of electrostatic and hydrophobic interactions to the adsorption of proteins by aluminum-containing adjuvants. *Vaccine.* 1995 Jan;13(1):41–4.

62. Garg A, Dewangan HK. Nanoparticles as adjuvants in vaccine delivery. *Crit Rev Ther Drug Carrier Syst*. 2020;37(2):183–204.
63. Mahony D, Cavallaro AS, Stahr F, Mahony TJ, Qiao SZ, Mitter N. Mesoporous silica nanoparticles act as a self-adjuvant for ovalbumin model antigen in mice. *Small*. 2013;9:3138–46.
64. Perez-Potti A, Rodríguez-Pérez M, Polo E, Pelaz B, Del Pino P. Nanoparticle-based immunotherapeutics: from the properties of nanocores to the differential effects of administration routes. *Adv Drug Deliv Rev*. 2023 Apr 28;197:114829.
65. Lombardo D, Kiselev MA. Methods of liposomes preparation: formation and control factors of versatile nanocarriers for biomedical and nanomedicine application. *Pharmaceutics*. 2022 Feb 28;14(3):543.
66. Rosalia RA, Cruz LJ, van Duikeren S, Tromp AT, Silva AL, Jiskoot W, de Gruijl T, Löwik C, Oostendorp J, van der Burg SH, Ossendorp F. CD40-targeted dendritic cell delivery of PLGA-nanoparticle vaccines induce potent anti-tumor responses. *Biomaterials*. 2015 Feb; 40:88–97.
67. Das J, Han JW, Choi Y-J, Song H, Cho S-G, Park C. Cationic lipid-nanoceria hybrids, a novel nonviral vector-mediated gene delivery into mammalian cells: investigation of the cellular uptake mechanism. *Sci Rep*. 2016; 6:29197.
68. Choo YW, Kang M, Kim HY, Han J, Kang S, Lee J-R. M1 macrophage-derived nanovesicles potentiate the anticancer efficacy of immune checkpoint inhibitors. *ACS Nano*. 2018;12:8977–93.
69. Slütter, BA. Challenges and opportunities in nasal subunit vaccine delivery: mechanistic studies using ovalbumin as a model antigen. *J Control Release*. 2010 Apr 19;143(2):207–14.
70. Hu X, Wu T, Bao Y, Zhang Z. Nanotechnology-based therapeutic modality to boost anti-tumor immunity and collapse tumor defense. *J Control Release*. 2017;256:26–45.
71. Dykman LA, Staroverov SA, Fomin AS, Khanadeev VA, Khlebtsov BN, Bogatyrev VA. Gold nanoparticles as an adjuvant: influence of size, shape, and technique of combination with CpG on antibody production. *Int Immunopharmacol*. 2018;54:163–8.
72. Est-Witte SE, Livingston NK, Omotoso MO, Green JJ, Schneck JP. Nanoparticles for generating antigen-specific T cells for immunotherapy. *Semi Immunol*. 2021; 56: 1–10. doi:10.1016/j.smim.2021.101541
73. Wen Z, Liu F, Chen Q, Xu Y, Li H, Sun S. Recent development in biodegradable nanovehicle delivery system-assisted immunotherapy. *Biomater Sci*. 2019;7(11):4414–43.
74. Sharma P, Kumar P, Sharma R. Natural killer cells – their role in tumour immunosurveillance. *J Clin Diagn Res*. 2017 Aug;11(8): BE01–05.
75. Brittenden J, Heys SD, Ross J, Eremin O. Natural killer cells and cancer. Cancer: Interdiscipl Int J Am Cancer Soc. 1996 Apr 1;77(7):1226–43.
76. Rastogi I, Jeon D, Moseman JE, Muralidhar A, Potluri HK, McNeel DG. Role of B cells as antigen-presenting cells. *Front Immunol*. 2022 Sep 8;13:954936.
77. Catacchio I, Scattone A, Silvestris N, Mangia A. Immune prophets of lung cancer: the prognostic and predictive landscape of cellular and molecular immune markers. *Transl Oncol*. 2018 Jun 1;11(3):825–35.
78. Shahverdi M, Masoumi J, Ghorbaninezhad F, Shajari N, Hajizadeh F, Hassanian H, Alizadeh N, Jafarlou M, Baradaran B. The modulatory role of dendritic cell-T cell cross-talk in breast cancer: challenges and prospects. *Adv Med Sci*. 2022 Sep 1;67(2):353.
79. Debele TA, Yeh CF, Su WP. Cancer immunotherapy and application of nanoparticles in cancers immunotherapy as the delivery of immunotherapeutic agents and as the immunomodulators. *Cancers (Basel)*. 2020 Dec 15;12(12):3773.
80. Sanità G, Carrese B, Lamberti A. Nanoparticle surface functionalization: how to improve biocompatibility and cellular internalization. *Front Mol Biosci*. 2020 Nov 26; 7:587012.
81. Xu M, Han X, Xiong H, Gao Y, Xu B, Zhu G, Li J. Cancer nanomedicine: emerging strategies and therapeutic potentials. *Molecules*. 2023 Jun 30;28(13):5145.
82. Smyth MJ, Ngiow SF, Ribas A, Teng MW. Combination cancer immunotherapies tailored to the tumour microenvironment. *Nature Rev Clin Oncol*. 2016 Mar;13(3):143–58.

6 Opportunities and Difficulties for Anticancer Nanomedicines Based on Polymer–Drug Conjugates in Concurrent/Combination Treatment

6.1 INTRODUCTION

Cancer remains one of the most formidable challenges in the realm of healthcare, necessitating innovative and multifaceted approaches for effective treatment. Among the promising strategies, nanomedicine has emerged as a groundbreaking field, offering unique solutions to enhance therapeutic outcomes. Within this domain, polymer–drug conjugates stand out as a versatile platform with significant potential for anticancer interventions. Many of these technologies exhibit reduced toxicity and, as a result, an enhanced therapeutic profile due to their increased selectivity for a single target. Liposomes, microparticles, as well as PEGylated proteins, are widely known, whereas the conjugates of polymer–drug are projected to enter the market soon [1–5].

Although DDS are routinely utilized for administering an individual therapeutic agent, there is currently a lack of research into the use of DDS to administer "cocktails" of medications. Conjunction therapy is a common practice in cancer treatment, and it has been shown to enhance the therapeutic profile when used in combination with other therapeutic agents [6].

Polymer–drug conjugates have been shown in many groundbreaking investigations during the past 5 years to be an effective delivery system for pharmaceutical mixtures. To begin, we will go over the basics of how combination therapy is used to treat cancer. Using the term conjugates of "polymer–drug for combination treatment," the present state of the topic is examined, with a focus on clinical research. Finally, we will go through the drawbacks and issues with the strategy and draw some broad conclusions. Figure 6.1 depicts an illustration of cancer in the human body.

6.2 CONCURRENT ADMINISTRATION OF THERAPIES

In the dynamic landscape of modern healthcare, the simultaneous administration of multiple therapeutic interventions has gained prominence as a strategy to enhance treatment efficacy and address the complexities of various diseases. This approach, known as concurrent administration of therapies, represents a paradigm shift in medical practice, especially in fields where a comprehensive and synergistic approach is crucial. This introduction explores the rationale behind concurrent therapy, emphasizing its potential advantages in improving patient outcomes. Concurrent administration of therapies is becoming more significant for a better-extended prognosis as well as a reduction in adverse effects because of the molecular complexity of many illnesses. When it comes to the treatment of an illness, "combination therapy" often refers to the concurrent administration of two or

DOI: 10.1201/9781003451020-6

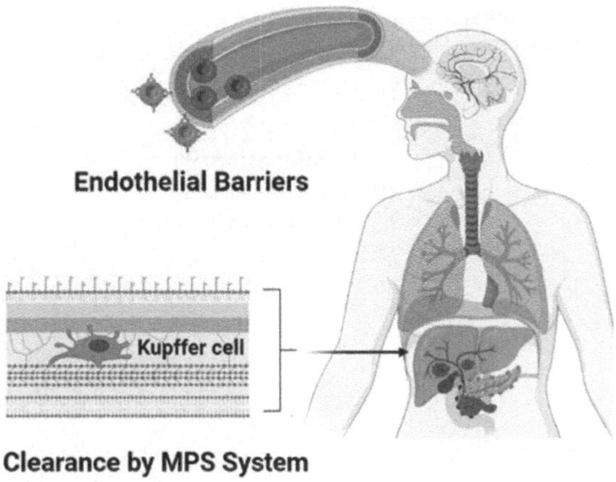

FIGURE 6.1 An illustration of cancer in the human body.

more two drugs that are pharmacologically active or to the conjugation between distinct modalities of therapy (e.g., chemotherapy plus radiation). To achieve greater therapeutic impact and maybe overcome mechanisms of resistance, multiagent treatment, as opposed to single agent, can regulate many signaling pathways in sick cells [7].

Malaria, HIV/AIDS, and cancer are just a few of the disorders that are often treated using a mix of drugs. HAART, for example, has been a crucial part of HIV therapy since it was initially launched in 1999 [8]. Combination treatment is the primary technique for preventing the development of resistance to antimalaria medications in the case of malaria. As a consequence of the disease's selection and subsequent spread of mutant parasites with lower treatment sensitivity, resistance develops. The odds of success are increased by the administration of many medications targeting various biochemical targets [9]. It is only starting to be examined in different disorders, like multiple sclerosis (MS), but with enormous hopes for relapsing–remitting MS patients. Mount Sinai School of Medicine (CombiRx) is now enrolling people to study the combination of interferon beta-1a (Avonex, Rebif®) as well as glatiramer acetate (Copaxone®) in the treatment of multiple sclerosis. Some early trials have revealed the obvious benefits of combination treatment over monotherapy in diabetes [10]. Glucagon-like peptide-1 (GLP-1) plus gastrin, yet not GLP-1 or only gastrin, restored the normal glycemic levels for diabetic NOD mice by elevating the mass of the pancreatic cell and decreasing the autoimmune response [11].

Because of its outstanding therapeutic efficacy and relevance to the chapter, cancer combination treatment is discussed separately in the section that follows.

6.2.1 Concurrent Treatment for Cancer

Cancer, a relentless adversary to human health, demands innovative and comprehensive treatment approaches to improve patient outcomes. In recent years, the concept of concurrent treatment has garnered significant attention as a promising strategy in the fight against cancer. Concurrent treatment involves the simultaneous administration of multiple therapeutic modalities, aiming to target various aspects of the disease and enhance the overall efficacy of the intervention. Concurrent therapy is deep rooted in the treatment of cancer as depicted in Figure 6.2 [6]. Chemotherapeutic treatments are usually accompanied by significant side effects however the administration of various agents with varied targets and toxicity profiles might increase the therapeutic index either via greater effectiveness or equivalent efficacy and lower toxicity can raise the therapeutic index.

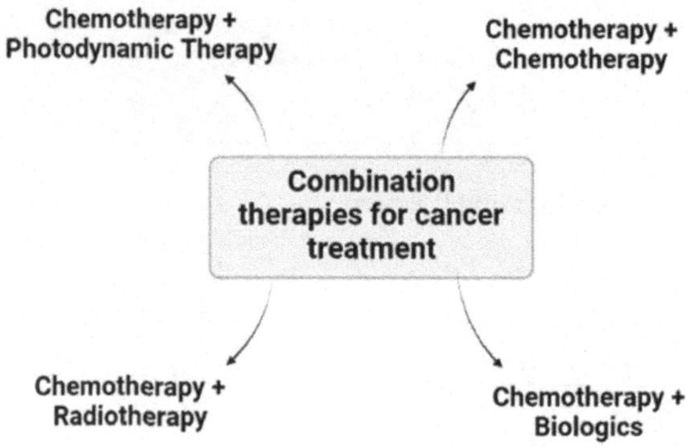

FIGURE 6.2 Combination therapy for cancer.

6.2.2 Concurrent Small Molecule Chemotherapy

In the relentless pursuit of effective cancer treatment, the concurrent use of small-molecule chemotherapy has emerged as a compelling strategy, aiming to tackle the heterogeneity and adaptability of cancer cells. Small molecule chemotherapy agents, characterized by their molecular size, have long been central to cancer therapeutics. The concept of concurrent treatment involves administering multiple small-molecule chemotherapy agents simultaneously, harnessing their distinct mechanisms of action to create a comprehensive and synergistic approach. From "Concurrent empiricism" in the 1940s through to "enlightened empiricism," with considerable advances in survival rates for children with leukemia as well as Hodgkin's disease, up to the present, a sufficiently scientific treatment method has been attained, the rationale for combination chemotherapy has developed through time. Biochemical synergy, non-over-lapping toxicity, elevation in fractional cell death, non-cross-resistant agents, and tumor cell dynamics [12] are just some of the factors that have been used to guide the progression.

Daunorubicin (DNA intercalator) and ara-C (inhibitor of DNA polymerase) are examples of complementary inhibition in the treatment of acute nonlymphocytic leukemia, where the conjugation interferes in DNA repair and synthesis. Additionally, in colorectal cancer, leucovorin (LV) before 5-fluorouracil (5-FU) significantly enhanced the 5-FU capacity for binding as well as inhibiting the activity of thymidylate synthetase [12, 13].

Anthracyline-based cancer therapy combinations include AC (adriamycin and cyclophosphamide), methotrexate-based combinations such as CMF (cyclophosphamide, methotrexate, 5-FU), CAF (cyclophosphamide, adriamycin, 5-FU); as well as CMFVP (cyclophosphamide, methotrexate, 5-fluorouracil, vincristine, prednisolone), along with preen multiagent therapy or changes to conventional regimens are now being investigated [14]. To elevate responsiveness, decrease side effects, as well as maximize therapeutic effectiveness, new methods of delivery are being tested. Patients suffering from advanced stomach cancer were treated using paclitaxel, 5-fluorouracil, folinic acid, as well as cisplatin in phase II research. Outcomes revealed that weekly treatment of paclitaxel maintained the therapeutic effectiveness of three weekly administrations and reduced adverse effects [15, 16].

If you have advanced cancer, you may use combination chemotherapy as palliative or adjuvant therapy before or after surgery to decrease tumor bulk, eliminate unresectable metastasis, or eradicate undetected micrometastasis [17].

6.2.3 Concurrent Therapy Based on the Endocrine System

The intricate interplay of hormones and regulatory signaling within the endocrine system plays a pivotal role in maintaining homeostasis and influencing various physiological processes. Leveraging the complexity of the endocrine system, concurrent therapy based on endocrine modulation has emerged as a promising avenue in medical interventions. This approach involves simultaneously targeting multiple hormonal pathways to address disorders and diseases, particularly in the context of endocrine-related conditions. Breast as well as prostate cancers are of special relevance for combinational treatment. Hormone therapy may be used to treat prostate and breast cancers in the same way as other solid tumors could be treated by surgery, radiation, chemotherapy, or conjugation of the three. Since the 1980s, clinical trials that combined endocrine as well as chemotherapy treatments have been conducted [18].

Recent studies have demonstrated the efficacy of endocrine therapy and bisphosphonate therapy (zoledronic acid) in the treatment of breast cancer, and new medicinal agents have been added to multiagent regimens. It is a two-pronged reason for the pairing. It is anticipated that the reduction of estrogen causes bone loss and that zoledronic acid will counteract that loss. Zoledronic acid has been shown in the Z-FAST study to decrease bone loss related to aromatase inhibitors in postmenopausal breast cancer patients, making it an effective medication for preventing bone loss as well as fractures in that patient group [19]. The CALGB 79809 study also yielded similar outcomes [20]. Various clinical trials intended to validate the antitumor effect of zoledronic acid, which had previously surfaced in preclinical as well as clinical research, in addition to bone protection experiments. 1803 premenopausal breast cancer patients were studied in a major clinical study evaluating the consequence of endocrine treatment (goserelin plus anastrozole or tamoxifen) by including or not including zoledronic acid [21]. Patients who received zoledronic acid and endocrine treatment at the start of that study had considerably longer disease-free as well as relapse-free survival at 5 years. These beneficial outcomes were ascribed by the authors to zoledronic acid's antimetastatic characteristics and emphasized the significance of the combination [22].

6.2.4 Concurrent Therapies Based on Monoclonal Antibodies

In the relentless pursuit of precision medicine, the combination of therapies based on monoclonal antibodies has emerged as a transformative approach in the field of medical interventions. Monoclonal antibodies, with their exquisite specificity and targeted action, have revolutionized the treatment landscape for various diseases, including cancer, autoimmune disorders, and infectious diseases. This introduction explores the evolving paradigm of combined therapies, where the synergistic use of multiple monoclonal antibodies holds the promise of enhancing therapeutic outcomes and overcoming the challenges associated with single-agent treatments. Antibodies that have been produced using monoclonal antibodies have become popular cancer treatments since their introduction to the market. For treating HER2-positive breast cancer, the monoclonal antibody trastuzumab (Herceptin®) is usually coupled with chemotherapy [23]. The use of various monoclonal antibodies, like rituximab (Rituxan®) [24] or bevacizumab (Avastin®) [25], is studied in conjunction with standard chemotherapy for treating advanced breast tumors, including colorectal cancer or NSCLC [26, 27]. The fact that bevacizumab was the initial antiangiogenic medicine accepted for sale by the US Food and Drug Administration (FDA) makes it of special significance (February 2004). To treat metastatic colorectal cancer, metastatic breast cancer, and non-small cell lung cancer, bevacizumab is now used in conjugation with chemotherapeutic drugs like 5-fluorouracil, carboplatin, or paclitaxel. As an example, in a randomized phase III study, individuals with metastatic breast cancer who received paclitaxel plus bevacizumab had a longer time without progression than those who received the other treatment [27]. Bevacizumab got expedited approval from the FDA in February 2008 for utilization in conjunction with paclitaxel chemotherapy for treating metastatic breast cancer.

More than a dozen clinical studies are evaluating the effectiveness of antiangiogenic medicines in conjunction with conventional chemotherapy as well as small-molecule inhibitors of particular cellular pathways, including erlotinib (Tarceva). As a result, several phase III studies failed in enhancing all-inclusive survival, despite the strong justification for the combination. At least some of these outcomes may be related to the lack of knowledge about the molecular pathways underlying the illness, which is evident in these unsatisfactory results [28].

Clinical trials are now being conducted to establish viable medication complexes and/or identify subpopulations of patients for whom these treatments may be beneficial, as was done with trastuzumab as well as HER2-positive cancer.

6.3 EXPLORATORY INVESTIGATION OF INNOVATIVE APPROACHES

Further preclinical research into novel combinations may lead to new therapeutic regimens in the future and give insight into the cellular processes that control responsiveness to therapy in tandem with the clinical research now underway. For the first time, Riganti and colleagues have developed a two-drug combination treatment that can restore chemotherapy resistance in mice by correcting misregulations in cell growth and death patterns. A combination of doxorubicin and rapamycin was used to treat animals. The combination of rapamycin and doxorubicin (Dox) resulted in total tumor remission, but mice treated with either medication alone seldom achieved complete remission [29]. Rapamycin restores cancer cell programmed death, and Dox triggers it, therefore the combination depends on precise control of certain biochemical pathways. In addition, a novel strategy for designing sensible medication combinations has been proposed [30]. The experts recommend that antigens produced by chemotherapy be recognized and targeted. When the chemotherapeutic medication CPT-11 (irinotecan) was administered to a xenograft model of colorectal cancer, LY6D/E46 antigen was induced in that model. Then, monomethyl auristatin, an antitubular drug, was conjugated to monoclonal antibodies targeting the antigen. For total tumor regression, the combination of immunoconjugate-irinotecan was the only treatment that worked [30]. A rationally planned combination may be created with the use of the technology even if it is still in preclinical development [31].

6.3.1 Encountered Numerous Therapeutic Approaches

Combining chemotherapy with radiation has also increased response as well as survival rates in patients suffering from cancer, in addition to combining two or more bioactive drugs. Recent research is examining the application of radiation therapy in combination with innovative drugs and/or therapeutic approaches. Such a combination is well-established and commonly utilized. Radiation treatment and a PSA-based vaccination are being tested in a randomized phase II trial by the National Cancer Institute in patients with prostate cancer (PCa) [32]. The objective was to boost patients' immune systems to maximize the effects of radiotherapy in light of preclinical findings that radiation therapy can alter tumor cells making them more susceptible to the body's immunological response [33]. An experimental vaccination for prostate cancer patients receiving radiation treatment was safe and well tolerated in research, with the vast majority of patients responding to the vaccine with an immune response specific to PSA [32].

Combination therapy is priced higher than monotherapies in the short term, but as was previously mentioned, the right drug combinations can have significant positive effects, including reduced treatment failure rates, case fatality ratios, slowed drug resistance development, and even long-term cost savings [34–37]. It is envisaged that knowledge of the underlying molecular pathways will let combination therapy play an even greater role in cancer treatment in the future [38–40]. Using DDS for multiagent treatment to guarantee that medication mixtures are delivered to the target location at the same time is an intriguing prospect from this perspective. The utilization of polymer conjugates for this purpose will be thoroughly examined in the next section.

6.3.2 Combination Therapy using Drug–Polymer Conjugates

The landscape of modern therapeutics is continually evolving, seeking innovative strategies to enhance the effectiveness of drug delivery and improve patient outcomes. Combination therapy, utilizing drug–polymer conjugates, represents a pioneering approach in this quest for more efficacious

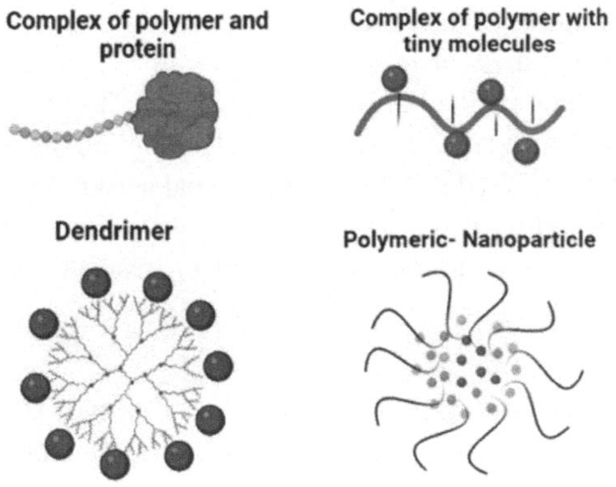

FIGURE 6.3 Conjugates of polymers and drugs for combination therapy.

medical interventions. By fusing the versatility of polymers with the pharmacological potency of drugs, this form of combination therapy aims to address the complexities of various diseases and optimize treatment regimens. Polymer–drug conjugates are pharmaceutical compounds in which the medication is covalently linked to a polymeric carrier via a biodegradable link. The idea was first proposed in the 1970s, and explored preclinically in the 1980s, entering the clinical pipeline in the 1990s [41–44]. A polyglutamic acid-paclitaxel combination (CT-2103 or OPAXIO®) is expected to hit the market soon [5, 45, 46], and more than a dozen polymer–drug conjugates have currently been investigated in clinical trials. Cell therapeutics submitted a request for OPAXIO® to treat non-small cell lung cancer (NSCLC) patients in March 2008 [47]. Over the parent-free medication, polymer–drug combinations have the following benefits: (a) passive tumor targeting via the EPR effect (increased permeability as well as retention); (b) less harmful effects; and (c) better solubility in biological fluids [38]. Drug resistance mechanisms are inhibited [48] and immunostimulatory effects are induced [49, 50]. The usage of polymer–drug combinations comprising only one agent has been extensively explored over the past few years, but their applications for combination therapy have just recently been expanded [41–43, 51, 52]. Figure 6.3 shows conjugates of polymers and drugs for combination therapy.

6.4 THE NOTION OF UTILIZING POLYMER–DRUG CONJUGATES IN COMBINATION THERAPIES

In the dynamic landscape of modern medicine, the integration of innovative strategies is paramount for advancing therapeutic efficacy, particularly in the treatment of complex diseases. The notion of utilizing polymer–drug conjugates in combination therapies stands at the forefront of this evolution, offering a promising avenue to enhance treatment outcomes. By combining the unique attributes of polymers with the therapeutic potential of drugs, this approach aims to address the multifaceted challenges posed by diseases and optimize the synergistic effects of different therapeutic modalities. Combining synthetic pharmaceuticals and synthetic polymers can be used to treat a variety of illnesses, including diabetes and cancer:

- Type 1: polymer–drug conjugate (PDC) and free drug. In the strategy, polymer–drug combinations containing a single agent are administered along with a low molecular weight medicament or another type of treatment (such as radiotherapy).
- Type 2: a drug combination and a polymer–drug conjugate are mixed. In the second method of therapy, polymer–drug conjugates with a single medicinal component are mixed.

- Type 3: a multimedication polymeric delivery system in one. Two or more medications are connected by a single polymer carrier.
- Type 4: polymer-directed enzyme prodrug therapy (PDEPT) and enzyme liposome treatment (PDEPT) (PELT). The fourth type of system (PELT) combines a polymer–drug conjugate with a polymer–enzyme conjugate (PDEPT) or a liposomal system with a polymer–phospholipase conjugate (PDEPT). The drug is released after the drug–polymer linker is broken (in PDEPT) or the liposomal system is compromised (in PELT), respectively, by the polymer–enzyme conjugate.

6.4.1 Administration of a Low Molecular Weight Pharmaceutical or an Alternative Form of Treatment in Combination with a Polymer–Drug Conjugation

Since injections of medication combinations are frequently used in anticancer treatments, evaluating polymer–drug conjugates in addition to free medications was a logical next step. Platines were used in clinical research to evaluate the PGA–paclitaxel conjugate. Forty-three patients suffering from advanced solid tumors were included in phase I research that used 75 mg/m^2 of cis-platin with increasing dosages of PGA-paclitaxel. PGA paclitaxel toxicity, maximum tolerated dosage (MTD), and pharmacokinetics were all assessed, as is customary in phase I research. However, in resistant individuals, that combination was shown to be effective [53]. PGA-paclitaxel and carboplatin were tested in phase I research on 22 patients suffering from advanced solid tumors [54]. The maximum tolerable dose was 225 mg/mL, and three partial reactions were noted. Patients who had received previous unsuccessful paclitaxel therapy were shocked to observe some outcomes. Based on promising results from earlier trials, the phase III clinical study STELLAR 3 compared PGA-paclitaxel with carboplatin and paclitaxel + carboplatin in 400 patients with NSCLC cancer as well as poor performance status. Patients' survival did not improve, although the conjugate combination was shown to be less toxic [54]. After a retrospective data analysis revealed that the anticancer activity of PGA-paclitaxel might be influenced by estrogen levels, Cell Therapeutics Inc. is now attending female patients who have advanced NSCLC as well as baseline oestradiol levels higher than 25 pg/mL, again comparing carboplatin plus PGA-paclitaxel or plus paclitaxel [5]. Several clinical studies have demonstrated the value of a polymer–drug complex when used with another therapeutic substance given as a free medication. In other words, it is challenging to assess the increased therapeutic effectiveness of that combination when compared with monotherapy because there was no direct comparison to just one treatment (such as the conjugate alone). Clinical experiments have also combined the use of polymer–drug conjugates and radiation. Phase I study to evaluate the efficacy of PGA paclitaxel and radiation was conducted in 21 individuals with oesophageal as well as gastric cancer. At 80 mg/m^2, it was determined that the combination was safe and had a maximum tolerated dose (MTD). Additionally, 33% of patients with locoregional illness had a full clinical response [55]. Chemotherapy and radiation treatment are often used in conjunction in clinical practice. Polymer–drug conjugates have been shown to accumulate in tumor tissue without any external assistance because of the leaky vasculature of the tumor (EPR effect). Polymer–drug conjugate irradiation is an intriguing option because of the potential influence on tumor vasculature that radiation treatment may have on the EPR effect.

Early clinical studies demonstrated greater activity if polymer–drug conjugates were used in conjunction with radiation [56]. Lammers *et al.* recently conducted comprehensive preclinical research on the influence of radiation on macromolecule accumulation in tumors. According to a preliminary investigation, irradiation increased the passive targeting of polyHPMA of various molecular weights as well as an HPMA copolymer–Dox complex [57].

Researchers discovered that the targeting of tumors was improved when mice were administered radiation before receiving HPMA copolymers comprising imaging agents along with HPMA copolymer–drug conjugates. As a result, both of the tested drugs (polymer-bound Dox and polymer-bound gemcitabine) had improved therapeutic indices [58].

6.4.2 A Combination of Drug–Polymer Conjugates

In the relentless pursuit of advancing therapeutic modalities, the integration of drug–polymer conjugates has emerged as a groundbreaking strategy, offering a versatile and dynamic platform for medical interventions. This introduction explores the innovative paradigm of a combination of drug–polymer conjugates, representing a fusion of pharmaceutical and polymer science to enhance the effectiveness of therapeutic agents. By leveraging the unique properties of both drugs and polymers, this approach seeks to optimize drug delivery, improve bioavailability, and address the intricate challenges associated with various diseases. Another choice is to mix several polymer–drug conjugates, each of which contains a single active pharmaceutical ingredient. Preclinical studies have been done, however clinical trials have not yet taken place [59].

Kopeek and associates investigated polymer–drug conjugates combining Dox as well as mesochlorin e6 and discovered that the pairing was more efficient than either conjugate individually. It has been shown that active targeting with the antibody OV-TL16 produces even greater results. As an example of how the method might be used in practice, the authors recently applied it to an ovarian cancer cell line by administering HPMA copolymer–SOS and HPMA copolymer–mesochlorin e6 monoethylenediamine sequentially, as well as found synergistic effects [60]. PEG–zinc protoporphyrin (ZnPP, a heme oxygenase inhibitor) as well as PEG–D-amino acid oxidase (DAO) conjugates were tested for their medicinal effects (DAO). PEG-ZnPP significantly reduced tumor formation in animal studies, followed by PEG-DAO and D-proline [61]. With just the conjugate, the effect could not be observed. The proapoptotic drug delivery system disclosed by Khandare and coworkers includes camptothecin (CPT), BH3 domain peptide, as well as luteinizing hormone release hormone [62]. The research team examined the efficacy of integrating such elements in cells from human ovarian cancer to determine the usefulness of doing so.

Proapoptotic activity increased when CPT-PEG-BH3 as well as CPT-PEG-LHRH were combined [63].

6.4.3 An Individual Polymeric Carrier Capable of Transporting Many Medications

The concept of an individual polymeric carrier capable of transporting multiple medications has emerged as a transformative approach in pharmaceutical sciences. This introduction explores the innovative paradigm of a singular polymeric carrier designed to transport and deliver a diverse range of medications simultaneously. Such carriers, often referred to as multi-drug-loaded polymeric platforms, hold great promise in overcoming challenges associated with traditional drug delivery methods and enhancing the efficacy of therapeutic interventions. Even though numerous researches have produced polymer–drug conjugates that include both a targeting residue and a medicament, two or more drugs have only been combined inside one polymeric carrier in the last 4 years [64, 65]. The technique differs considerably from polymer–drug conjugates in that both agents are designed to elicit a pharmacological reaction rather than just one, as opposed to polymer–drug conjugates that contain an active component as well as an extra targeting group. It is possible to provide both medications at the same time by conjugating the drugs to an individual carrier.

First, of its kind, the HPMA copolymer–AGM–Dox compound (HPMA copolymer–AGM–Dox) included a combination of endocrine treatment and chemotherapy (Dox) [66]. In the molecule, which featured a peptidyl linker designed to be cleaved in the lysosomal region in tumor cells, AGM and Dox exhibited w/w drug loadings of approximately 5% and 7%, respectively. That substance has an anticancer effect, according to *in vitro* investigations on breast tumor cell lines. It was intriguing to observe that the polymer conjugate that included both drugs was more potent than the combination of two polymer combinations that each contained a distinct medicament. That increased activity may be influenced by several factors, such as drug release rate, conjugate structure in solution, and maybe activation of particular biological pathways (induction of apoptosis, for example, downregulation of Bcl-2 protein) [67, 68].

In other instances, PEG (NO) was used to combine the anticancer drug EPI with the diffused messenger nitric oxide. The issue of PEG's maximal loading capability of two drug molecules in each chain was effectively solved by affixing a dendronized construct to one PEG chain terminal [69]. Using the particular method, a significant increase in NO loading (up to eight molecules in each chain) and two chemically distinct termini (a carboxylic acid for NO conjugation as well as a hydroxyl group for EPI conjugation) were also achieved. That combination is of particular relevance since EPI and NO produce pharmacological reactions that are partially tissue-dependent. Opposite to tumor cells, NO balances cardiotoxicity brought on by EPI in cardiomyocytes [70]. By combining the two drugs on a single chain, the advantages of the combination are maximized since they are distributed equally throughout the body. The PEG–NO–EPI combination showed antitumor action *in vivo* but was less cardiotoxic [70, 71]. Additionally, Minko and colleagues used a PEG polymer branched to expand on the previously disclosed PEG conjugate and promising results by combining multiple conjugates [62].

The researchers created a six-branched conjugate with equal amounts of CPT, BH3, and LHRH. When compared to monotherapy, the multicomponent drug was shown to have a stronger antitumor effect *in vivo* and to be a hundred times more cytotoxic than single conjugates *in vitro* [63, 72]. TNP-470 (Caplostatin), the first polymer–drug combination to contain an antiangiogenic agent, was developed by Miller *et al.* and Satchi-Fainaro *et al.* [73, 74] and is now being preclinically developed by SynDevRx, Inc. [75]. The authors then designed an HPMA copolymer comprising TNP-470 as well as alendronate based on that single drug system [76]. Alendronate serves as both a pharmacologically active drug and a targeted moiety in the combination. The human osteosarcoma model showed almost full tumor shrinkage when treatment with the combination compound was administered *in vitro*, confirming the combination's antiangiogenic and antitumor characteristics [76]. Alendronate and paclitaxel were incorporated into an HPMA copolymer carrier in a separate investigation. Potential therapeutic options for bone metastases are suggested by anticancer and antiangiogenic activity against prostate as well as breast cancer cells *in vitro* [77].

Two additional HPMA copolymer-based combination conjugates have been created in recent years. We examined *in vivo* the ability of one combination to deliver Gemcitabine (Gem) and Dox, two chemotherapy drugs, to tumor tissue [78]. When tested *in vivo* in a cancer rat model, HPMA-Gem-Dox was more effective than a combination of two polymer conjugates, each carrying a single drug, and even more effective than the conjunction of the free medications [66]. Compared to controls, HPMA–Gem–Dox also reduced angiogenesis as well as increased apoptosis. The anticancer drug Dox and the anti-inflammatory drug dexamethasone (DEX) were combined in an HPMA copolymer in the other conjugate [79]. The authors created a collection of conjugates that included only Dox, only DEX, or both at once. More biological research examining the conjugate's effect is needed to confirm the therapeutic usefulness of the combination. Last but not least, Kwon and associates developed a system based on polymer–drug conjugates as well as polymeric micelles [80]. Poly(ethylene glycol)–poly (aspartate hydrazide) block copolymers were produced, as well as Dox plus the phosphatidylinositol–3 kinase inhibitor wortmannin (WOR) were added either individually or in conjugation, at varying ratios of the drug, to the polymer. Micellar structures were formed by the conjugates, according to chemicophysical experiments. The quantity of medication required to induce biological activity was shown to be lowered when both agents were delivered through the micellar method [80]. Figure 6.4 shows a drug combination carried by a single polymeric carrier.

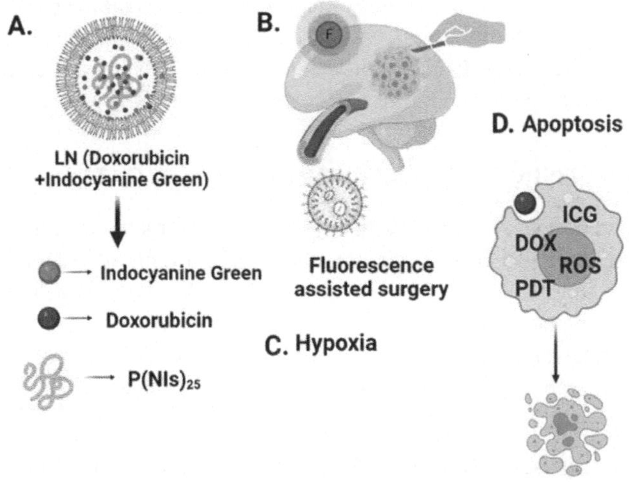

FIGURE 6.4 Drug combination carried by a single polymeric carrier.

6.5 POLYMER-ENZYME LIPOSOME THERAPY (PELT) AND POLYMER-DIRECTED ENZYME PRODRUG THERAPY (PDEPT)

In the realm of advanced therapeutic strategies, two innovative approaches—polymer-enzyme liposome therapy (PELT) and polymer-directed enzyme prodrug therapy (PDEPT)—have emerged as promising paradigms that integrate polymer science, liposomal delivery, and enzymatic activation for targeted and potent medical interventions. These methodologies signify a convergence of bioengineering and pharmacology, capitalizing on the unique attributes of polymers, liposomes, and enzymes to enhance the precision and efficacy of therapeutic interventions. A polymer conjugate-based method, polymer-directed enzyme prodrug treatment has two components. To achieve tumor-targeted medication release, that method combines a polymer–drug combination with a polymer–enzyme conjugate. The enzyme from the second conjugate is indeed meant to scavenge the linker that links a drug with the polymer in the initial conjugation [81]. HPMA copolymer–Dox along with HPMA copolymer–cathepsin B (Figure 6.3) were the first model compounds investigated for their anticancer efficacy in phase II clinical trials. If cathepsin B is exposed to HPMA copolymer–Dox, its activation would depend on its intracellular movement, cellular absorption rate, and of course, the content of the enzyme encountered. The use of a polymer–cathepsin B conjugates ensured that the medicine would be released at the tumor location, regardless of the conditions stated above. An area under the curve (AUC) about four times greater compared to what is achieved with the HPMA copolymer–Dox individually was found in preclinical investigations using the HPMA–cathepsin B combination [81]. It was found that the approach might be improved upon even more via follow-up research. Gly–Gly–cephalosporin linkage was used to connect Dox with HPMA, which is sensitive to non-mammalian enzyme-lactamase but not cathepsin [82]. An increase in survival time and a reduction in tumor development rate were seen in the mice treated with the PDEPT combination. There was no indication of toxicity for the PDEPT combination, however non-human proteins may trigger immunological responses. After optimization, PDEPT has considerable therapeutic promise, and additional investigations using catalytic antibodies have shown its utility [83]. A common strategy for extending proteins' time in circulation and lowering their immunogenicity is polymer–protein conjugation.

Similar tactics are used in liposome treatment (PELT) [84], but, a polymer–enzyme combination is given to cause liposome disintegration as well as the successive release of the medication from the liposomes [85, 86]. Study results showed the efficacy of the strategy using HPMA copolymer-phospholipase C as well as liposomal formulation Doxil (HPMA-PLC). Recently, a dextrin–phospholipase A2 combination was discovered in a lab somewhere else. Both as an anticancer drug and as part of a PELT approach were tested using the combination. The new conjugate's potential will be confirmed in future *in vivo* research [87].

6.6 PROBLEMS IN USING POLYMER–DRUG CONJUGATES IN COMBINATION

While polymer–drug conjugates offer a promising avenue for targeted drug delivery and enhanced therapeutic outcomes, their use in combination therapies presents a nuanced landscape marked by both opportunities and challenges. This introduction explores the complexities and problems associated with employing polymer–drug conjugates in combination strategies, addressing the need for a comprehensive understanding of the intricacies involved. Multiagent polymeric chains provide new opportunities for therapeutics, but they also present new problems.

6.6.1 Determining the Most Suitable Medication Ratios and Combinations

Numerous drug combinations are founded on the idea that by focusing on different routes, therapeutic efficacy may be increased and toxicity reduced, as previously said. Several successful combinations have verified the truth of the assertion, although other investigations have fallen short of the early hopes [28]. Finding the right combination of medications to deliver them effectively together is thus an important and not minor consideration. It is necessary to conduct a comprehensive biological examination based on a thorough knowledge of the underlying molecular pathways.

It is difficult to determine the appropriate dosage in multiagent systems since the relative ratios between each component might affect activity. The effect of various drug ratios on the biological activity of polymer–drug conjugates has not yet been thoroughly investigated. Celator Technologies Inc., a Canadian business, has devised a rigorous way to evaluate alternative medication ratios in its liposomal technology [88]. CPX-1 (irinotecan: floxuridine), as well as CPX-351 (irinotecan: floxuridine), are two liposomal formulations nowadays being tested in phase II clinical studies (cytarabine: daunorubicin). When it comes to developing combination polymer–drug conjugates, it is believed that a similar strategy will be used.

6.6.2 Drug Release Kinetics

The field of drug delivery has witnessed a paradigm shift with the advent of polymer–drug conjugates, where polymers serve as carriers for therapeutic agents. Understanding and manipulating drug release kinetics in the context of combination therapies involving polymer–drug conjugates are critical aspects in optimizing treatment outcomes. This introduction explores the intricate dynamics of drug release kinetics within polymer–drug conjugates when employed in combination strategies. It is generally accepted that the release of the medication from the carrier is necessary for polymer–drug combinations to have anticancer effects. Therefore, a suitable linker must be robust in circulation as well as cleaved by enzyme or chemical means at the site of the tumor. Following significant 1980's research comparing peptidyl linkers to selectively cleave in the lysosomal compartment, HPMA copolymer-GFLG-Dox was created and clinically tested [89]. The action of the conjugates was demonstrated to be influenced by the release rates of several peptidyl linkers. Another finding showed that the linker's biodegradability was influenced by the medication attached. A time-dependent release of the drug was found when the tetrapeptide GG had been attached to Dox, but not when melphalan was attached [90].

In polymer–drug conjugates including more than one agent, the existence of an additional agent affects drug release. Even for a single kind of linker. Drug release rates in HPMA copolymer–GFLG–Dox–AGM were compared to those in HPMA copolymer–GFLG–Dox alone by Vicent *et al.*

[66]. The existence of AGM from the HPMA copolymer–GFLG–AGM did not have an impact on the release of Dox via the HPMA copolymer–GFLG–Dox. The HPMA copolymer–GFLG–Dox–AGM, on the other hand, showed a distinct release profile. According to scientists, that kind of variation might account for some of the observed variations in biological behavior [66]. Krakovicova and colleagues found a different circumstance when they contrasted the expulsion of DEX from HPMA copolymer–DEX and HPMA copolymer–Dox–DEX. There was no association between Dox with DEX release quantity, although there was a correlation between DEX release rate as well as the quantity of Dox on the polymer [79].

The importance of *in vitro* investigations that confirm medication release and quantify the quantity and rate of drug release cannot be overstated. When constructing conjugates, it is crucial to take relative drug release rate as well as sequential drug release (which drug is first released) into account because complexity rises when more than one agent is coupled [67, 68].

6.6.3 Capacity for Loading

The capacity for loading drugs within polymer–drug conjugates represents a critical aspect of combination therapies, offering a platform to optimize therapeutic efficacy and address the complexities of various diseases. This introduction delves into the intricate considerations surrounding the loading capacity of drugs in polymer–drug conjugates when employed in combination therapies, emphasizing the pivotal role this parameter plays in achieving desired therapeutic outcomes. To ensure effective drug delivery to the tumor location, polymer–drug conjugates have always needed a polymer carrier with the right loading capacity.

Multiagent treatments need carriers with substantial carrying capacities, making the research even more critical. When linear polymers were first investigated as drug carriers, several of them only had a limited ability to carry drugs. Contrarily, only a few monomers containing functional groups that are appropriate for drug conjugation (usually at a molar ratio of 10%) are found in HPMA copolymers, which have been the subject of previous research [89, 90]. Other linear polymers with higher carrying capacities have recently been investigated. Additionally, the PGA-based conjugates show notable drug loading (37% PGA-Paclitaxel [46] and 33%-35% PGA-Camptothecin [91]) since PGA may potentially transport one drug molecule per monomer. Additionally, innovative polymeric structures including dendrimers [92, 93], hyperbranched polymers [94], and hybrid macromolecular structures [95] are being investigated in addition to the more traditional linear polymer structure. These novel architectures exhibit customized functions at the surface end group, quasi-monodispersed nanoscale geometry or monodispersed, and reduced flexibility as compared to linear random coil polymers, in addition to having a high carrying capacity. These are just a few of the many advantages these new architectures offer over traditional ones. These systems' toxicity and biocompatibility have been questioned, which calls for further research. About the distribution of medications [96], however, it is obvious that these novel structures have significant potential.

6.7 *In Vitro–In Vivo* Correlation

Newly created polymer–drug conjugates are frequently examined for anticancer activity *in vitro* using established viability tests on cancer cells. Polymer–drug conjugates should not be screened *in vitro* as the EPR effect, which can only be observed *in vivo*, is crucial to the effectiveness of these molecules because a polymer–drug combination must first be swallowed by endocytosis, transported to the proper cellular compartment, and then enzymatically or chemically activated (i.e., drug released), the start of action is substantially delayed than for a free drug. As a result, the conjugated drug becomes more active compared to the free drug *in vitro*, although *in vivo* research has demonstrated the opposite trend [89]. In light of these considerations, there is debate over the significance of *in vitro* testing as well as their capacity to forecast *in vivo* behavior. *In vitro* prescreening has obvious advantages in terms of ethics and cost, but there are further benefits, notably in the case of combination treatments, which are polymer-based. It is probable to detect any potential benefits of combining two medications into an individual drug carrier at a young stage since it is possible to assess the relative activity of different polymer–drug conjugates *in vitro*. Also, it is possible to carry out a comprehensive study of several medication ratios, which would not be viable at a later stagnation period. At long last, tests may be conducted to illustrate how these systems work, such as studying how drugs are released or how they stimulate or stop certain cellular processes (66) (e.g., apoptosis [97], or angiogenesis [73]).

6.7.1 Physical and Chemical Characterization

Lastly, the characterization of these nanoconstructs in terms of their physicochemical properties is an important concern, even if it is not necessary to meet tight regulatory standards [98]. Polymer–drug conjugates are more difficult to understand than tiny molecules. Several factors combine to make these systems fundamentally diverse. Polydisperse polymers are the most common kind of polymer carrier. Although batch-to-batch repeatability is guaranteed by optimizing reaction conditions, covalent attachment of a drug to the carrier can frequently be a random process [99]. In many cases, the site of attachment remains unpredictable and undirected. Further complications arise when a second medicine is attached to the same carrier. It is thus difficult to get an accurate physicochemical profile [100]. In contrast, a complete characterization is required for the development of medications from such substances and their ultimate commercialization. Comprehensive chemical–physical characterization of these compounds may also support the understanding of their biological behavior and help generate rationally designed following generations [101].

Various techniques, including NMR, IR, HPLC, and GPC [102, 103], have been employed in the past to characterize polymer–drug conjugates. Polymer–drug conjugates have recently been subjected to sophisticated methodologies for the first time, allowing researchers to get a deeper grasp of this emerging technology. Clarifying the structural characteristics of these hybrid macromolecules in solution has shown to be a helpful application of SANS [104, 105] in addition to how they influence their biological behavior [106]. For example, static light scattering (QELS) and dynamic light scattering (DLS) [107] are regarded as methods for determining the size (hydrodynamic radius (Rh)) and absolute Mw of these hybrid macromolecules. Macromolecular structures as well as their intermolecular interactions can be characterized using NMR technologies' excellent spatial and temporal resolution.

The molecular size, binding state, or aggregation of a compound may be determined using NMR spectroscopy, as can the drug loading, heterogeneity, and purity of the sample. Furthermore, NOESY and TOCSY have been used to show drug integrity and covalent attachment to the polymer in a 1D and 2D 1H manner [108–110].

6.7.2 Developments in Clinical Practice

To show the efficacy of these combination products in the clinical setting, further rigorous testing is required. Additionally, it must be demonstrated that the clinical benefits are linked to the enhanced drug delivery method rather than just the additive or synergistic effects of the parent medications administered as separate therapeutic entities [111]. Therefore, it is necessary to demonstrate the effectiveness of merging two or more agents into a single delivery mechanism compared to giving the free drugs orally. Combination products are expected to cost much more to produce than existing pharmaceuticals because of the difficulty in organizing clinical trials and the ethical difficulties that arise as a result [112]. When it comes to extending the patent life of blockbuster pharmaceuticals via the use of combination therapies, pharmaceutical corporations may see it as a potential opportunity.

6.8 CONCLUSIONS

More recent research has looked at the possibility of first-generation polymer–drug conjugates being used as drug delivery platforms for combination treatment. As a result, this early research revealed surprising therapeutic effects but also highlighted new questions about "system design." Research on the effects of drug combinations on cellular and molecular systems is essential for rationally developing novel treatments.

REFERENCES

[1] Holz E, Darwish M, Tesar DB, Shatz-Binder W. A review of protein-and peptide-based chemical conjugates: past, present, and future. *Pharmaceutics*. 2023 Feb 10;15(2):600.

[2] Pacheco C, Baiao A, Ding T, Cui W, Sarmento B. Recent advances in long-acting drug delivery systems for an anticancer drug. *Adv Drug Deliv Rev*. 2023 Feb 4;194:114724.

[3] Bajwa N, Mahal S, Singh PA, Jyoti K, Dewangan P, Madan J, Baldi A. Chapter -15 Drug–polymer conjugates: challenges, opportunities, and prospects in clinical trials. in Jitender Madan, Ashish Baldi, Monika Chaudhary, Neetu Chopra (Eds.). *Polymer Drug Conjugates*. 2023:389–469. ISBN 9780323916639; https://doi.org/10.1016/B978-0-323-91663-9.00011-4

[4] Veronese FM, Harris JME. Peptide and protein PEGylation III: advances in chemistry and clinical applications. *Adv Drug Deliv Rev*. 2008;60:1–88 (whole volume).

[5] Manandhar S, Sjöholm E, Bobacka J, Rosenholm JM, Bansal KK. Polymer-drug conjugates as nanotheranostic agents. *J Nanotheranostics*. 2021;2(1):63–81.

[6] Gee JMW, Howell A, Gullick WJ, Benz CC, Sutherland RL, Santen RJ, Martin, Ciardiello F, Miller WR, Dowsett M, Barrett-Lee P, Robertson JFR, Johnston SR, Jones HE, Wakeling AE, Duncan R, Nicholson RI. Consensus statement Endocrin. *Rel Cancer*. 2005;12:S1–S7.

[7] Broxterman HJ, Georgopapadakou NH. Anticancer therapeutics: "addictive" targets, multi-targeted drugs, new drug combinations. *Drug Resis Update*. 2005;8:183–97.

[8] de Gaetano Donati K, Rabagliati R, Iacoviello L, Cauda R. HIV infection, HAART, and endothelial adhesion molecules: current perspectives. *Lancet Infect Dis*. 2004;4:213–22.

[9] Mitchell MJ, Billingsley MM, Haley RM, Wechsler ME, Peppas NA, Langer R. Engineering precision nanoparticles for drug delivery. *Nat Rev Drug Discov*. 2021 Feb;20(2):101–24.

[10] Ji L, Chan JCN, Yu M, Yoon KH, Kim SG, Choi SH, Huang CN, Te Tu S, Wang CY, Paldánius PM, Sheu WHH. Early combination versus initial metformin monotherapy in the management of newly diagnosed type 2 diabetes: an East Asian perspective. *Diabetes Obes Metab*. 2021;23(1):3–17.

[11] Suarez-Pinzon WL, Power RF, Yan Y, Wasserfall C, Atkinson M, Rabinovitch A. Combination therapy with glucagon-like peptide-1 and gastrin restores normoglycemia in diabetic NOD mice. *Diabetes*. 2008; 57:3281–88.

[12] Vodenkova S, Buchler T, Cervena K, Veskrnova V, Vodicka P, Vymetalkova V. 5-fluorouracil and other fluoropyrimidines in colorectal cancer: past, present and future. *Pharmacol Ther*. 2020 Feb 1;206:107447.

[13] Kumar A, Singh AK, Singh H, Thareja S, Kumar P. Regulation of thymidylate synthase: an approach to overcome 5-FU resistance in colorectal cancer. *Med Oncol*. 2022 Oct 29;40(1):3.

[14] Muggia F. Platinum compounds 30 years after the introduction of cisplatin: implications for the treatment of ovarian cancer act. *Gyn Oncol*. 2009; 112:275–81.

[15] Berhoune M, Banu E, Scotte F, Prognon P, Oudard S, Bonan B. Therapeutic strategy for the treatment of metastatic non-small cell lung cancer. *Ann Pharmacother*. 2008; 42:1640–52.

[16] Honecker F, Kollmannsberger C, Quietzsch D, Haag C, Schroeder M, Spott C, Hartmann JT, Baronius W, Hempel V, Kanz L, Bokemeyer C. Phase II study of weekly paclitaxel plus 24-h continuous infusion 5-fluorouracil, folinic acid and 3-weekly cisplatin for the treatment of patients with advanced gastric cancer. *Anticancer Drugs*. 2002;13:497–503.

[17] Akeson M, Zetterqvist B-M, Dahllöf K, Brännström M, Horvath G. Effect of adjuvant paclitaxel and carboplatin for advanced stage epithelial ovarian cancer: a population-based cohort study of all patients in western Sweden with long-term follow-up. *Acta Obstet Gynecol Scand*. 2008; 87:1343–52.

[18] Pearson OH, Hubay CA, Gordon NH, Marshall JS, Crowe JP, Arafah BM, McGuire W. Endocrine versus endocrine plus five-drug chemotherapy in postmenopausal women with stage II estrogen receptor–positive breast cancer. *Cancer.* 1989; 64:1819–23.
[19] Logman JFS, Heeg BMS, Botteman MF, Kaura S, van Hout BA. Economic evaluation of zoledronic acid for the prevention of osteoporotic fractures in postmenopausal women with early-stage breast cancer receiving aromatase inhibitors in the UK. *Ann Oncol.* 2010;21(7):1529–36. doi:10.1093/annonc/mdp560.
[20] Greco F, Vicent MJ. Combination therapy: opportunities and challenges for polymer–drug conjugates as anticancer nanomedicines. *Adv Drug Deliv Rev.* 2009 Nov 12;61(13):1203–13.
[21] Gnant M, Mlineritsch B, Schippinger W, Luschin-Ebengreuth G, Poestlberger S, Menzel C, Jakesz R, Kubista E, Marth C, Greil R, On behalf of the ABCSG. Adjuvant ovarian suppression combined with tamoxifen or anastrozole, alone or in combination with zoledronic acid, in premenopausal women with hormoneresponsive, stage I and II breast cancer: first efficacy results from ABCSG-12. *J Clin Oncol.* 2008;26(May 20 suppl., abstr LBA4):LBA4–LBA4.
[22] Gnant M, Mlineritsch B, Schippinger W, Luschin-Ebengreuth G, Poestlberger S, Menzel C, Jakesz R, Kubista E, Marth C, Greil R, On behalf of the ABCSG. Adjuvant endocrine therapy plus zoledronic acid in premenopausal women with early-stage breast cancer: 5-year follow-up of the ABCSG-12 bone-mineral density substudy. *Lancet Oncol.* 2008;9:679–691.
[23] Metro G, Mottolese M, Fabi A. HER-2-positive metastatic breast cancer: trastuzumab and beyond. *Expert Opin Pharmacother.* 2008;9:2583–601.
[24] Ritchie GE, Fernando M, Goldstein D. Rituximab to treat gemcitabine-induced hemolytic–uremic syndrome (HUS) in pancreatic adenocarcinoma: a case series and literature review. *Cancer Chemother Pharmacol.* 2017 Jan;79:1–7.
[25] Van Poppel H. Treatment of advanced and metastatic renal cancer: a revolution? *Eur Urol Suppl.* 2009;8:483–88.
[26] Rugo HS, Bevacizumab in the treatment of breast cancer: rationale and current data. *Oncologist.* 2004;9(Suppl 1):43–9.
[27] Delaloge S, Perol D, Courtyard C, Brain E, Asselain B, Bachelot T, Debled M, Dieras V, Campone M, Levy C, Jacot W. Paclitaxel plus bevacizumab or paclitaxel as first-line treatment for HER2-negative metastatic breast cancer in a multicenter national observational study. *Ann Oncol.* 2016 Sep 1;27(9):1725–32.
[28] Jones D. Avastin–Tarceva combination fails in lung cancer. Nat *Biotechnol.* 2009;27:108–09.
[29] Riganti C, Contino M. New strategies to overcome resistance to chemotherapy and immune system in cancer. *Int J Mol Sci.* 2019;20(19): 4783.
[30] Lane D, Designer combination therapy for cancer. Nat *Biotechnol.* 2006;24:163–64.
[31] Steiner M, Neri D. Antibody-radionuclide conjugates for cancer therapy: historical considerations and new trends. *Clin Cancer Res.* 2011 Oct 15;17(20):6406–16.
[32] Gulley JL, Arlen PM, Bastian A, Morin S, Marte J, Beetham P, Tsang K-Y, Yokokawa J, Hodge JW, Menard C, Camphausen K, Coleman N, Sullivan F, Steinberg SM, William JS. Combining a recombinant cancer vaccine with standard definitive radiotherapy in patients with localized prostate cancer. *Clin Cancer Res.* 2005;11:3353–62.
[33] Chakraborty M, Abrams SI, Coleman CN, Camphausen K, Schlom J, Hodge JW. External beam radiation of tumors alters the phenotype of tumor cells to render them susceptible to vaccine-mediated T-cell killing. *Cancer Res.* 2004;64:4328–37.
[34] Ringsdorf H. Structure and properties of pharmacologically active polymers. *J Polym Sci Polym Symp.* 1975;51:135–53.
[35] Duncan R, Seymour LCW, Scarlett L, Lloyd JB, Rejmanova P, Kopeček J. Fate of N-(2-hydroxypropyl) methacrylamide copolymers with pendant galactosamine residues after intravenous administration to rats. *Biochim Biophys Acta.* 1986;880:62–71.
[36] Duncan R, Seymour LW, O'Hare KB, Flanagan P, Wedge S, Ulbrich K, Strohalm J, Subr V, Spreafico F, Grandi M, Ripamonti M, Farao M, Suarato A. Preclinical evaluation of polymer-bound doxorubicin. *J Control Release.* 1992;19:331–46.
[37] Ekladious I, Colson YL, Grinstaff MW. Polymer–drug conjugate therapeutics: advances, insights, and prospects. *Nat Rev Drug Discov.* 2019 Apr;18(4):273–94.

[38] Meerum Terwogt JM, ten Bokkel Huinink WW, Schellens JHM, Schot M, Mandjes I, Zurlo M, Rocchetti M, Rosing H, Beijnen KJH. Phase I clinical and pharmacokinetic study of PNU166945, a novel water-soluble polymer conjugated prodrug of paclitaxel. *Anticancer Drug Des.* 2001;12:315–23.
[39] Howell SB. The design and development of the tumor-targeting nanopolymer dach platinum conjugate AP5346 (Prolindac™). In: Bonetti A, Leone R, Muggia FM, Howell SB (Eds.). Platinum and other heavy metal compounds in cancer chemotherapy. (pp. 33–39). Cancer Drug Discovery and Development. 2009;Humana Press, Totowa, NJ. https://doi.org/10.1007/978-1-60327-459-3_5.
[40] Bayat Mokhtari R, Homayouni TS, Baluch N, Morgatskaya E, Kumar S, Das B, Yeger H. Combination therapy in combating cancer. *Oncotarget.* 2017;8(23):38022–43.
[41] Duncan R. Polymer conjugates as anticancer nanomedicines. *Nat Rev Cancer.* 2006;6:688–701.
[42] Vicent MJ, Duncan R. Polymer conjugates: nanosized medicines for treating cancer. *Trends Biotechnol.* 2006;24:39–47.
[43] Seifu MF, Nath LK. Polymer-drug conjugates: novel carriers for cancer chemotherapy. *Polymer Plastics Technol Mater.* 2019 Jan 22;58(2):158–71.
[44] Li C, Wallace S. Polymer–drug conjugates: recent development in clinical oncology. Adv *Drug Deliv Rev.* 2008;60:886–98.
[45] Chipman SD, Oldham FB, Pezzoni G, Singer JW. Biological and clinical characterization of paclitaxel poliglumex (PPX, CT-2103), a macromolecular polymer–drug conjugate. *Int J Nanomed.* 2006;1:375–83.
[46] Singer JW, Paclitaxel poliglumex (XYOTAX™, CT-2103): a macromolecular taxane. *J Control Release.* 2005;109:120–6.
[47] Xu H, Ma H, Yang P, Zhang X, Wu X, Yin W, Wang H, Xu D. Targeted polymer-drug conjugates: current progress and future perspective. *Colloids Surf B: Biointerfaces.* 2015 Dec 1;136:729–34.
[48] Minko T, Kopečková P, Pozharov V, Kopeček J. HPMA copolymer bound adriamycin overcomes MDR1 gene encoded resistance in a human ovarian carcinoma cell line. *J Control Release.* 1998;54:223–33.
[49] Ríhová B, Strohalm J, Prausová J, Kubácková K, Jelínková M, Rozprimová L, Sírová M, Plocová D, Etrych T, Subr V, Mrkvan T, Kovár M, Ulbrich K. Cytostatic and immune mobilizing activities of polymer-bound drugs: experimental and first clinical data. *J Control Release.* 2003;28:1–16.
[50] Kostková H, Etrych T, Říhová B, Ulbrich K. Synergistic effect of HPMA copolymer-bound doxorubicin and dexamethasone in vivo on mouse lymphomas. *J Bioactive Compat Polymers.* 2011 May;26(3):270–86.
[51] Greco F, Vicent MJ. Polymer–drug conjugates: current status and future trends. *Front Biosci.* 2008;13:2744–56.
[52] Haag R, Kratz F. Polymer therapeutics: concepts and applications. Angew *Chem Int Ed.* 2006;45:1198–215.
[53] Verschraegen CF, Skubitz K, Daud A, Kudelka AP, Rabinowitz I, Allievi C, Eisenfeld A, Singer JW, Oldham FB. A phase I and pharmacokinetic study of paclitaxel poliglumex and cisplatin in patients with advanced solid tumors. Cancer Chemother *Pharmacol.* 2009;63:903–10.
[54] O'Brien ME, Socinski MA, Popovich AY, Bondarenko IN, Tomova A, Bilynsky BT, Hotko YS, Ganul VL, Kostinsky IY, Eisenfeld AJ, Sandalic L. Randomized phase III trial comparing single-agent paclitaxel Poliglumex (CT-2103, PPX) with single-agent gemcitabine or vinorelbine for the treatment of PS 2 patients with chemotherapy-naive advanced non-small cell lung cancer. *J Thor Oncol.* 2008 Jul 1;3(7):728–34.
[55] Dipetrillo TA, Milas L, Evans D. Paclitaxel poliglumex (PPX–xyotax) and concurrent radiation for esophageal and gastric cancer—a phase I study. *J Clin Oncol.* 2006;29:376–79.
[56] Ke S, Milas L, Charnsangavej C, Wallace S, Li C. Potentiation of radioresponse by polymer–drug conjugates. *J Control Release.* 2001;74:237–42.
[57] Lammers T, Peschke P, Kühnlein R, Subr V, Ulbrich K, Debus J, Huber P, Hennink W, Storm G. Effect of radiotherapy and hyperthermia on the tumor accumulation of HPMA copolymer-based drug delivery systems. *J Control Release.* 2007;117:333–41.
[58] K Iyer A, He J, M Amiji M. Image-guided nanosystems for targeted delivery in cancer therapy. Curr Med Chem. 2012 Jul 1;19(19):3230–40.

[59] Shiah JG, Sun Y, Kopečková P, Peterson CM, Straight RC, Kopeček J. Combination chemotherapy and photodynamic therapy of targetable N-(2-hydroxypropyl) methacrylamide copolymer–doxorubicin/mesochlorin e(6)–OV–TL 16 antibody immunoconjugates. *J Control Release*. 2001;74:249–53.
[60] Kopeček J. Polymer-drug conjugates origins, progress to date and future directions. *Adv Drug Deliv Rev*. 2013;65(1):49–59.
[61] Fang J, Sawa T, Akaike T, Greish K, Maeda H. Enhancement of chemotherapeutic response of tumor cells by a heme oxygenase inhibitor, pegylated zinc protoporphyrin. *Int J Cancer*. 2004;109:1–8.
[62] Khandare JJ, Chandna P, Wang Y, Pozharov VP, Minko T. Novel polymeric prodrug with multivalent components for cancer therapy. *J Pharmacol Exp Ther*. 2006 Jun 1;317(3):929–37.
[63] Khandare J, Minko T. Polymer–drug conjugates: progress in polymeric prodrugs Prog. *Polym Sci*. 2006;31:359–97.
[64] Seymour LW, Ferry D, Anderson D, Julyan P, Poyner R, Doran J, Young A, Burtles S, Kerr D. Hepatic drug targeting: phase I evaluation of polymer-bound doxorubicin. *J Clin Oncol*. 2002;20:1668–76.
[65] Haas M, Kato Y, Haverdings RF, Moolenaar F, Suzuki K, de Zeeuw D, Sugiyama Y, Meijer DK. Delivery of drugs and antisense oligonucleotides to the proximal tubular cell of the kidney using macromolecular and pro-drug approaches. Drug Target: Organ Specific Strategies. 2001 Jul 12;12:121–55.
[66] Vicent MJ, Greco F, Paul A, Griffiths PC, Nicholson RI, Duncan R. Polymer therapeutics designed for combination therapy of hormone-dependent cancer. *Angew Chem Int Ed*. 2005;44:4061–66.
[67] Greco F, Vicent MJ, Penning NA, Nicholson RI, Duncan R. HPMA copolymer– aminoglutethimide conjugates inhibit aromatase in MCF-7 cell lines. *J Drug Target*. 2005;13:459–70.
[68] Greco F, Vicent MJ, Gee S, Jones AT, Gee J, Nicholson RI, Duncan R. The mechanism of enhanced cytotoxicity of HPMA copolymer–DOX–AGM in breast cancer cells. *J Control Release*. 2007;117:28–39.
[69] Nakamura H, Koziolová E, Chytil P, Tsukigawa K, Fang J, Haratake M, Ulbrich K, Etrych T, Maeda H. Pronounced cellular uptake of pirarubicin versus that of other anthracyclines: comparison of HPMA copolymer conjugates of pirarubicin and doxorubicin. Mol Pharm. 2016 Dec 5;13(12):4106–15.
[70] Santucci L, Mencarelli A, Renga B. Nitric oxide modulates proapoptotic and antiapoptotic properties of chemotherapy agents: the case of NO–pegylated epirubicin. *FASEB J*. 2006;20:765–73.
[71] Santucci L, Mencarelli A, Renga B, Ceccobelli D, Pasut G, Veronese F, Distrutti E, Fiorucci MD. Cardiac safety and anti-tumoral activity of a new nitric oxide derivative of pegylated epirubicin in mice. *Anticancer Drugs*. 2007;18:1081–91.
[72] Chandna P, Saad M, Wang Y, et al. Targeted proapoptotic anticancer drug delivery system. *Mol Pharm*. 2007;4(5):668–78. doi:10.1021/mp070053o
[73] Miller K, Eldar-Boock A, Polyak D, Segal E, Benayoun L, Shaked Y, Satchi-Fainaro R. Antiangiogenic antitumor activity of HPMA copolymer–paclitaxel–alendronate conjugate on breast cancer bone metastasis mouse model. Mol Pharm. 2011 Aug 1;8(4):1052–62.
[74] Satchi-Fainaro R, Mamluk R, Wang L, Short SM, Nagy JA, Feng D, Dvorak AM, Dvorak HF, Puder M, Mukhopadhyay D, Folkman J. Inhibition of vessel permeability by TNP-470 and its polymer conjugate, calpastatin. *Cancer Cell*. 2005;7:251–61.
[75] Lammers T. Improving the efficacy of combined modality anticancer therapy using HPMA copolymer-based nanomedicine formulations. *Adv Drug Deliv Rev*. 2010 Feb 17;62(2):203–30.
[76] Segal E, Pan H, Ofek P, Udagawa T, Kopečková P, Kopeček J, Satchi-Fainaro R. Targeting angiogenesis-dependent calcified neoplasms using combined polymer therapeutics. *PLoS ONE*. 2009;4(4):e5233.
[77] Miller K, Erez R, Segal E, Shabat D, Satchi-Fainaro R. Targeting bone metastases with a novel bi-specific anticancer and anti-angiogenic polymer–alendronate– taxane conjugate. Angew *Chem Int Ed*. 2009;48:2949–54.
[78] Chytil P, Koziolová E, Etrych T, Ulbrich K. HPMA copolymer–drug conjugates with controlled tumor-specific drug release. *Macromol Biosci*. 2018 Jan;18(1):1700209.
[79] Krakovicova H, Etrych T, Ulbrich K. HPMA-based polymer conjugates with drug combination. *Eur J Pharm Sci*. 2009;37:405–12.
[80] Bae Y, Diezi TA, Zhao A, Kwon GS. Mixed polymeric micelles for combination cancer chemotherapy through the concurrent delivery of multiple chemotherapeutic agents. *J Control Release*. 2007;122:324–30.
[81] Satchi R, Connors TA, Duncan R. PDEPT: polymer-directed enzyme prodrug therapy I. HPMA copolymer–cathepsin B and PK1 as a model combination. *Br J Cancer*. 2001;85:1070–6.

[82] Satchi-Fainaro R, Hailu H, Davies JW, Summerford C, Duncan R. PDEPT: polymer-directed enzyme prodrug therapy. 2. HPMA copolymer–beta-lactamase and HPMA copolymer–C–Dox as a model combination. Bioconjug *Chem.* 2003;14:797–804.
[83] Satchi-Fainaro R, Wrasidlo W, Lode HN, Shabat D. Synthesis and characterization of a catalytic antibody-HPMA copolymer-conjugate as a tool for tumor-selective prodrug activation. Bioorg *Med Chem.* 2002;10:3023–9.
[84] Duncan R, Gac-Breton S, Keane R, Musila R, Sat YN, Satchi R, Searle F. Polymer–drug conjugates, PDEPT and PELT: basic principles for design and transfer from the laboratory to clinic. *J Control Release.* 2001;74:135–46.
[85] Ferguson EL, Scomparin A, Hailu H, Satchi-Fainaro R. HPMA copolymer–phospholipase C and dextrin–phospholipase A2 as model triggers for polymer enzyme liposome therapy (PELT). *J Drug Target.* 2017;25(9–10):818–28. https://doi.org/10.1080/1061186X.2017.1358726
[86] Ferguson EL, Schmaljohann D, Duncan R. Polymer–phospholipase conjugates as novel anti-cancer agents: dextrin–phospholipase A2. *Proc 33rd Annual Mtg Control Release Soc.* 2006;33:660.
[87] Ferguson EL, Duncan R, Investigating a dextrin–phospholipase A2 conjugate as a trigger for polymer enzyme liposome therapy (PELT). Cardiff University. https://research.cardiff.ac.uk/converis/portal/detail/Project/2571087;jsessionid=9zc48lAI7lEelWrhSkZbhwMZ9jeokJgbXPot4O5-.cu?lang=cy_CY (last accessed on 20 August 2023).
[88] Leung AWY, Amador C, Wang LC, Mody UV, Bally MB. What drives innovation: The Canadian touch on liposomal therapeutics. *Pharmaceutics.* 2019;11(3):124.
[89] Pang X, Du HL, Zhang HQ, Zhai YJ, Zhai GX. Polymer–drug conjugates: present state of play and future perspectives. Drug Discov Today. 2013 Dec 1;18(23–24):1316–22.
[90] Duncan R, Hume IC, Yardley HJ, Flanagan PA, Ulbrich K, V .Subr, Strohalm J. Macromolecular prodrugs for use in targeted cancer chemotherapy: melphalan covalently coupled to N-(2-hydroxypropyl) methacrylamide copolymers. *J Control. Release.* 1991;16:121–36.
[91] Bhatt R, de Vries P, Tulinsky J, Bellamy G, Baker B, Singer JW, Klein P. Synthesis and in vivo antitumor activity of poly(L-glutamic acid) conjugates of 20 (S)-camptothecin. *J Med Chem.* 2003;46:190–93.
[92] Jain NK, Asthana A. Dendritic systems in drug delivery applications. Expert Opin *Drug Deliv.* 2007;4:495–512.
[93] Li X, Naeem A, Xiao S, Hu L, Zhang J, Zheng Q. Safety challenges and application strategies for the use of dendrimers in medicine. *Pharmaceutics.* 2022 Jun 17;14(6):1292.
[94] Kainthan RK, Hester SR, Levin. In vitro biological evaluation of high molecular weight hyperbranched polyglycerols. *Biomaterials.* 2007;28:4581–90.
[95] Mishra MK, Kobayashi S (Eds.). *Star and Hyperbranched Polymers*, Marcel Dekker, New York. 1999.
[96] Duncan R, Izzo L. Dendrimer biocompatibility and toxicity. *Adv Drug Deliv Rev.* 2005;57:2215–37.
[97] Vicent MJ, Polymer–drug conjugates as modulators of cellular apoptosis. *AAPS J.* 2007;9:E200–07.
[98] Abdellatif AA, Mohammed HA, Khan RA, Singh V, Bouazzaoui A, Yusuf M, Akhtar N, Khan M, Al-Subaiyel A, Mohammed SA, Al-Omar MS. Nano-scale delivery: A comprehensive review of nano-structured devices, preparative techniques, site-specificity designs, biomedical applications, commercial products, and references to safety, cellular uptake, and organ toxicity. *Nanotechnol Rev.* 2021 Oct 21;10(1):1493–559.
[99] Greco F, Vicent MJ. Combination therapy: opportunities and challenges for polymer–drug conjugates as anticancer nanomedicines. *Adv Drug Deliv Rev.* 2009 Nov 12;61(13):1203–13.
[100] Stater EP, Sonay AY, Hart C, Grimm J. The ancillary effects of nanoparticles and their implications for nanomedicine. Nat Nanotechnol. 2021 Nov;16(11):1180–94.
[101] Yang B, Chen Y, Shi J. Reactive oxygen species (ROS)-based nanomedicine. *Chem Rev.* 2019 Apr 11;119(8):4881–985.
[102] Schluter AD. A covalent chemistry approach to giant macromolecules with cylindrical shape and an engineerable interior and surface. Top *Curr Chem.* 2005;245:151–91.
[103] Vicent MJ, Dieudonne L,Carbajo RJ, Pineda-Lucena A. Polymer conjugates as therapeutics: future trends, challenges and opportunities. *Expert Opin Drug Deliv.* 2008;5:593–614.
[104] Griffiths PC, Paul A, Khayat Z, Wan KW, King SM, Grillo I, Schweins R, Ferruti P, Franchini J, Duncan R. Understanding the mechanism of action of poly(amidoamine)s as endosmotic polymers: correlation of physicochemical and biological properties. *Biomacromolecules.* 2004;5:1422–27.

[105] Paul A, Vicent MJ, Duncan R. Using small-angle neutron scattering to study the solution conformation of N-(2-hydroxypropyl)methacrylamide copolymer– doxorubicin conjugates. *Biomacromolecules.* 2007;8:1573–79.
[106] Vicent MJ, Pérez-Payá E. Poly-L-glutamic acid (PGA) aided inhibitors of apoptotic protease activating factor 1 (Apaf-1): an antiapoptotic polymeric nanomedicine. *J Med Chem.* 2006;49:3763–65.
[107] Pinciroli V, Rizzo V, Angelucci F, Tato M, Vigevani A. 1 H-NMR of polymer conjugates with the anticancer drug doxorubicin. Magn *Reson Chem.* 1997;35:2–8.
[108] Hentschel J, ten Cate MGJ, Borner HG. Peptide-guided organization of peptide–polymer conjugates: expanding the approach from oligo- to polymers. *Macromolecules.* 2007;40:9224–32.
[109] Klee JE. Review: mass spectrometry of step-growth polymers. *Eur J Mass Spectrom.* 2005;11:591–610.
[110] Mendichi R, Rizzo V, Gigli M, Schieroni AG. Fractionation and characterization of a conjugate between a polymeric drug-carrier and the antitumor drug camptothecin. Bioconjug *Chem.* 2002;13:1253–58.
[111] Chou R, Gordon DB, de Leon-Casasola OA, Rosenberg JM, Bickler S, Brennan T, Carter T, Cassidy CL, Chittenden EH, Degenhardt E, Griffith S. Management of postoperative pain: a clinical practice guideline from the American Pain Society, the American Society of Regional Anesthesia and Pain Medicine, and the American Society of Anesthesiologists' committee on regional anesthesia, executive committee, and administrative council. *J Pain.* 2016 Feb 1;17(2):131–57.
[112] Paul SM, Mytelka DS, Dunwiddie CT, Persinger CC, Munos BH, Lindborg SR, Schacht AL. How to improve R&D productivity: the pharmaceutical industry's grand challenge. *Nat Rev Drug Discov.* 2010 Mar;9(3):203–14.

7 siRNA Therapeutic Nanocarriers for the Treatment of Cancer

7.1 INTRODUCTION

The field of cancer therapeutics has witnessed remarkable advancements in recent years, with a particular focus on innovative approaches that aim to target the underlying molecular mechanisms driving malignancy. Small interfering RNA (siRNA) has emerged as a promising tool in this endeavor, offering a precise and customizable means to silence specific genes implicated in cancer progression. However, the therapeutic application of siRNA faces challenges related to its stability, efficient delivery, and targeted release within the complex biological milieu. All across the globe, cancer is a huge public health issue. By 2020, the world's cancer incidence is projected to have doubled, with 15 million new cases of the disease diagnosed annually. The three most popular cancer treatments now are surgery, chemotherapy, as well as radiation therapy. Non-targeted therapy, on the other hand, is often ineffective and may have adverse consequences on organs as well as tissues. Various novel tumor therapies are being created as a result of these factors. Gene therapy utilizing RNAi [1] is one of these therapies. Gene mutations are the primary cause of cancer. Combining oncogene-activating mutations as well as the absence of tumor suppressor gene activity may lead to cell proliferation in an uncontrolled manner and death [2–4]. A large number of important genes, known as "driver genes," have been discovered [5, 6].

Suppression of certain genes using siRNA therapies may be useful in the treatment of cancer [7, 8]. Because siRNA therapy may target a wide range of cancer-related genes, it has a significant advantage over traditional cancer therapies in that it does not have to worry about the druggability of its protein products. siRNA therapy may be able to cure previously untreatable tumors. Plants were the first to discover RNAi. According to research done in worms in 1998 by Andrew Z. Fire along with Craig C. Mello, a double-stranded RNA (dsRNA) inhibits gene activity more efficiently than single-stranded RNA and experimented with the interfering effects of dsRNA transfection on mammalian cells. In 2010, Davis *et al.* published their findings on the first human systemic injection of a targeted siRNA delivery nanocarrier. Fire and Mello discovered double-stranded RNA1 in 2006, and they both shared the Nobel Prize for their work [9]. Gene silencing and the therapy of previously incurable malignancies are two possible therapeutic uses for RNAi. Despite numerous successful preclinical studies, only some numbers of siRNA-targeted nanocarriers (NCs) are permitted for use in clinical settings.

MicroRNA (miRNA) as well as small interfering RNA (siRNA) are two varieties of small RNA molecules. Processing of the two varieties of short RNA differs just slightly, as well as the reported lengths for siRNA and miRNA, respectively, are 21 to 23 and 18 to 25 nucleotides. The primary distinction is how they work. In general, complete complementarity between siRNA and mRNA is required for siRNA to target its transcripts, although less perfection is required for

DOI: 10.1201/9781003451020-7

miRNA. Several distinct transcripts may be targeted by a single miRNA. For example, siRNAs normally halt gene expression after transcription by degrading the mRNA of their target genes, whereas miRNAs typically mute their targets by repressing their translation. Posttranscriptional gene silencing and transcriptional gene silencing are the two primary phases of the siRNA-mediated gene silencing process [10, 11]. Both exert a distinct restraint on the subject's behavior. Direct sequence-specific cleavage, which inhibits translation along with, as a result, degradation, is one of two methods for post-transcriptional gene silencing. Direct cleavage specific to sequence may be explained as follows: when the dicer ribonuclease enzyme breaks down endogenous dsRNA into short, double-stranded fragments of an average of 21 to 23 base pairs in length, it can detect the 2-nucleotide overhangs at the 3′ ends. As a result of cleavage, siRNAs are produced. A passenger strand plus a guide strand are joined by an active protein complex (RISC) to form the RNA-induced silencing complex. With its 5′ ends at base 10 and its 3′ ends at base 11, the guide strand directs its silencing enzyme argonaute-2 toward a target gene and cuts it in half between bases 10 and 11. Thus, siRNA may disrupt the mRNA translation pathway [12–15]. Using complementary complexing with the 3′UTR of miRNA-targeted mRNAs, through mediating protein translation inhibition and/or facilitating degradation, the miRNA-controlled gene silencing pathway affects the stability of mRNA [16]. Figure 7.1 shows MiRNA and siRNA RNAi mechanisms.

Anticancer medication development has several challenging hurdles, including various genetic alterations, the intricacy of cancer progression, and the variety of the tumor microenvironment. Cancer medication therapy is also plagued by multiple drug resistance and severe systemic toxicity. Combining two or more anticancer drugs may be a useful approach because of their cumulative or synergistic effects. Clinical trials using combination therapies may benefit from high-throughput screening to narrow down the field of potential participants. It is possible to better optimize favorable medication interactions by using the process of drug synergy except for randomly selecting drug conjugations. Numerous combinations of siRNA and chemotherapy have lately attracted significant research interest. The use of siRNA to inhibit MDR-related proteins has shown promising results in reversing MDR. Simultaneous administration of small-molecule therapies and siRNA in MDR cell lines may boost the efficacy of chemotherapy. Other disorders may potentially benefit from the application of siRNA as a therapeutic agent. Because siRNA does not need genome integration and can be inexpensively manufactured, it is an intriguing therapeutic option. siRNA's ability to transport siRNA to its intended target remains a key obstacle to its application as a therapeutic agent. For RNAi to be used in therapeutics, researchers must first figure out a safe way to transport the tiny siRNA to the intended organ(s). siRNA must be protected from degradation and filtered out by the kidneys, as well as from exiting blood arteries so that it may enter target tissues. Unfortunately, it has turned out to be a much tougher issue than anticipated. By providing a comprehensive overview,

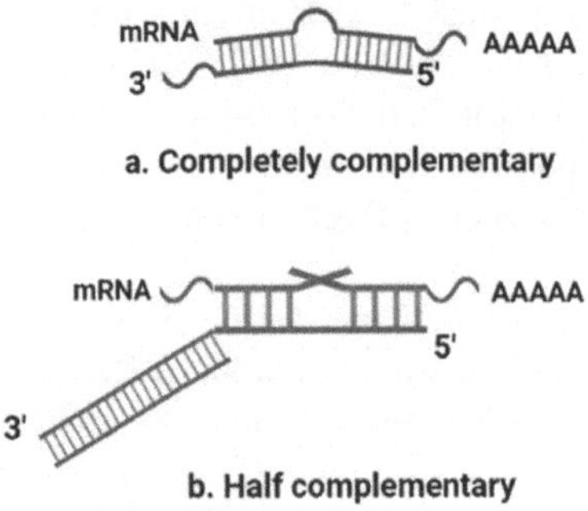

FIGURE 7.1 miRNA and siRNA RNAi mechanisms.

we aim to underscore the significance of siRNA therapeutic nanocarriers as a cutting-edge approach in the ongoing quest for more precise and potent cancer therapies.

7.2 THE BENEFITS AND DIFFICULTIES OF DELIVERING SIRNA FOR CANCER PREVENTION AND TREATMENT

As we navigate the complex landscape of cancer prevention and treatment, the emergence of small interfering RNA (siRNA) has ignited a new wave of optimism. siRNA holds tremendous potential for selectively silencing genes associated with cancer development, presenting a revolutionary avenue for therapeutic intervention. However, the translation of this promise into effective clinical outcomes faces a myriad of challenges, chief among them being the delivery of siRNA to target tissues. In comparison with chemotherapeutic anticancer medications, siRNA anticancer therapies have benefits, notably in the treatment of untreatable cancers. To begin with, it is quite secure. As a result, siRNA avoids the mutation and teratogenic concerns that are frequent in gene therapy by acting on post-translational gene expression. Third, the effectiveness of siRNA is exceptional. Fourth, an individual cell with only a few duplicates of siRNA may significantly reduce gene expression. The freedom in target selection that a siRNA offers when compared to other smaller molecule drugs or treatments based on antibodies, as well as the specificity that comes from complementary base pairing, are its two main advantages. Silencing cancer-promoting genes using a targeted siRNA1 may be used as a primary method for treating cancer. Table 7.1 outlines and discusses the principal difficulties in delivering siRNA to cancer cells [16].

Delivering siRNA to target cells is hampered by several roadblocks that must be overcome. Under physiological circumstances, siRNA is not stable. In the blood, serum nucleases can efficiently break down the siRNA. The plasma membrane, which prevents large hydrophilic or charged molecules from passing through, is the initial obstacle to nuclear drug delivery [17, 18]. Initial endosomes, which mix with sorting endosomes and subsequently transfer their contents to endosomes behind, are primarily responsible for the transport of siRNA into cells. The endosomal compartments are acidic, whereas the cytoplasm or intracellular space (pH 7.4) is neutral (pH 5.0 to 6.2) are very acidic [19]. Acidification takes place at pH 4.5, which is achieved when the endosome is moved to the lysosomes [20]. They include nucleases that help to degrade siRNA.

Systemic injection of siRNA is the best method for delivering it to cancer cells since it can pass the boundaries of the human body. When administered intravenously, endogenous nucleases quickly degrade siRNA, which is then eliminated by the kidney or picked up by the process of phagocytes as well as aggregated along with serum protein [21].

TABLE 7.1
Significant Barriers Impede the Transportation of Small Interfering RNA (siRNA) to Cancer Cells

Delivery Location	Delivery Challenges for siRNA Nanocarriers
Circulation	Because of non-specific interactivities to serum proteins, nanocarrier disintegration, dissociation, or aggregation occurs. Clearance of particles smaller than 6–10 nm by the kidneys. The toxicity of nanocarriers may be caused.
Tissue	Permeation of the endothelium. The target tissue is reached from the bloodstream.
Extracellular	Diffusion and stability outside of the cell. Nanocarriers may be damaged by tissue microenvironment distinctions in pH, ions, or enzymes, resulting in dissociation before cellular entrance.
Intracellular	The endosomal compartment has been breached and you have escaped. Release of siRNA payload after dissociation from the nanocarrier in the cytoplasm.
Integrative immunity	Immune activation as well as cytokine generation in the laboratory and animals.

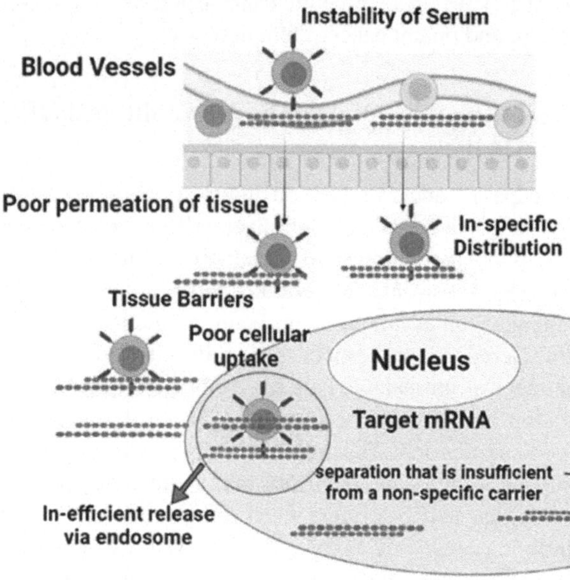

FIGURE 7.2 Obstacles that siRNA faces after being delivered systemically upon its administration.

The nuclease activity in blood or tissues is a major hurdle for given siRNA. A 3′ exonuclease is the most prevalent nuclease in plasma. Plasma is capable of cleaving internucleotide bond cleavage as well. In serum, unaltered siRNA possesses a half-life of a few minutes to an hour [22]. The kidneys are critical in the removal of siRNA. According to several animal studies, siRNA had the maximum uptake in the kidney [23]. *In vivo*, injection of siRNA (RES) encounters major challenges due to renal clearance, degradation of the circulating nuclease, and siRNA absorption via the reticuloendothelial system. Phagocytic cells in the RES, like circulating monocytes as well as tissue macrophages, eliminate foreign pathogens, cell debris, and necrotic tissue [24]. The most prevalent macrophages in the liver as well as the spleen, which receive a lot of blood flow, are Kupffer cells. Figure 7.2 describes the obstacles to the intracellular and extracellular delivery of siRNA nanocarriers to cancer cells.

Following systemic injection, siRNA is found in high amounts in many organs. siRNA taken after i.v. (intravenous) injection on the tail vein or i.p. (intraperitoneal) injection occurred at 4 hours [25]. As an anionic, double-stranded, and hydrophilic RNA called siRNA, it is difficult for cells to take up free siRNAs. As a result, siRNA's hydrophilicity and negative charge make it difficult for it to pass biological membranes. It is also necessary to use an appropriate carrier for siRNA to enter cells. The off-target reactions of siRNA include mediation of unintended transcripts dependent on sequence via partial sequence complementarity to their 3′ UTRs, plus broad impacts on miRNA processing as well as functioning through saturating the endogenous RNAi machinery by exogenous siRNA. These effects make it more difficult to understand the therapeutic benefits of siRNA [26]. When RNAi screens were used to find new components of signal transduction pathways, remarkable off-target effects were discovered [27]. TGF-b receptor 1, as well as 2 (TGFBR1 and TGFBR2), are recognized upstream pathway components that all is targeted by siRNA and decrease levels of mRNA through miRNA-like off-target effects [27]. Global regulation of genes by endogenous miRNA could be disrupted by transfection of siRNAs. It is possible that siRNA will not be as safe as first thought. *In vitro* along with *in vivo*, higher doses of siRNA are shown to activate innate immune responses, stimulate immunological responses, repress immune responses, and produce cytokines [28, 29]. TLR3, TLR7, and TLR8 [26, 30–32] are among the TLRs (toll-like receptors) implicated in siRNA recognition [30]. A sequence-independent activation of TLR3 signaling has been discovered via siRNA. When it comes to the identification of siRNAs, TLR7 and TLR8 preferentially identify certain RNA sequences such as UG dinucleotides plus the 50-UGU30 pattern. As a result, more research into the sequencing issue surrounding siRNA-mediated immune activation is required. NLRs and the inflammasome, two intracellular receptors that stimulate innate immune responses, are also involved in the immunological interactions of nanocarriers [33]. New siRNA distribution methods are required to overcome these challenges and fully exploit the siRNA's enormous therapeutic potential. siRNA needs to be chemically altered and administered without endangering the organism. Polymers, aptamers, lipids, peptides, antibodies, and other tiny molecules are being utilized to overcome the issues of *in vivo* distribution of siRNA-based nanocarriers. High-throughput screening has been used to rationally design several preclinical systems that have proven to be very effective. Endo/lysosomal vesicles, rather than nuclei, are the primary destinations of current drug delivery vehicles. For medications to be effective, they must first enter the cytoplasm and then enter the nucleus [34]. Many intracellular resistance mechanisms, including upregulation of drug efflux pumps (e.g., P-gp), metabolism of the drug as well as its detoxification, drug deactivation as well as drug sequestering in acidic compartments, limiting the number of cytosolic drugs that can enter cancer cell nuclei. Only a tiny portion of the medicine injected inside the cytosol enters the nucleus in cancer cells, which are resistant to drugs [35, 36]. For instance, only 5% to 10% of the DNA fractions contained cisplatin, whereas 75% to 85% of the drug was associated with proteins. The median amount of an administered dosage (ID) that reaches specific tumors, according to a recent meta-analysis of preclinical data on delivery systems based on nanocarriers for cancer issued over the last decade, is roughly 0.7% [9, 37]. As a result, cellular internalization, which requires binding to and passing through the cell membrane, is the last stage in drug delivery.

An excellent strategy to increase the efficacy of therapy in siRNA-mediated treatments has emerged as an effective nuclear drug delivery technique. A gold siRNA delivery method based on nanoparticles for long-term silencing of genes in tumor cells, for example, was recently described [38]. The nuclear-targeted nanocarrier significantly decreased TK1 mRNA expression in comparison to the non-targeted nanocarrier. For more than 30 days, the nuclear-targeted siRNA effectively decreased TK1 protein expression, as well as TK1 mRNA expression. When it comes to long-term gene silencing, nuclear targeting outperforms cytoplasmic targeting in a study. Nuclear-targeted nanocarrier therapy decreased cell proliferation and tumor growth *in vivo*, which is an important finding [38].

Nanocarriers, in contrast to low molecular weight medicines, are ingested via endocytosis rather than passive diffusion. Endocytic compartments include early and late endosomes; as they proceed through the endocytic pathway they meet increasingly more acidic regions as they reach lysosomal compartments. As the acidic pH and associated enzymes in these areas are present, the carriers release medicines into the cytosol and nucleus.

7.3 CHARACTERIZATION OF SIRNA NANOCARRIERS FOR PRECISE DELIVERY OF MEDICINE TO CANCER CELLS AND THEIR POTENTIAL FOR USE IN CLINICAL APPLICATIONS

In the relentless pursuit of more effective cancer treatments, the utilization of small interfering RNA (siRNA) as a therapeutic modality has emerged as a promising strategy. One of the critical challenges in harnessing the full potential of siRNA lies in the development of nanocarriers capable of precise and efficient delivery to cancer cells. The characterization of these siRNA nanocarriers represents a crucial step in bridging the gap between theoretical promise and clinical application. This introduction aims to navigate the landscape of siRNA nanocarriers, focusing on their characterization methods and the implications of their unique properties for targeted medicine delivery to cancer cells. Cancer cells provide several challenges for siRNA delivery systems, and these challenges must be taken into consideration while designing a delivery system. Simultaneous delivery of large, negatively charged siRNA molecules (13 kDa), which are required for efficient distribution across cancer cell membranes, has proved to be very challenging [39]. So, siRNA delivery systems must be created to meet the following criteria: (a) serum stability, (b) immune evasion, (c) mitigation of interactions between non-cancerous cells and serum proteins (d), resistance to renal clearance (e), enhancement of vascular permeability (f), cell entry as well as endosome escape (g), and low toxicity. To treat cancer, patients should get a systemic dose of 21, 39 siRNA. However, when siRNA is administered into the blood, its natural immune system as well as serum nucleases swiftly break it down. Chemical alteration of the siRNA structure is a frequent solution to these issues. 2′-O-methyl plus 2′-deoxy-2’fluoro groups, sealed or unsealed nucleic acids, and phosphorothioate connections are the most typical alterations to chemicals [40]. The natural immune system's ability to recognize siRNA may be thwarted by careful siRNA sequence and structure design. Chemical modifications are less successful than nanoparticles that contain siRNA at securing siRNA from deterioration and immune detection [40, 41]. Several different blood components may interfere with the transfer of siRNA to cancer cells in a variety of ways. Nanoparticles having a high positive charge on their surface might induce erythrocytes to clump together in an undesirable way [42]. However, that kind of association between serum proteins as well as nanoparticles may potentially facilitate the uptake of cancer cells [43, 44].

As a result of their interaction with lipids in the serum, hepatocytes that take up the lipids may take up liposomal delivery systems and siRNA that have been conjugated to lipophilic molecules [43].

Delivered nanoparticles are tagged for mononuclear phagocytosis when they are coated with serum opsonin proteins (MPS) [21, 44]. The MPS absorbs nanoparticles from the bloodstream as a result of osmolysis, which is the main method of nanoparticle removal from the bloodstream. Using polyethylene glycol as a surface shield for the distribution of nanoparticles is the most effective and widely utilized technique for minimizing interactions with serum proteins (PEG) [21, 45].

When delivery nanoparticles are coated with polyethylene glycol (PEG), non-target tissues, such as the innate immune system, are less likely to interact with the nanoparticles. To stabilize and safeguard nanoparticles, PEG encases them in a protective barrier [46]. The stabilization and protection qualities of PEG may be improved for specific delivery systems by changing the PEG chain length. PEGylated nanocarriers, alternatively, are restricted by undesirable effects such as activation of the complement system, which may cause hypersensitivity responses and even anaphylaxis. The liver, spleen, kidney, and lung are just a few of the organs that may remove siRNA from the circulation once it has been administered systemically. The most frequent route to elimination is through the kidneys. Water and smaller molecules can enter the nascent urine via renal glomeruli, whereas bigger molecules remain in the bloodstream [47, 48]. Molecules smaller than 50 kDa are often eliminated by the kidney and pass via a hole in the barrier to glomerular filtration that is approximately 8 nm wide [49]. Because siRNA is so little, it may be excreted in the urine [39]. The nanoparticle's size may be raised sufficiently to escape glomerular filtration by combining siRNA with synthetic materials [50]. The majority of delivery methods are intended to be greater than 20 nm in size [51]. Triantennary N-acetylgalactosamine (GalNAc) conjugates and dynamic polyconjugates (DPC; 10 nm) [52] are two highly efficient delivery methods. The EPR effect, which boosts permeability and retention, causes nanoparticles of sizes between tens and hundreds of nanometers to passively aggregate in tumors at a faster rate compared to the healthy tissues. That is mostly due to the aberrant arrangement and architecture of newly generated tumor vasculature. Numerous nanosized drug delivery strategies, involving dendrimers, liposomes, micelles, as well as inorganic hybrid particles, have been created for treating cancer [53]. The majority of siRNA distribution strategies use the endocytosis mechanism, which allows siRNA to enter cells. Several delivery systems use targeting ligands to boost the pace of cellular absorption by specifically binding to receptors on the targeted cells to start receptor-mediated endocytosis [53, 54]. If serum proteins stick to the surface of nanoparticles, ligand-receptor binding may be hindered [55]. Endocytosis and non-endocytic

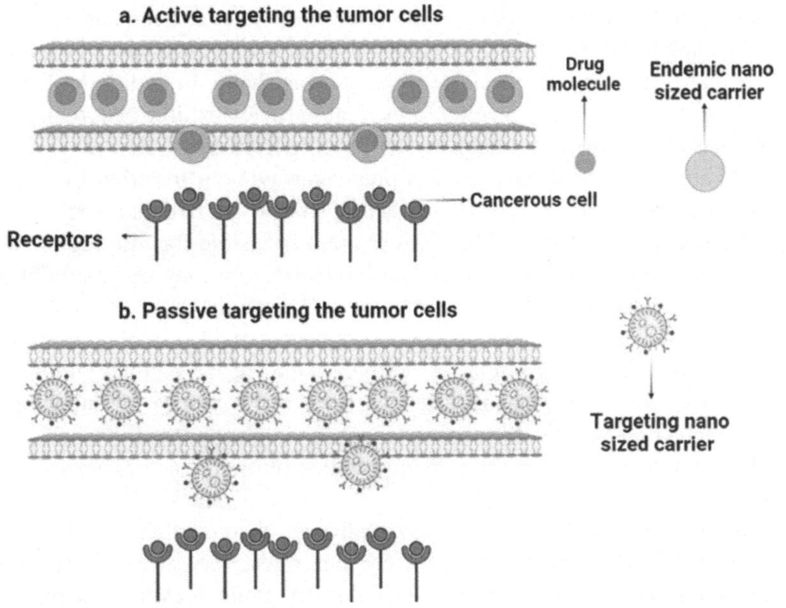

FIGURE 7.3 Receptor-mediated transport of nanoformulations to tumor cells can occur through both (a) active and (b) passive mechanisms.

processes are used in other systems to stimulate cell absorption of cell-penetrating peptides [56]. As early endosomes merge with mature late endosomes, endocytosed components are transported into membrane-bound endocytic vesicles. The release of siRNA from endosomes may be triggered by delivery methods that use components engineered to become membrane-disrupting in a low pH environment [56, 57]. Many siRNA delivery strategies use an endosomal release process that is currently poorly understood. The most crucial aspect of any delivery technique of siRNA is low toxicity. Even the most effective siRNA delivery method will be useless if it causes substantial toxicity in the body and the cells overall. Viral vectors, which were one of the initial vehicles to be investigated for siRNA delivery, may result in hazardous levels of toxicity [58]. To reduce immune system activation or inhibition, a significant range of alternate delivery systems of nucleic acid are developed employing synthetic lipids and polymers. Biodegradability is often required for the clearance of compounds with a higher molecular weight. Cytotoxicity may be reduced by using high molecular mass polycations, polymers with intracellularly cleavable links, and biodegradable polymers [59]. Figure 7.3 depicts a diagram showing the receptor-mediated (a) passive and (b) active transport of nanoformulations to tumor cells.

7.4 NANOCARRIERS' DIMENSIONS, FORM, AND CHARGE

In the realm of drug delivery, the design and characteristics of nanocarriers play a pivotal role in determining the success of therapeutic interventions. Among these key attributes, the dimensions, form, and charge of nanocarriers stand out as critical factors influencing their behavior within biological systems. Understanding and optimizing these features are essential steps toward achieving effective drug delivery, with particular significance in the context of nanomedicine. The size and shape of nanocarriers, ranging from nanoparticles to liposomes, profoundly influence their interactions with biological entities and cellular uptake. Additionally, the charge of these carriers holds sway over their stability, biodistribution, and the ability to traverse cellular membranes. By unraveling the complexities of these characteristics, we aim to shed light on their significance in the design of next-generation nanocarrier systems and their potential to revolutionize drug delivery in the realm of nanomedicine. Nanoparticle biodistribution is influenced by a variety of variables, including particle size, surface charge, elasticity as well as shape. In addition to liposomes, gold nanoparticles, as well as polymeric micelles, spherical particles exhibit diverse sizes and *in vivo* fates. EPR effect has been shown for nanoparticles ranging from 100–200 nm in size that extravasate via tumor-expanded vascular fenestrations plus getaway from filtration by the liver as well as spleen. Nanoparticles are stuck in the liver and spleen in greater numbers when they reach sizes greater than or equal to 150 nm. The kidneys are responsible for filtering out nanoparticles less than 5 nm in size [60]. Pharmacokinetic and biodistribution may be greatly affected by the nanoparticle's geometry, which includes cylindrical and discoidal geometries. Because of their distinct flow properties, dissimilar nanoparticle shapes have variable circulation lifetimes and cell membrane interactions, which in turn impact macrophage uptake and biodistribution [61]. Because of the special surface chemistry of nanoparticles, their charge affects opsonization, circulation time, as well as interaction with MPS organ-resident macrophages, with particles that are positively charged becoming more susceptible to sequestration through macrophages within the lungs, spleen plus liver.

If the nanoparticles are neutral or just slightly negatively charged, there is less buildup in these organs and longer periods for circulation [60, 10]. Systems of delivery smaller than 100 nm in diameter can be captured in the mononuclear phagocyte system, while delivery systems larger than 50 kDa can be eliminated by filtering [61].

The optimal systemic delivery vehicle, according to Bedi *et al.*, is 10–50 nm in size. According to Wang and colleagues, a size ranging from 10–100 nm is ideal [62, 63]. Particles smaller than 100 nm in diameter have been shown to increase tissue absorption and transfection effectiveness, according to other studies [10, 64]. While that might be the case, other investigators have demonstrated that, with some exceptions [65–69], delivery techniques smaller than 200 nm allow effective tissue as well as cell absorption [70]. According to Hirota and Terada along with their colleagues, the ideal particle size range for cellular absorption is different depending on the type of cancer cell. Particles with a diameter of 50 nm or less are often acceptable [71]. The flexibility and shape of the nanocarrier may have a remarkable impact on the behavior of the particles and cellular uptake. According to Young *et al.*, rod-shaped items have a broader contact surface, which blocks neighboring receptor sites, which causes endocytosis rates to be higher for spherical objects [72].

Spherical particles have the highest rates of internalization and absorption, according to Li *et al.*, since their energy barrier for membrane bending is less than that of non-spherical systems [73]. He and Park discovered that they are prone to stick to cells plus be taken up by malignant cells when compared with geometries with a smaller facet ratio as well as sharply angular properties [74]. The effects of different shapes on receptor-mediated endocytosis as well as phagocytosis were investigated by researchers Richards with Endres utilizing one-dimensional as well as two-dimensional physical models to clarify the differences in the cellular internalization of variously shaped nanocarriers. According to their findings, orientation has an important effect on the rate of internalization. The quickest internalization is possible for non-spherical shapes [75]. Positive charged particles are more readily absorbed compared to negative charged ones, hence a delivery system's surface charge has a considerable impact on its uptake. It is possible to calculate the surface charge using the zeta potential.

Electrostatic repulsive interactions between particles are measured by zeta potential, which implies stability if the value is larger than zero. By increasing electrostatic interactivities among the positively charged surface of the particle and the negatively charged membrane of the cell in delivery techniques with higher positive zeta potentials, cellular uptake is improved [67, 76]. However, certain delivery methods have been shown to have negative zeta potentials. Even though they should be attracted to positively charged particles, cells could absorb negatively charged particles in positively charged locations to neutralize them and bend the membrane, leading to endocytosis. Tumors typically prefer to accept delivery vehicles having a positive charge as well as having a higher cellular absorption than those having a negative or neutral charge [76, 77]. For particles with no surface charge, cellular uptake was the lowest.

Some researchers have proposed that cationic polymers, like poloxamers and polyethylene oxide, be attached via receptor-mediated endocytosis to improve selectivity and cell absorption [65–78]. A delivery system has to first enter the cell and then travel via the cell membrane to escape the cell. It is possible to modify the characteristics of nanocarrier systems for delivery to improve endosomal-lysosomal escape. One well-known method for reaching the objective is the proton sponge effect. The acidification of the endosomes may be prevented by buffering the pH of the endosomes [67, 77, 79–81]. To reduce the pH, cells will pump more protons into endosomes, followed by chloride ions and water inflow as a result of the increased ionic concentration. A rise in osmotic pressure eventually leads the endosome to enlarge and burst, spilling its contents into the cytoplasm.

Due to their potent pH buffering capabilities over a wide pH range, lipopolyamines, polyamidoamine dendrimers, as well as polyethyleneimine have all been demonstrated to display the proton sponge effect (PEI). pKa values for polymers with secondary or tertiary amine groups are frequently close to or at endosomal levels [82]. By protonating these polymers, endosome acidification could be decreased. PEI is renowned for its wide range of uses and applications due to its powerful pH buffering capacity, capacity to condense siRNAs in nanoscale complexes, and capacity to transfect cells *in vitro* as well as *in vivo* [67]. Despite that, reports of PEI's hazardous effects, which are regulated by its molecular weight, have kept it from being widely used in clinical settings. PEI's transfection effectiveness rises with increasing molecular weight, but so does non-specific toxicity. Low molecular weight PEI, on the other hand, is less poisonous and less effective in transfecting cells. According to Essex *et al.*, the chemical coupling of PEI to dioleoyl phosphatidylethanolamine (DOPE) enhanced the intracellular transfection efficiency of siRNA with low levels of cytotoxicity. Chitosan as well as polylysine are two examples of polypeptides that do not act as pH buffers in polymers [83]. By introducing histidine or functional groups, polypeptides like GALA, endosome-disruptive peptides that are sensitive to pH, can be made better. Another escape pathway is the fusion of cationic polymers, peptides, as well as cationic lipids like DOPE, which destabilizes the cellular membrane. siRNAs must first undergo several tests before they can serve as therapeutic agents. These capabilities include the capacity to prevent nucleic acid molecules from degrading during systemic delivery, to withstand an extended circulation without renal filtration, to accumulate in a patient's tissue of interest, to enter target cells via a particular uptake mechanism, to initiate cell uptake via endocytosis, and, finally, to escape the cell's endosomal cation [84, 85]. A delivery technique should have the following qualities: biocompatibility, biodegradability, non-toxicity, and immunogenicity.

7.5 THE METHOD OF GENE SILENCING USING SMALL INTERFERING RNA (SIRNA)

The method of gene silencing through small interfering RNA (siRNA) has emerged as a transformative approach in the field of molecular biology and therapeutic research. Harnessing the cell's own machinery, siRNA provides a powerful means to selectively silence target genes, offering unprecedented precision in modulating gene expression. This introduction explores the fundamental principles underlying the method of gene silencing using siRNA, highlighting its significance in unraveling gene function and its therapeutic potential for various genetic disorders, including cancer and viral infections. To get siRNA to its target, a delivery technique must first get through the cell membrane as well as steer clear of the endocytic pathway. To create the ideal delivery system, it is essential to have a complete grasp of how cellular transport functions. A bilayer of phospholipids that is permeable in a selective manner makes up the cell membrane. On the surface of the membrane, it has a hydrophilic, polar phosphate head, while on the inside, it has two hydrophobic (non-polar) fatty acid tails. As a general rule, molecules that are smaller and more hydrophobic tend to move more quickly across the lipid bilayer [84, 86]. Endocytosis is the primary mode of transport through the membrane of the cell. For phagocytosis (cell eating) as well as pinocytosis (cell drinking), particle size is a significant element in determining the manner of absorption, with particle size being the primary determinant [84]. As the cell membrane stretches outwards, the phagosome is formed, which may then merge with a lysosomal membrane for digestion. Bacteria and cellular debris may be cleared via phagocytosis, which is accomplished by monocytes, neutrophils, macrophages, and endothelial cells that operate to remove particles with diameters bigger than 0.5 m. Macrophages can ingest polystyrene spherical particles coated with IgG that vary in size from 200 to 2 nm [87]. Drug and RNA delivery techniques in the size range are deemed ineffective [88]. Pinocytosis captures particles from 50 nm–5 m in size, which occurs in practically every cell, including cancer cells. The plasma membrane's envelope folds inward when particles imported by pinocytosis come into touch with the membrane's external surface. A vesicle is created when the membrane is entirely enclosed, and it contains both extracellular fluid and the recently imported particles. Pinocytosis is mediated by one of three mechanisms: receptor-mediated endocytosis, receptor-independent endocytosis, or micropinocytosis, all of which are discussed below. When a particle binds to a particular receptor, it is preferentially taken up by the endocytosis machinery. Both clathrin-mediated endocytosis and caveolin-mediated endocytosis may be subdivided into two basic categories: (a) the cell membrane protein clathrin-initiated endocytosis; and (b) caveolin, a protein that binds cholesterol, causes endocytosis.

Particles less than 50 nm may be endocytosed without clathrin or caveolin receptors being involved. 72 micropinocytosis is the preferred method of cell entrance for particles smaller than 5 nm. Macropinosomes take up particles in a non-selective manner in that procedure [88–90]. To manage size, delivery is also a consideration. Nanosystems may be active or passive, depending on their design. Proteins, peptides, and tiny molecules may be used to adorn the vehicle surface for active transport and stimulate receptor-mediated endocytosis. Biophysical features such as size, shape, and zeta potential need to be manipulated when designing passive transport delivery systems [91]. Once an endocytosis vehicle has passed the cell membrane, it stays in the endosome until it is recycled or destroyed and enters the endocytic process. The pH of the endosome is critical in that process. Cells use hydrolytic enzymes to break down the ingested chemical in an increasingly acidic environment. Following are the steps in which the procedure takes place: an early endosome is a sorting organelle that is positioned in the cell's periphery and is responsible for receiving the majority of particles that enter the cell via its surface. Their pH ranges from 0 to 6, which is considered somewhat acidic. From here, a large number of the molecules either get exocytosed or sorted into late endosomes; (b) the late endosomes then get the endocytosed materials from the earliest endosomes via transport carriers or Rab conversion [92].

The primary function of lysosomes, the final endocytic compartment, is to disassemble waste products, carbohydrates, proteins, lipids, as well as other macromolecular components into their component subunits. An ATP-dependent proton pump that moves across the membrane makes them acidic.

Lysosomes are comprised of degradative hydrolytic enzymes that are active under an acidic region. The particle and its payload will degrade if the delivery method is unable to exit that compartment. Instead of exposing the contents of a delivery mechanism to the lysosomal degradation enzymes, it is preferable if the contents are released via the acidic endosomal compartment. The challenges of leaving late endosomes as well as being exposed to selective cytoplasmic disintegration must be solved for siRNA methods of delivery inside the cell to be effective. Even a 0.1% escape of siRNA may be sufficient due to the siRNA's ability to increase inside the cell. Non-dividing cells may only need to be dosed every 6 months, or possibly once a year if they are receiving siRNAs.

7.6 APPROACHES FOR ADMINISTERING SIRNA THERAPEUTICS TO CANCER CELLS

The development of small interfering RNA (siRNA) as a therapeutic modality has ushered in a new era of precision medicine, particularly in the context of cancer treatment. However, the successful translation of siRNA therapeutics from bench to bedside necessitates effective delivery strategies tailored to navigate the complexities of the human body. This introduction explores the diverse approaches employed for administering siRNA therapeutics to cancer cells, highlighting the challenges and innovations that underscore this critical facet of targeted cancer therapy. The utilization of targeted delivery strategies for cancer medicines has considerably increased during the past few decades. Out of a large number of successful preclinical trials, only a small number of passive targeted NCs (around 20) have received clinical usage approval. Clinical studies have shown no improvement in any of the currently targeted NCs. Targeted delivery techniques have had limited clinical translation and effectiveness in clinical trials, thus iti s critical to examine the underlying concepts to figure out why. The creation of innovative actively targeted NCs requires consideration of several criteria and concerns. We have covered several possible directions for the creation of cancer-targeting siRNA techniques below. The first step is to get the cancer properly diagnosed as soon as possible. The next step is to develop a cancer model that has been diagnosed and to characterize tumor markers. If you know how to create and manufacture the right kind of nanocarrier for your specific needs, you can ensure that your medicine and siRNA can enter the target cell, overcome any obstacles, and eventually reach their intended destination. There are numerous procedures involved in the characterization of the nanocarrier, such as physico-chemical, *in vitro*, as well as *in vivo* testing. Overexpressed proteins and genes may be used as cancer targets. The next step is to select a suitable targeting ligand that will accurately adhere to the target chosen as well as to identify the perfect ligand density and drug concentration, which was done after *in vitro* cytotoxicity, efficacy, and immunogenicity experiments. Figure 7.4 depicts siRNA-targeted approaches to cancer treatment and prevention,

Efficacy biodistribution and toxicity testing will be conducted in the following phase. Imaging modalities and effectiveness studies should be used to optimize the density of the target ligands *in vitro* plus *in vivo*. Whether using a single or two distinct antibodies, gold nanoparticles are known to

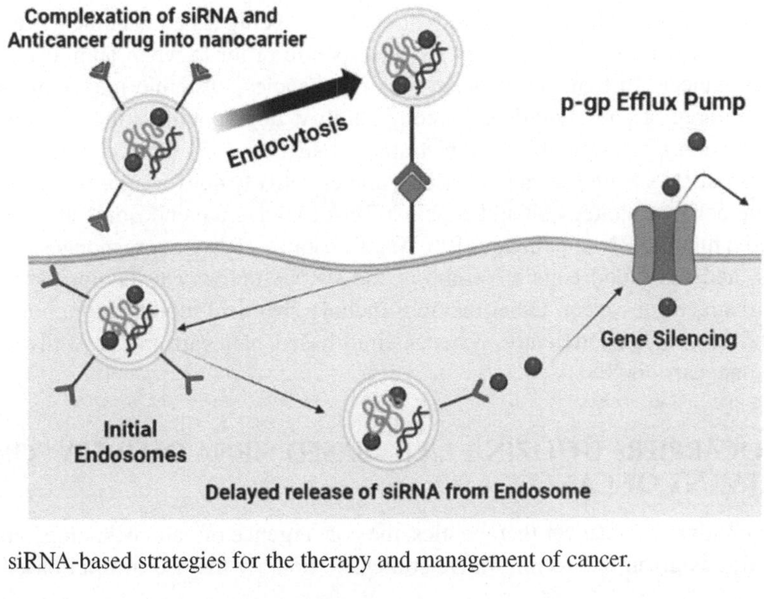

FIGURE 7.4 siRNA-based strategies for the therapy and management of cancer.

have a variety of effects *in vitro* as well as *in vivo* [93]. Determining the EPR impact is critical for deciding on whether to administer the medication locally or systemically. Depending on the EPR, local administration may be used, whereas systemic administration is preferable for high EPRs. As a result, EPR-targeted NCs may not be adequate to achieve substantial tumor targeting. However, rapid quantitative EPR imaging methods are thus essential for assessing the EPR impact and selecting individuals who are most likely to react to EPR-based cancer therapy. Actively focused delivery has the benefit of being able to target scattered areas of the body. Hematological malignancies and metastatic cancers might be revolutionized by the use of active targeted delivery when EPR is not an option.

The impact of a protein corona in a cell environment on biological distribution, targeting, therapeutic efficacy, and toxicity must be taken into consideration when developing NCs that are passively or actively targeted. Improved methods are needed to generate a nanocarrier that can be controlled and predicted biologically. Controlled and targeted administration may be improved with the use of stimuli-responsive nanocarriers. Patients with solid tumors, hematological malignancies, and cancers that have spread are predicted to benefit from the use of these techniques. Exogenous cell or exosome-mediated distribution of nanocarriers delivering medicines or immune-modulating payloads in malignancies is one method of avoiding the EPR effect. Despite many preclinical studies demonstrating the therapeutic potential of nanocarriers, only a small number of clinical trials using tailored delivery systems have been successful. To achieve clinical success with targeted delivery, an appropriate approach must still be devised. Figure 7.4 depicts the siRNA-targeted techniques for cancer prevention and treatment.

7.7 DESIGNING SIRNA MOLECULES WITH HIGH THERAPEUTIC SIGNIFICANCE FOR APPLICATION AS NANOCARRIERS FOR THE DELIVERY OF DRUGS

In the dynamic landscape of molecular therapeutics, the integration of small interfering RNA (siRNA) holds immense promise, particularly when harnessed as a cornerstone in the design of nanocarriers for drug delivery. The strategic fusion of siRNA with nanocarriers not only enables precise gene modulation but also opens avenues for targeted and controlled release of therapeutic drugs [94]. This explores the intricate process of designing siRNA molecules with high therapeutic significance, emphasizing their pivotal role as nanocarriers for drug delivery applications. There have been several methods described for delivering siRNA to cancer cells' cytoplasms. Most of them are suitable for *in vitro* use. Alternatively, *in vivo*, results are less encouraging. To circumvent the complexities of systemic distribution, the bulk of siRNA treatments now being tested in clinical trials are supplied specifically to diseased areas. siRNA still has therapeutic promise when administered directly or locally to treat cancer. To treat the majority of malignancies, systemic means of siRNA administration are required. There should be biocompatibility, degradability, and non-immunogenicity requirements for an *in vivo* systemic administration of siRNAs [95]. It needs to have the capability of protecting the siRNA from serum nucleases while effectively delivering it to the target cells. Not to mention, the delivery strategy should enable siRNA to leave the endosome and get to the RNAi apparatus, activating the RNAi pathways [96, 97]. Exosomes, RNA microsponges, oligonucleotide nanoparticles, and red blood cells are some of the siRNA delivery technologies currently being used for the treatment of cancer. Other methods include chemical modification, polymer-mediated delivery systems, conjugate delivery systems, lipid-based nanocarriers, as well as extracellular vehicle (EV) nanocarriers [98].

7.8 NANOCARRIERS UTILIZING LIPID-BASED SIRNA DELIVERY FOR THE TREATMENT OF CANCER

In the pursuit of advancing cancer therapeutics, the convergence of nanotechnology and RNA interference (RNAi) has given rise to innovative strategies, notably the use of lipid-based nanocarriers for delivering small interfering RNA (siRNA). This synergistic approach holds immense potential for revolutionizing cancer treatment by harnessing the precision of siRNA-mediated gene silencing and the versatile delivery capabilities of lipid-based nanocarriers [99]. This explores the intricate interplay of these components, shedding light on their collaborative role in shaping the landscape of cancer therapy. Employing cationic lipid formulations like Lipofectamine 2000 as well as Lipofectamine RNAimax *in vitro*, siRNA transfection efficiency can be enhanced by tens of thousands [100]. During liposome transfection, negatively charged nucleic acids electrostatically interact with the positively charged lipids. When they are coupled, lipoplexes [101–103] form on their own. Because all biological membranes have a negative surface charge, electronegative or neutral liposomes have greater biocompatibility and exhibit better pharmacokinetics compared to cationic liposomes. It has been demonstrated that the neutral lipid DOPC (1,2-dioleoylsn-glycero-3-phosphatidylcholine) improves the effectiveness of siRNA entrapment. In an orthotopic ovarian cancer model, Landen *et al.*'s DOPC-encapsulated siRNA liposome that targets EphA2 was very effective at reducing EphA2 expression 48 hours after therapy [104]. At the M.D. Anderson Cancer Center, a DOPC-encapsulated siRNA liposome (siRNA-EphA2-DOPC) is being tested in ongoing phase I clinical investigations. Cationic liposomes continue to be the best choice because neutral or electronegative liposomes are difficult for cells to absorb. For instance, cationic liposomes are created using the lipid dioleoyl-phosphatidylethanolamine (DOTAP) when the siRNA is negatively charged [105].

In a mouse sepsis model, liposomes containing cationic DOTAP were used for delivering siTNF- and lessening the lethal response to injection of lipopolysaccharide [106]. To try to maintain a total positive charge on the surface for adsorption via the membrane of the cell and minimize the potential clearance created by a positive charge, the ratio of nitrogen to phosphate (N/P) typically ranges between 2 and 3. By coating liposomes, the lipid-anchored PEG may decrease particle size, [107] stop aggregation during storage, [108] elevate circulatory half-life, and [109] block absorption by RES, red blood cells, as well as macrophages. PEG is however occasionally a good option since its steric as well as charge effects secure the liposomes from leaving the endosomes. Numerous investigations are conducted to improve the effectiveness of PEGylated nanoparticles, involving the addition of connections sensitive to pH connecting PEG to the liposome. It has been proven that pH-sensitive PEG enhanced with ionic contacts, like the HEMA-modified PEG liposome, is especially effective at modifying PEG length as well as density. At neutral pH, the copolymer of PEG carries a net negative charge while the DOPE as well as cholesterol inside the liposomal central core possess a net positive charge. The protonation of PEG by endosomal protonation of imidazole as well as methacrylic acid residues outcomes in PEG release along with positively charged liposomal membrane exposure. The liposome is then successfully able to interact with the endosome along with escape [108]. Atu027, a lipoplexed siRNA drug, has been used to treat lymph node metastases in animal models of prostate, pancreatic, as well as various types of lung metastasis [109]. Silence Therapeutics (located in London, UK) evaluated Atu027 in phase I research. According to preliminary findings [110], Atu027 was well tolerated up to a dosage of 0.18 mg/kg and did not have any negative effects. The most well-known type of lipid-based nanocarrier for clinical investigations is the SNALP (stable nucleic acid-lipid particle). They are lipid nanoparticles that deliver siRNA to the cells for which they are designed. The diameter of SNALPs is about 120 nm. They have assisted in the *in vivo* administration of therapeutic siRNAs to animals.

A lipid bilayer made up of conjugation of cationic as well as fusogenic lipids and enveloped with diffusible polyethylene glycol is a component of SNALPs [111]. SNALPs are highly accessible due to EPR-mediated extended blood circulation duration, which leads to a buildup of SNALPs at vascular leakage sites, particularly cancer development sites. siRNA is delivered into cancer cells by SNALPs once they have been accumulated in cancer cells. The hepatitis B virus, dyslipidemia, and Ebola (Zaire) have all been treated using SNALPs [112]. The extent of the subcutaneous tumors was reduced by 75% with SNALP-siPlk1 therapy [113]. 2010 saw the first trials of Plk1-targeting siRNA encapsulated by SNALP (TKM080301) in adult-age patients having solid tumors and lymphomas. Alnylam Pharmaceuticals formulated a dual-targeted siRNA drug ALNVSP02, a SNALP-formulated siRNA targeting VEGF as well as KSP. Phase I research for the management of advanced liver cancer was started in April of the year 2009. In the initial six-dose cohorts, it was depicted that ALNVSP02 was typically tolerated well at the highest permissible dosage of 1.25 mg/kg [114]. It has been demonstrated that siRNA may be effectively delivered by lipid-like lipidoid nanoparticles (LNPs) made of cholesterol as well as PEG-modified lipids [110]. Akinc and coworkers, who developed a unique chemical technique for quickly synthesizing a large library of lipidoids [115], significantly enhanced SNALP-mediated transport. One of the highly potent lipidoid drugs was 98N12-5 lipidoid-based siRNA formulation, which lowered ApoB or FVII factor expression in hepatocytes in non-human primate plus mouse models by 75–90% [116]. In non-human primates, the therapeutic value of RNAi-mediated gene silencing is being demonstrated. That innovative new class of siRNA NCs, which relies on the cationic lipids of tumor cells, is still a long way from being approved for use in clinical trials and commercialization. Lipid-based siRNA NCs possess the capacity to be toxic and to immediately elicit an immune response [117].

7.9 CONCLUSION

The issues with siRNA-based NC distribution *in vivo* have been addressed by using polymers, small molecules, peptides, antibodies, lipids, aptamers, exosomes, and red blood cells, among other things. High-throughput screens have been used to rationally design several successful preclinical systems. Recently, Patisiran was approved for usage following a lengthy clinical investigation. That is an encouraging development. A few more siRNA-based medications are awaiting approval shortly in the pipeline. siRNA clinical trials have taken longer than expected to develop. Many years have been devoted to developing nanoparticles that can protect siRNAs from destruction as they travel through the circulation to their intended target organ. The ability of siRNA to amplify itself in the cell has been shown. An escape rate of 0.1% may be enough. Once siRNAs have entered the cells, patients might have to take them every 6 months or longer to maintain their condition. It is necessary to develop new techniques for making NCs with predictable and controllable biological characteristics. It is conceivable to develop NC delivery methods that help cancer drugs get beyond the endosome-lysosome barrier. By combining stimuli-responsive NC elements with the relevant components, it is possible to prevent the untimely release of systems that deliver into endosomal-lysosomal compartments. Patients with solid tumors, hematological malignancies, and cancers that have spread are predicted to benefit from the use of these techniques. Exogenous cells or the exosome-regulated delivery of nanocarriers is one method of delivering siRNA treatments to tumors. Because there are significant differences between preclinical as well as clinical requirements for drug development, it is challenging for siRNA therapies to reach the clinic. The rate of success of siRNA drugs when used to treat cancer will most likely increase if concurrent preclinical evaluation of siRNA-based drugs, good laboratory practice (GLP) consideration, a decrease of the variance between *in vitro* results as well as *in vivo* outcomes, and consideration for clinical acceptance standards in drug products are all taken into account.

REFERENCES

1. Tian Z, Liang G, Cui K, Liang Y, Wang Q, Lv S, Cheng X, Zhang L. Insight into the prospects for RNAi therapy of cancer. Front Pharmacol. 2021 Mar 16;12:644718.
2. Lee EY, Muller WJ. Oncogenes and tumor suppressor genes. *Cold Spring Harb Perspect Biol.* 2010 Oct;2(10):a003236.
3. McLeod HL. Cancer pharmacogenomics: early promise, but concerted effort needed. *Science.* 2013;339:1563–66.
4. Suva ML, Riggi N, Bernstein BE. Epigenetic reprogramming in cancer. *Science.* 2013; 339:1567–70.

5. Farooqi AA, Rehman ZU, Muntane J. Antisense therapeutics in oncology: current status. *OncoTargets Ther*. 2014 Nov 3;7:2035–42.
6. Walther W, Schlag PM. Current status of gene therapy for cancer. *Curr Opin Oncol*. 2013;25:659–64.
7. Bora RS, Gupta D, Mukkur TK, Saini KS. RNA interference therapeutics for cancer: challenges and opportunities. Mol *Med Rep*. 2012;6:9–15.
8. Gitlin L, Karelsky S, Andino R. Short interfering RNA confers intracellular antiviral immunity in human cells. *Nature*. 2002 Jul 25;418(6896):430–4.
9. Davis SS. Biomedical applications of nanotechnology—implications for drug targeting and gene therapy. *Trends Biotechnol*. 1997;15(6): 217–24.
10. Tatiparti K, Sau S, Kashaw SK, Iyer AK. siRNA delivery strategies: a comprehensive review of recent development. *Nanomaterials*. 2017;7:77.
11. Castanotto D, Rossi JJ. The promises and pitfalls of RNA-interference-based therapeutics. *Nature*. 2009;457:426–33.
12. Ipsaro JJ, Joshua-Tor L. From guide to target: molecular insights into eukaryotic RNA-interference machinery. *Nat Struct Mol Biol*. 2015 Jan;22(1):20–8.
13. Martinez J, Patkaniowska A, Urlaub H, Lührmann R, Tuschl T. Single-stranded antisense siRNAs guide target RNA cleavage in RNAi. *Cell*. 2002;110:563–74.
14. Meister G, Tuschl T. Mechanisms of gene silencing by double-stranded RNA. *Nature*. 2004;431:343–49.
15. Gao H, Cheng R, A. Santos H. Nanoparticle-mediated siRNA delivery systems for cancer therapy. *View*. 2021 Jun;2(3):20200111.
16. Ahmadzada T, Reid G, McKenzie DR. Fundamentals of siRNA and miRNA therapeutics a review of targeted nanoparticle delivery systems in breast cancer. *Biophys Rev*. 2018;10:69–86.
17. Deepthi A, Raju S, Kalyani A, Udaya KM, Vanaja A. Targeted drug delivery to the nucleus and its potential role in cancer chemotherapy. *J Pharm Sci Res*. 2013;5(2):48–56.
18. Wagstaff KM, Jans DA. Protein transduction: cell-penetrating peptides and their therapeutic applications. *Curr Med Chem*. 2006;13:1371–87.
19. Ohkuma S, Poole B. Fluorescence probe measurement of the intralysosomal pH in living cells and the perturbation of pH by various agents. *Proc Natl Acad Sci*. 1978;75: 3327–31.
20. Gavrilov K, Saltzman WM. Therapeutic siRNA: principles, challenges, and strategies. *Yale J Biol Med*. 2012 Jun;85(2):187.
21. Alexis F, Pridgen E, Molnar LK, et al. Factors affecting the clearance and biodistribution of polymeric nanoparticles. *Mol Pharm*. 2008;5:505–15.
22. Layzer JM, McCaffrey AP, Tanner AK, et al. In vivo activity of nuclease-resistant siRNAs. *RNA*. 2004;10: 766–71.
23. Van de Water FM, Boerman OC, Wouterse AC, et al. Intravenously administered short interfering RNA accumulates in the kidney and selectively suppresses gene function in renal proximal tubules. *Drug Metab Dispos*. 2006;34:1393–7.
24. Fleming BD, Mosser DM. Regulatory macrophages: setting the threshold for therapy. *Eur J Immunol*. 2011 Sep;41(9):2498–502.
25. Larson SD, Jackson LN, Chen LA, et al. Effectiveness of siRNA uptake in target tissues by various delivery methods. *Surgery*. 2007;142:262–9.
26. Jackson AL, Linsley PS. Recognizing and avoiding siRNA off-target effects for target identification and therapeutic application. *Nat Rev Drug Discov*. 2010;9:57e67.
27. Kern F, Krammes L, Danz K, Diener C, Kehl T, Küchler O, Fehlmann T, Kahraman M, Rheinheimer S, Aparicio-Puerta E, Wagner S. Validation of human microRNA target pathways enables evaluation of target prediction tools. *Nucleic Acids Res*. 2021 Jan 11;49(1):127–44.
28. Hornung V, Guenthner-Biller M, Bourquin C, et al. Sequence-specific potent induction of IFN-a by short interfering RNA in plasmacytoid dendritic cells through TLR7. *Nat Med*. 2005;11:263–70.
29. Judge AD, Sood V, Shaw JR, et al. Sequence-dependent stimulation of the mammalian innate immune response by synthetic siRNA. *Nat Biotechnol*. 2005;23:457–62.
30. Kariko K, Bhuyan P, Capodici J, et al. Small interfering RNAs mediate sequence-independent gene suppression and induce immune activation by signaling through toll-like receptor 3. *J Immunol*. 2004;172: 6545–9.
31. Marques JT, Williams BR. Activation of the mammalian immune system by siRNAs. *Nat Biotechnol*. 2005;23:1399–405.

32. Tanji H, Ohto U, Shibata T, Taoka M, Yamauchi Y, Isobe T, Miyake K, Shimizu T. Toll-like receptor 8 senses degradation products of single-stranded RNA. *Nat Struct Mol Biol*. 2015 Feb;22(2):109–15.
33. Iwasaki A, Medzhitov R. Toll-like receptor control of the adaptive immune responses. *Nat Immunol*. 2004;5:987–95.
34. Rajendran L, Knolker HJ, Simons K. Subcellular targeting strategies for drug design and delivery. *Nat Rev Drug Discov*. 2010; 9(1):29–42.
35. Burrow SM, Phoenix DA, Wainwright M, Tobin MJ. Intracellular localization studies of doxorubicin and Victoria Blue BO in EMT6-S and EMT6-R cells using confocal microscopy. *Cytotechnology*. 2002;39(1):15–25.
36. Duvvuri M, Krise JP. Intracellular drug sequestration events associated with the emergence of multidrug resistance: a mechanistic review. *Front Biosci*. 2005;10:1499–509.
37. Drozdov AS, Nikitin PI, Rozenberg JM. A systematic review of cancer targeting by nanoparticles revealed a global association between accumulation in tumors and the spleen. *Int J Mol Sci*. 2021 Dec 1;22(23):13011.
38. Li N, Yang H, Yu Z, Li Y, Pan W, Wang H, Tang B. Nuclear-targeted siRNA delivery for long-term gene silencing. *Chem Sci*. 2017;8:2816.
39. Kanasty R, Dorkin JR, Vegas A, Anderson D. Delivery materials for siRNA therapeutics. *Nat Mater*. 2013 Nov;12(11):967–77.
40. Deleavey GF, Damha MJ. Designing chemically modified oligonucleotides for targeted gene silencing. *Chem Biol*. 2012;19:937–54.
41. Wang AZ, Langer R, Farokhzad OC. Nanoparticle delivery of cancer drugs. *Annu Rev Med*. 2012;63:185–98.
42. Malek A, Merkel O, Fink L, et al. In vivo pharmacokinetics, tissue distribution, and underlying mechanisms of various PEI (-PEG)/siRNA complexes. *Toxicol Appl Toxicol*. 2009;236:97–108.
43. Wolfrum C, Shi S, Jayaprakash KN, et al. Mechanisms and optimization of in vivo delivery of lipophilic siRNAs. *Nat Biotechnol*. 2007;25:1149–57.
44. Kim M, Jeong M, Hur S, Cho Y, Park J, Jung H, Seo Y, Woo HA, Nam KT, Lee K, Lee H. Engineered ionizable lipid nanoparticles for targeted delivery of RNA therapeutics into different types of cells in the liver. *Sci Adv*. 2021 Feb 26;7(9):eabf4398.
45. Romberg B, Hennink WE, Storm G. Sheddable coatings for long-circulating nanoparticles. *Pharm Res*. 2008;25:55–71.
46. Bazile D, Prud'homme C, Bassoullet MT, et al. Stealth Me. PEG-PLA nanoparticles avoid uptake by the mononuclear phagocyte system. *J Pharm Sci*. 1995;84:493–8.
47. Martina MS, Nicolas V, Wilhelm C, et al. The in vitro kinetics of the interactions between PEG-ylated magnetic-fluid loaded liposomes and macrophages. *Biomaterials*. 2007;28:4143–53.
48. Schlöndorff D, Wyatt CM, Campbell KN. Revisiting the determinants of the glomerular filtration barrier: what goes round must come round. *Kidney Int*. 2017 Sep 1;92(3):533–6.
49. Wartiovaara J, Ofverstedt LG, Khoshnoodi J, Nephrin strands contribute to a porous slit diaphragm scaffold as revealed by electron tomography. *J Clin Invest*. 2004;114:1475–83.
50. Rappaport J, Hanss B, Kopp JB, et al. Transport of phosphorothioate oligonucleotides in the kidney: implications for molecular therapy. *Kidney Int*. 1995;47:1462–69.
51. Lee H, Lytton-Jean AKR, Chen Y, et al. Molecularly self-assembled nucleic acid nanoparticles for targeted in vivo siRNA delivery. *Nat Nanotechnol*. 2012;7: 389–93.
52. Rozema DB, Lewis DL, Wakefield DH, et al. Dynamic PolyConjugates for targeted in vivo delivery of siRNA to hepatocytes. *Proc Natl Acad Sci*. 2007;104:12982–7.
53. Edis Z, Wang J, Waqas MK, Ijaz M, Ijaz M. Nanocarriers-mediated drug delivery systems for anticancer agents: an overview and perspectives. *Int J Nanomed*. 2021 Feb 17;16:1313–30.
54. Yu B, Zhao X, Lee LJ, et al. Targeted delivery systems for oligonucleotide therapeutics. *AAPS J*. 2009;11:195–203.
55. Salvati A, Pitek AS, Monopoli MP, et al. Transferrin-functionalized nanoparticles lose their targeting capabilities when a biomolecule corona adsorbs on the surface. *Nat Nanotechnol*. 2013;8:137–43.
56. Bolhassani A. Potential efficacy of cell-penetrating peptides for nucleic acid and drug delivery in cancer. *Biochim Biophys Acta-Rev Cancer*. 2011;1816:232–46.

57. Ulkoski D, Bak A, Wilson JT, Krishnamurthy VR. Recent advances in polymeric materials for the delivery of RNA therapeutics. *Expert Opin Drug Deliv.* 2019 Nov 2;16(11):1149–67.
58. Barquinero J, Eixarch H, Perez-Melgosa M. Retroviral vectors: new applications for an old tool. *Gene Ther.* 2004;11:S3–9.
59. Vandenbroucke RE, De Geest BG, Bonn_e S, et al. Prolonged gene silencing in hepatoma cells and primary hepatocytes after small interfering RNA delivery with biodegradable poly (b-amino esters). *J Gene Med.* 2008;10:783–94.
60. Elvin B, Haifa S, Mauro F. Principles of nanoparticle design for overcoming biological barriers to drug delivery. *Nat Biotechnol.* 2015;33(9):941–51.
61. Nazanin H, Samantha G, Hongbin H, Gang B. The effect of nanoparticle size on in vivo pharmacokinetics and cellular interaction. *Nanomedicine (Lond.).* 2016;11(6):673–92.
62. Ryu YC, Kim KA, Kim BC, Wang HM, Hwang BH. Novel fusion peptide-mediated siRNA delivery using self-assembled nanocomplex. *J Nanobiotechnol.* 2021 Dec;19(1):1–8.
63. Wang K, Kievit FM, Zhang M. Nanoparticles for cancer gene therapy: recent advances, challenges, and strategies. *Pharmacol Res.* 2016;114:56–66.
64. Jing H, Cheng W, Li S, Wu B, Leng X, Xu S, et al. Novel cell-penetrating peptide-loaded nanobubbles synergized with ultrasound irradiation enhance EGFR siRNA delivery for triple-negative breast cancer therapy. *Colloids Surf B Biointerfaces.* 2016;146:387–95.
65. Rosenblum D, Joshi N, Tao W, Karp JM, Peer D. Progress and challenges towards targeted delivery of cancer therapeutics. *Nat Commun.* 2018;9:1410.
66. Draz MS, Fang BA, Zhang P, Hu Z, Gu S, Weng KC, et al. Nanoparticle-mediated systemic delivery of siRNA for treatment of cancers and viral infections. *Theranostics.* 2014;4(9):872–92.
67. Chen M, Wang L, Wang F, Li F, Xia W, Gu H, Chen Y. Quick synthesis of a novel combinatorial delivery system of siRNA and doxorubicin for a synergistic anticancer effect. *Int J Nanomed.* 2019 May 15;14:3557–69.
68. Govindarajan S, Sivakumar J, Garimidi P, Rangaraj N, Kumar JM, Rao NM, et al. Targeting human epidermal growth factor receptor 2 by a cell-penetrating peptide–affibody bioconjugate. *Biomaterials.* 2012;33(8):2570–82.
69. Ngamcherdtrakul W, Morry J, Gu S, Castro DJ, Goodyear SM, Sangvanich T, et al. Cationic polymer-modified mesoporous silica nanoparticles for targeted siRNA delivery to HER2+ breast cancer. *Adv Funct Mater.* 2015;25(18):2646–59.
70. Shin JH, Shin DH, Kim JS. Let-7 miRNA and CDK4 siRNA co-encapsulated in Herceptin-conjugated liposome for breast cancer stem cells. *Asian J Pharm Sci.* 2020 Jul 1;15(4):472–81.
71. Hirota K, Terada H. Endocytosis of particle formulations by macrophages and its application to clinical treatment. In Ceresa B (ed), *Molecular regulation of endocytosis.* 2012. InTech.
72. Young SWS, Stenzel M, Yang J. Nanoparticle-siRNA: a potential cancer therapy? *Crit Rev Oncol Hematol.* 2016;98:159–69.
73. Li Y, Kröger M, Liu WK. Shape effect in cellular uptake of PEGylated nanoparticles: comparison between sphere, rod, cube, and disk. *Nanoscale.* 2015;7(40):16631–46.
74. He Y, Park K. Effects of the microparticle shape on cellular uptake. *Mol Pharm.* 2016 13(7):2164.
75. Richards DM, Endres RG. Target shape dependence in a simple model of receptor-mediated endocytosis and phagocytosis. *Proc Natl Acad Sci U S A.* 2016;113(22):6113–18.
76. Honary S, Zahir F. Effect of zeta potential on the properties of nano-drug delivery systems—a review (part 2). *Trop J Pharm Res.* 2013;12(2):265–73.
77. Arnold AE, Czupiel P, Shoichet M. Engineered polymeric nanoparticles to guide the cellular internalization and trafficking of small interfering ribonucleic acids. *J Control Release.* 2017;259:3–15.
78. Sun H, Yarovoy I, Capeling M, Cheng C. Polymers in the co-delivery of siRNA and anticancer drugs for the treatment of drug-resistant cancers. *Polymeric Gene Deliv Syst.* 2018;375(2):329–58.
79. Behr JP. The proton sponge: a trick to enter cells the viruses did not exploit. *Chimia.* 1997;51:34–6.
80. Gujrati M, Vaidya A, Lu ZR. Multifunctional pH-sensitive amino lipids for siRNA delivery. *Bioconjug Chem.* 2016;27(1):19–35.
81. Li J, Xue S, Mao Z-W. Nanoparticle delivery systems for siRNA-based therapeutics. *J Mater Chem B.* 2016;4(41):6620–39.
82. Liang W, Lam JKW. Endosomal escape pathways for non-viral nucleic acid delivery systems. In Ceresa B (ed), *Molecular regulation of endocytosis.* 2012. InTech.

83. Mendes LP, Sarisozen C, Luther E, Pan J, Torchilin VP. Surface-engineered polyethyleneimine-modified liposomes as novel carriers of siRNA and chemotherapeutics for combination treatment of drug-resistant cancers. *Drug Deliv*. 2019 Jan 1;26(1):443–58.
84. Prokop A. *Intracellular delivery: fundamentals and applications* (Vol. 5). Springer. 2011: 1–154.
85. Pittella F, Kataoka K. Polymeric micelles for siRNA delivery. In Howard, K. (eds.). *RNA interference from biology to therapeutics*. Advances in Delivery Science and Technology (pp. 161–184). Springer, Boston, MA. 2013. https://doi.org/10.1007/978-1-4614-4744-3_8
86. Alberts B, Johnson A, Lewis J, Raff M, Roberts K, Walter P. Principles of membrane transport. In *Molecular biology of the cell* (4th ed). 2002. Science, New York.
87. Trivedi V, Zhang SC, Castoreno AB, Stockinger W, Shieh EC, Vyas JM, Frickel EM, Nohturfft A. Immunoglobulin G signaling activates lysosome/phagosome docking. *Proc Natl Acad Sci*. 2006 Nov 28;103(48):18226–31.
88. Bulbake U, Doppalapudi S, Kommineni N, Khan W. Liposomal formulations in clinical use: an updated review. *Pharmaceutics* 2017;9(2):12.
89. Finlay J, Roberts CM, Lowe G, Loeza J, Rossi JJ, Glackin CA. RNA-based TWIST1 inhibition via dendrimer complex to reduce breast cancer cell metastasis. *Biomed Res Int*. 2015;2015:382745.
90. Fan W, Wang X, Ding B, Cai H,Wang X, Fan Y, et al.Thioaptamer conjugated CD44-targeted delivery system for the treatment of breast cancer in vitro and in vivo. *J Drug Target*. 2016; 24(4):359–71.
91. Roberts TC, Ezzat K, El Andaloussi S, Weinberg MS. Synthetic siRNA delivery: progress and prospects. In Shum K, Rossi J. (Eds.) *SiRNA delivery methods. Methods in molecular biology* (vol. 1364, pp. 291–310). Humana Press, New York, NY. 2016. https://doi.org/10.1007/978-1-4939-3112-5_23
92. Poteryaev D, Datta S, Ackema K, Zerial M, Spang A. Identification of the switch in early-to-late endosome transition. *Cell*. 2010;141(3):497–508.
93. Colombo M, et al. Tumour homing and therapeutic effect of colloidal nanoparticles depend on the number of attached antibodies. *Nat Commun*. 2016;7:13818.
94. Dong Y, Siegwart DJ, Anderson DG. Strategies, design, and chemistry in siRNA delivery systems. Adv Drug Deliv Rev. 2019 Apr 1;144:133–47.
95. Sajid MI, Moazzam M, Kato S, Yeseom Cho K, Tiwari RK. Overcoming barriers for siRNA therapeutics: from bench to bedside. *Pharmaceuticals*. 2020 Oct 7;13(10):294.
96. Kanasty R, Dorkin JR, Vegas A, et al. Delivery materials for siRNA therapeutics. *Nat Mater*. 2013;12:967–77.
97. Juliano RL. The delivery of therapeutic oligonucleotides. *Nucleic Acids Res*. 2016 Aug 19;44(14):6518–48.
98. Subhan MA, Torchilin VP. Efficient nanocarriers of siRNA therapeutics for cancer treatment. *Transl Res*. 2019 Dec 1;214:62–91.
99. Ebrahimi N, Manavi MS, Nazari A, Momayezi A, Faghihkhorasani F, Abdulwahid AH, Rezaei-Tazangi F, Kavei M, Rezaei R, Mobarak H, Aref AR. Nano-scale delivery systems for siRNA delivery in cancer therapy: new era of gene therapy empowered by nanotechnology. *Environ Res*. 2023 Oct 4;239(Pt 2):117263.
100. Santel A, Aleku M, Keil O, et al. A novel siRNA-lipoplex technology for RNA interference in the mouse vascular endothelium. *Gene Ther*. 2006;1:1222–34.
101. Hayes ME, Drummond DC, Hong K, et al. Assembly of nucleic acid-lipid nanoparticles from aqueous-organic monophases. *Biochim Biophys Acta Biomembr*. 2006;1758:429–442.
102. Khoury M, Louis-Plence P, Escriou V, et al. Efficient new cationic liposome formulation for systemic delivery of small interfering RNA silencing tumor necrosis factor-a in experimental arthritis. *Arthritis Rheum* 2006;54:1867–77.
103. Zuhorn IS, Oberle V, Visser WH, et al. Phase behavior of cationic amphiphiles and their mixtures with helper lipids influences lipoplex shape, DNA translocation, and transfection efficiency. *Biophys J*. 2002;83:2096–108.
104. Wagner MJ, Mitra R, McArthur MJ, Baze W, Barnhart K, Wu SY, Rodriguez-Aguayo C, Zhang X, Coleman RL, Lopez-Berestein G, Sood AK. Preclinical mammalian safety studies of EPHARNA (DOPC nanoliposomal EphA2-targeted siRNA). *Mol Cancer Ther*. 2017 Jun 1;16(6):1114–23.
105. Wu SY, McMillan NA. Lipidic systems for in vivo siRNA delivery. *AAPS J*. 2009;11:639–52.

106. Sørensen DR, Leirdal M, Sioud M. Gene silencing by systemic delivery of synthetic siRNAs in adult mice. *J Mol Biol.* 2003;327:761–66.
107. Bao Y, Jin Y, Chivukula P, et al. Effect of PEGylation on biodistribution and gene silencing of siRNA/lipid nanoparticle complexes. *Pharm Res.* 2013;30:342–51.
108. Lin SY, Zhao WY, Tsai HC, et al. Sterically polymer-based liposomal complexes with dual-shell structure for enhancing the siRNA delivery. *Biomacromolecules.* 2012;13:664–75.
109. Schultheis B, Stromberg D, Santel A, Vank C, Gebhardt F, Keil O, Lange C, Giese K, Kaufmann J, Khan M, Drevs J. First-in-human phase I study of the liposomal RNA interference therapeutic Atu027 in patients with advanced solid tumors. *J Clin Oncol.* 2014 Dec 20;32(36):4141–8.
110. Strumberg D, Schultheis B, Traugott U, et al. Phase I clinical development of Atu027, a siRNA formulation targeting PKN3 in patients with advanced solid tumors. *Int J Clin Pharmacol Ther.* 2012;50:76.
111. Morrissey DV, Lockridge JA, Shaw L, et al. Potent and persistent in vivo anti-HBV activity of chemically modified siRNAs. *Nat Biotechnol.* 2005;23:1002–7.
112. Dong Y, Siegwart DJ, Anderson DG. Strategies, design, and chemistry in siRNA delivery systems. *Adv Drug Deliv Rev.* 2019 Apr 1;144:133–47.
113. Judge AD, Robbins M, Tavakoli I, et al. Confirming the RNA-mediated mechanism of action of siRNA-based cancer therapeutics in mice. *J Clin Invest.* 2009;119:661.
114. Yadav DN, Ali MS, Thanekar AM, Pogu SV, Rengan AK. Recent advancements in the design of nano delivery systems of siRNA for cancer therapy. *Mol Pharm.* 2022 Nov 21;19(12):4506–26.
115. Akinc A, Zumbuehl A, Goldberg M, et al. A combinatorial library of lipid-like materials for delivery of RNAi therapeutics. *Nat Biotechnol.* 2008;26: 561–69.
116. Gupta N, Rai DB, Jangid AK, Pooja D, Kulhari H. Nanomaterials-based siRNA delivery: routes of administration, hurdles and role of nanocarriers. In Singh, S., Maurya, P. (Eds.). *Nanotechnology in modern animal biotechnology,* (pp. 67–114). Springer, Singapore. 2019. https://doi.org/10.1007/978-981-13-6004-6_3.
117. Shajari N, Mansoori B, Davudian S, Mohammadi A, Baradaran B. Overcoming the challenges of siRNA delivery: nanoparticle strategies. Curr Drug Deliv. 2017 Feb 1;14(1):36–46.

8 Boosting Nanomedicine Efficacy with Hyperbaric Oxygen Therapy

8.1 INTRODUCTION

Nanomedicine is an interdisciplinary field that involves the application of nanotechnology in medicine, aiming to diagnose, treat, and prevent diseases at the molecular and cellular levels. Hyperbaric oxygen therapy (HBOT) is a medical treatment that involves breathing pure oxygen in a pressurized room or chamber, and it has been traditionally used for conditions like decompression sickness and chronic non-healing wounds. The intersection of nanomedicine and hyperbaric oxygen therapy presents an intriguing avenue for enhancing the efficacy of therapeutic interventions. Treatment with hyperbaric oxygen therapy necessitates subjecting patients to elevated atmospheric pressure and 100% oxygen concentrations. That pressure may be more than or equivalent to 1.4 atmospheres (atm) [1], as stated by the Undersea as well as Hyperbaric Medical Society (UHMS). However, for all currently accepted UHMS purposes, patients must be isolated in a pressured chamber of at least 2 ATA [2] and breathe near 100% oxygen.

In 1662, a British doctor named Henshaw used pressured air to treat patients, marking the first time such treatment had been used. Interestingly, it was performed nearly a century before John Priestly discovered oxygen and the Boyle-Mariotte law was developed to define the connection between the pressure as well as the volume of gas [3]. The subsequent route of HBOT in medical treatment was slowed by Lavoisier and Seguin's 1789 finding of potential O_2-derived deleterious effects at 100% concentrations. The "father of hyperbaric physiology," Paul Bert, first documented the physiological underpinnings of pressurized air inside the human body in 1872. He also identified the neurotoxic effects of oxygen in the human body, leading to the Paul Bert effect [4, 5]. Lorrain Smith then went on to describe the lung toxicity of oxygen. At the same time, it was asserted that the implementation of HBOT to the curing of decompression sickness in World War II divers was beneficial [6]. Since then, there have been several studies, and by the turn of the millennium, hundreds of HBOT-based clinics were constructed [7].

There are now 14 authorized uses for HBOT, covering a broad range of medical conditions from air embolism and severe anemia to viral infections and idiopathic sensory hearing loss. Additionally, the most current European Consensus Conference on Hyperbaric Medicine highlighted the use of HBOT as a primary method of treatment for some conditions with moderate to greater evidence (such as after carbon monoxide (CO) poisoning) as well as an alternate adjuvant to take into account in other circumstances with considerable amount of scientific evidence (such as diabetic foot) [8–10].

DOI: 10.1201/9781003451020-8

8.2 THE SIGNIFICANCE OF OXYGEN IN BIOLOGICAL ECOSYSTEMS

Oxygen holds paramount significance in biological ecosystems, serving as a fundamental element that underpins various essential processes. At the cellular level, oxygen is a linchpin of aerobic respiration, acting as the final electron acceptor in the electron transport chain and facilitating the production of ATP, the energy currency of cells. This process is vital for the metabolism of organic molecules, supporting the growth and development of organisms. Not only is oxygen crucial for the respiration of aerobic organisms, but it also plays a pivotal role in photosynthesis, where plants and certain microorganisms produce oxygen as a byproduct. Because it must be inhaled into the body rather than ingested, like all other nutrients [9], oxygen (O_2) is often overlooked. When it comes to the mitochondrial process known as "aerobic respiration," which is essential for human cell survival, oxygen is king. Here, oxidative phosphorylation, which ultimately leads to the creation of ATP, uses oxygen as an electron acceptor. Archaea and eubacteria, which need prokaryotic cells to breathe oxygen, formed an endosymbiotic relationship with an organism that could not breathe oxygen [10]. Since complex creatures evolved alongside O_2, it has become a critical ingredient for human cells [11], giving them an adaptive edge over cells that are unable to use it.

To deliver oxygen to the body, two independent processes—ventilation (where gases are transported via the environment to the bronchial tree) as well as diffusion (where an equilibrium is reached in the dispersion of O_2 amongst the alveolar space and the blood)—cooperate. Since there is a high concentration of carbon dioxide (CO_2) and a low partial pressure of oxygen (PO_2), gas exchange occurs in the region [12]. Since air pressure does not change, the oxygen flow is dependent on the volume and pressure differences between the chest wall and lungs [13]. Once oxygen enters the circulatory system, it is carried throughout the body in two forms: first, binding to hemoglobin (Hb) into the erythrocytes, and second, in a slightly dissolved form. The varying partial pressure of O_2 as well as the Hb oxygen saturation (SO_2), which is also reliant on other factors like temperature, PCO_2, alongside pH, among various others, lead to the generation of oxygen exchange among the microcirculatory vessels (which include not only the capillaries, but also arterioles as well as venules) and the other tissues which are left [14]. However, hypoxia, which occurs when tissues do not get enough oxygen, may show up. The low levels of oxygen inside the blood (Hypoxemia) might be the result of difficulty with ventilation, perfusion, or gas diffusion through the hemato-alveolar membrane. Tissue hypoxia may also result from insufficient blood flow (ischemia) or impaired oxygen delivery [15]. That is why cells have sensors called hypoxia-inducible factors (HIF) that, when exposed to low oxygen levels, bind to the hypoxia response element (HRE) and turn on a broad range of cellular functions [16]. On rare occasions, hypoxia may have beneficial effects on health, such as at early stages of development [17] or with intermittent exposures [18]. However, hypoxia often induces pathogenic stress for cells, which is linked to the onset as well as the progression of a wide range of disorders [19]. Therefore, oxygen has been considered a possible treatment agent for individuals enduring various acute or persistent/chronic diseases [20, 21]. Clinical therapy of hypoxia focuses on adjusting global hypoxemia and oxygen supply to tissues [22], while addressing cellular hypoxia is a potential but still developing strategy [23]. Because it raises oxygen levels inside the blood and tissues, hyperbaric oxygen therapy is a remarkable aid in dealing with hypoxia and associated problems [24]. Below, we will discuss the therapeutic foundations and unique aspects of HBOT, outlining the concepts and processes that underpin its effectiveness.

8.3 AN OVERVIEW OF HYPERBARIC OXYGEN THERAPY: RATIONALES FOR THERAPEUTICS

Hyperbaric oxygen therapy is a medical treatment that involves breathing pure oxygen in a pressurized room or chamber. The therapy is based on the principle that increasing the pressure around a patient allows their body to absorb a higher concentration of oxygen, leading to various therapeutic benefits.

The rationale for hyperbaric oxygen therapy is rooted in its ability to enhance oxygen delivery to tissues, influencing a range of physiological processes. One primary rationale for HBOT is its role in promoting wound healing and tissue repair. Elevated levels of oxygen under increased pressure stimulate angiogenesis, the formation of new blood vessels, which enhances the supply of oxygen and nutrients to damaged tissues. This is particularly beneficial for chronic wounds, non-healing ulcers, and conditions where compromised blood flow hampers the healing process. As was said up top, hyperbaric oxygen therapy involves supplying the patient with oxygen while also increasing the pressure. If just one patient is receiving the surgery or several patients, the chamber used will be either monoplane or multiple. When using compressed oxygen, the chambers are filled with the gas, whereas when using supplemental oxygen, patients breathe the gas in via a hood, face mask, or endotracheal tube [25]. Multiplace chambers appear to offer a superior examination of the necessary functions in instances of severely ill patients, even though monoplace chambers are similarly safe and well-accepted by patients [26, 27]. Estimated session lengths range from 1.5 to 2 hours, with administration occurring once to three times a day at dosages ranging from 20 to 60 therapeutic units per condition [28]. Two to three atmospheres of pressure are often used in the procedure. However, good outcomes have been found in several studies from 1.5 ATA (less than 2 ATA) for some circumstances [29, 30], even though all UHMS presently authorized indications call for a chamber pressured to at least 2 ATA [2]. Even though 6 atm are acceptable in specific procedures (for example, gas embolism therapy), little benefit is often observed from >3 atms since it may be linked with a variety of side consequences [31]. Furthermore, at pressures greater than 2.8 atm, additional gases such as helium, nitrogen, and ozone make it unsafe to breathe pure O_2. Alternatively, norm baric oxygen treatment (NBOT) uses oxygen at a pressure of 1 atmosphere. Since hyperbaric chambers are not required for NBOT, it is more affordable, less complicated to implement, and available at almost any hospital [32]. However, certain studies have shown that NBOT is not as effective as HBOT [33, 34], demonstrating the need for HBOT for specific situations. However, in cases when patients are unable to use HBOT due to a lack of available facilities, NBOT may be of vital importance.

There are three basic reasons why hyperbaric oxygen therapy works: according to the Boyle-Mariotte law as well as Henry's law, it lessens the size of bubbles of gas inside the blood [6]. Breathing 100% oxygen creates a positive gradient, favoring diffusion from the hyperoxic lungs to the hypoxic tissues. In other words, without the help of Hb, the supply of oxygen to blood (hyperoxemia) as well as tissues (hyperoxia) may be greatly increased by creating a hyperbaric atmosphere with pure oxygen [35]. Multiple pathological processes, such as wound healing, necrosis, or reperfusion injuries, may benefit from HBOT's usage in therapeutic therapy [36].

Hyperoxia is something to which humans have not adapted in the same way as hypoxia. Many of the mediators and cellular processes generated by hypoxia are also shared by exposure to intermittent hyperoxia. The hyperoxia–hypoxia paradox [37] describes the situation. It is important to note that it need not be seen as a defect. Short-term hyperoxia exposure, like the intermittent hypoxia that occurs naturally, may have beneficial effects on the cell. Hormesis, a fundamental concept in biology, is explained by establishing a relationship between the nature of the reaction and the magnitude of the administered dosage [38]. From a molecular standpoint, increased formation of reactive oxygen species (ROS) plus reactive nitrogen species (RNS) due to the large quantity of PO_2 present inside the tissues can have significant repercussions in cell signaling (RNS). These alterations cause a wide range of consequences in the body, involving increased production of growth factors, enhanced neovascularization, and immunomodulatory features [39, 40]. In addition, the ROS/RNS as well as the extracellular regulated kinases (ERK1/ERK2) pathway is responsible for the upregulation of HIF after HBOT [37, 41]. Similarly, DNA damage, oxidative stress, metabolic abnormalities, acute pulmonary injury, endothelial dysfunction, as well as neurotoxicity may all be brought on by hyperoxia's excessive generation of ROS and RNS [42]. Since hyperbaric oxygen therapy has the potential for both therapeutic and detrimental consequences, it is important to weigh

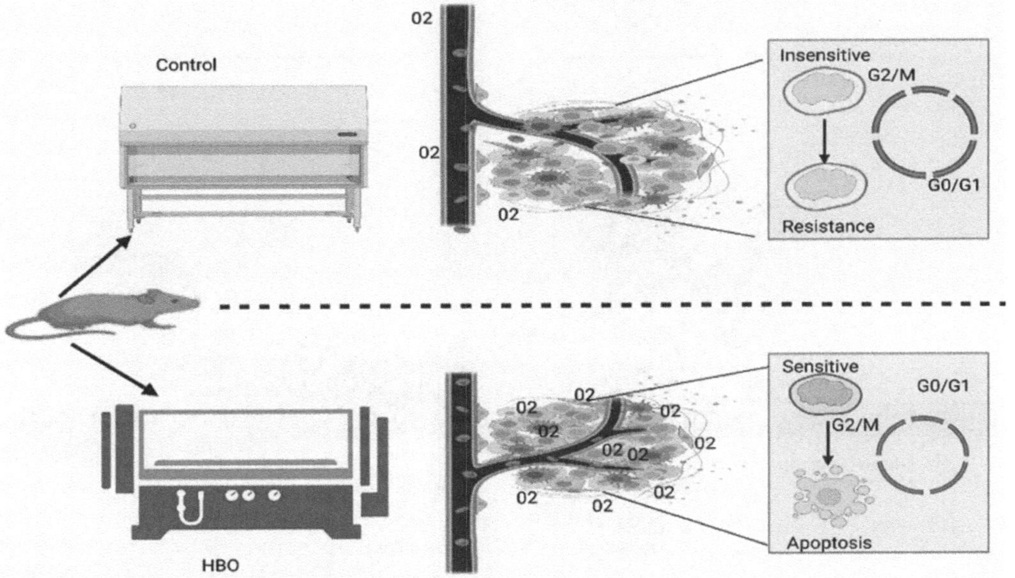

FIGURE 8.1 The figure demonstrates the main effects of pressurized O_2 delivery as well as the configuration and features of hyperbaric chambers.

these possibilities before making a clinical recommendation for or against HBOT [43]. The physical nature of HBOT makes it challenging to perform sufficient research and clinical trials to completely approve its usage. Apart from that, there are prediction models that might be employed in addition to identifying the patients who would benefit from the medication the most, taking into account other therapeutic techniques if required [44]. The main effects of pressurized O_2 delivery as well as the configuration and features of hyperbaric chambers are shown in Figure 8.1.

8.4 COMPARISON OF HBO AND VARIOUS STRATEGIES FOR TUMOR HYPOXIA

Hyperbaric oxygen therapy and various strategies for managing tumor hypoxia represent distinct approaches to addressing the challenges posed by oxygen-deficient microenvironments within solid tumors. HBOT involves exposing individuals to pure oxygen at increased atmospheric pressure, leading to a transient elevation in systemic oxygen levels and improved oxygen delivery to tissues. This approach finds applications in wound healing, decompression sickness, and certain non-cancerous conditions, with emerging exploration in oncology, particularly as an adjunct to radiation therapy. In contrast, alternative strategies, such as hypoxia-activated prodrugs and antiangiogenic agents, are designed specifically for cancer treatment. Hypoxia-activated prodrugs exploit the low oxygen conditions within tumors to selectively release active agents, while antiangiogenic agents aim to normalize tumor blood vessels, enhancing oxygen delivery. In addition to hyperbaric oxygen (HBO) treatment, several methods exist for treating tumor hypoxia. These include increasing intratumor blood flow, oxygen delivery through carriers, tumor-based oxygen production, and decreasing tumor oxygen consumption [45–50]. Here, we will look at these five approaches side by side and discuss the benefits and drawbacks of each. Oxygen carriers like modified hemoglobin (Hb) and perfluorochemicals are the most often employed methods for targeting malignancies with the treatment (PFC). There have been several organizations working on the tactic, and it has been evaluated carefully elsewhere [51]. The oxygen binding regions in the Hb protein or the oxygen

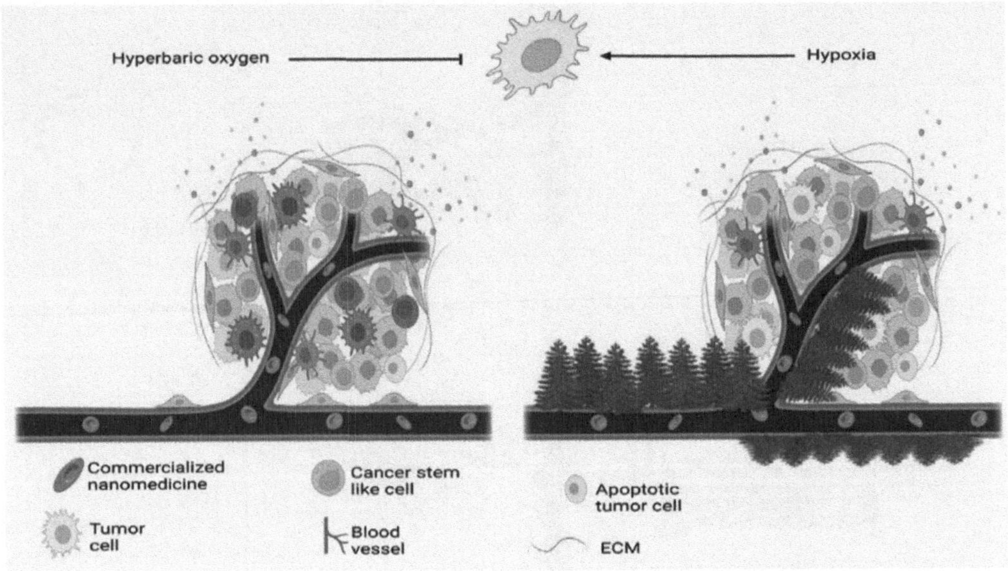

FIGURE 8.2 Cancer cells in hypoxia and hyperbaric oxygen are shown differently in the above diagram.

release to tumor tissue, however, are limitations of that approach. Through the use of pharmacological molecules, photothermal therapy, or enzymes (such as hyaluronidase, and HAase), tumor hypoxia may be alleviated [52]. For instance, Gong *et al.* demonstrated that HAase might degrade hyaluronic acid, the main component of tumor ECM, and enhance the density and effective area of the tumor's blood vessels, increasing the perfusion of the tumor and the therapeutic effect of PDT [53]. The method may boost the efficacy of cancer treatments like radiation and chemotherapy by maximizing the EPR impact of nanomedicine. However, the oxygen-binding capability of Hb in tumor blood arteries makes the method ineffective [54]. Also, the tumor tissue must have adequate quantities of the drug molecules, photothermal agents, and enzymes before treatment can begin.

By catalytically decomposing endogenous H_2O_2 with MnO_2 or catalase, *in situ*, the generation of oxygen inside the tumor is an approach to ameliorate tumor hypoxia (CAT). Let us use the following instance as an illustration. However, the low quantities of H_2O_2 present in tumor cells limit the technique's effectiveness [55].

Tumor hypoxia may also be alleviated by reducing the tumor's oxygen demand. Met-HCe6-liposomes were created by Song *et al.*, and their use enhanced tumor oxygenation by decreasing tumor cell oxygen consumption [56–60]. However, the oxygen level in tumor tissue is not raised by the method. Overall, these approaches have widespread implications for treating hypoxic solid tumors since they can alleviate tumor hypoxia and enhance a wide range of cancer treatments, like photodynamic therapy, chemotherapy, and radiation. Because of its straightforward operation, cheap cost, and many therapeutic uses, HBO offers more benefits than disadvantages, despite its well-documented and manageable side effects and paradoxes [61, 62]. The variance between hyperbaric oxygen as well as hypoxia cancer cells is depicted in Figure 8.2.

8.4.1 Applications of Hyperbaric Oxygen Therapy in the Treatment of Cancer

Hyperbaric oxygen therapy has shown promise in its applications for cancer treatment, particularly as a complementary approach to conventional therapies. One key avenue is its role in enhancing the effectiveness of radiation therapy. By exposing patients to pure oxygen at increased atmospheric pressure, HBOT aims to increase oxygen levels in tumor tissues, potentially sensitizing cancer cells to radiation. This synergy may lead to improved treatment outcomes, especially in cases where tumors exhibit hypoxia. Additionally, HBOT is explored as a postradiation therapy adjunct to support tissue recovery, mitigating the potential long-term side effects of radiation. In specific cancers, such as those affecting the head and neck, where osteoradionecrosis poses a risk, HBOT is considered for its preventive potential. Despite ongoing research and promising results, the use of HBOT in cancer treatment remains an evolving field, and careful consideration, guided by healthcare professionals, is crucial for its integration into comprehensive cancer care plans. At the turn of the twentieth century, researchers started looking at how oxygen may improve the effectiveness of radiotherapy for cancer. For the first time, hypoxia's ability to cause radio resistance and impact radiotherapy's therapeutic efficacy was verified by Gray *et al.* in 1953 [63, 64]. It was shown in 1986 that HBO might make malignancies of the head as well as neck more susceptible to radiation-based treatment. Since that time, researchers and clinicians have come to recognize HBO's potential as an adjunctive treatment for a wide range of cancers.

8.4.2 Application of HBO in Radiation Therapy

Hyperbaric oxygen therapy has demonstrated several applications in the context of radiation therapy, contributing to the overall management of radiation-induced complications and potentially enhancing treatment outcomes. One primary application is in the mitigation of radiation-induced tissue damage and improvement of wound healing. HBOT involves breathing pure oxygen in a pressurized environment, leading to increased oxygen levels in the bloodstream. In radiation therapy, this elevated oxygenation can aid in the recovery of damaged tissues by promoting angiogenesis and supporting the cellular processes crucial for effective wound healing. Radiotherapy is a mainstay of cancer treatment because it destroys cancer cells by irradiating their DNA and causing mutations. A double-strand break in the DNA molecule is only possible when radiation-induced DNA radicals are oxidized in the presence of molecules of oxygen. As a result, tumor cells are much less sensitive to radiation in a hypoxic TME. HBO was first employed for radiosensitization [65], and it has since been shown to be the most efficient approach for treating tissue hypoxia. It has been shown that HBO may have a dual purpose in radiation for cancer. To begin, it has radiation sensitizer applications. Second, it has therapeutic potential for mitigating radiation injury [66]. The curative impact in treating skin cancer as well as bladder cancer is inadequate [67], but HBO has been shown to elevate the therapeutic effectiveness of radiation for head as well as neck malignancies, cervical cancer, plus glioma in a series of clinical studies. It was shown that HBO increased the sensitivity of the patient to radiation when the radiation was administered less often but at a greater dosage [68]. HBOT is often administered before radiotherapy as adjuvant therapy for sensitizing radiotherapy; studies have shown that administering radiation 15 minutes after HBOT improves therapeutic efficacy and reduces collateral damage [69]. As a therapeutic agent, HBO may mitigate the harmful effects of radiation treatment in addition to its role as a radiotherapy sensitizer. Patients with prostate cancer who have had radiation treatment have been observed by Polom *et al.* to benefit greatly from HBO treatment for urinary and digestive system problems [70]. Researchers Craighead *et al.* have investigated the effectiveness of HBO in preventing or treating radiation-related injuries. They revealed that HBO might successfully treat or prevent radiation-related injuries [71]. HBOT is particularly considered in cases where patients develop radiation necrosis, a condition characterized by the death of healthy tissue due to radiation exposure. By providing a higher concentration of oxygen to affected tissues, HBOT may reduce inflammation, promote tissue repair, and alleviate symptoms associated with radiation necrosis, improving the overall quality of life for patients. Additionally, HBOT is explored as a preventive measure against osteoradionecrosis, a potential complication in head and neck cancer patients who undergo radiation therapy. The increased oxygen levels facilitated by HBOT contribute to improved vascularity and tissue oxygenation, reducing the risk of osteoradionecrosis and enhancing the resilience of bone tissues.

8.4.3 Utilizing HBO Therapy in Conjunction with Chemotherapy

The integration of hyperbaric oxygen therapy with chemotherapy represents a promising avenue in the comprehensive treatment of cancer. HBOT, characterized by the administration of pure oxygen at increased atmospheric pressure, holds the potential to address a critical challenge in cancer treatment—tumor hypoxia. By enhancing oxygenation within tumor tissues, HBO therapy may sensitize cancer cells to the effects of chemotherapy, overcoming resistance associated with hypoxic microenvironments. Improved oxygen levels not only optimize the action of certain chemotherapy agents but also contribute to mitigating treatment resistance. Moreover, HBO therapy's supportive role in wound healing and tissue recovery becomes particularly relevant in managing potential side effects of chemotherapy. The combination of HBO therapy and chemotherapy is an evolving strategy, with ongoing research focused on refining protocols, identifying optimal patient populations, and elucidating the underlying mechanisms. Tumor medication resistance and chemotherapy failure were both linked to hypoxia. The ways that hypoxia makes tumor cells resistant to anticancer medications can vary to some extent depending on the exact medications being used, but generally speaking, hypoxia makes tumor cells resistant to medications in the following ways [72]. First off, hypoxia lowers intracellular concentrations of chemotherapeutic agents by elevating the production of therapeutic drugs by the P-Glycoprotein (Pgp), a multidrug resistance protein. Second, hypoxia alters tumor cells' metabolic as well as signaling processes. Finally, hypoxia alters the redox state of tumor cells. Finally, hypoxia causes mutation and gene instability in tumor cells. By enhancing the hypoxic microenvironment of tumor tissues, HBO may increase the efficacy of chemotherapeutic medicines in killing cancer cells. Treating non-small cell lung cancer with hyperthermia, paclitaxel, and cisplatin was coupled with HBO by Ohguri *et al.* The findings demonstrated the combination therapy's potential to greatly extend patients' lives without causing serious adverse responses [73]. Stępień *et al.* found that the average retention length of cisplatin in patients with brain cancer was significantly prolonged by HBO when treating gliomas with cisplatin plus HBO [74]. HBO does increase the therapeutic impact of a wide range of chemotherapeutic drugs, according to several *in vivo* as well as *in vitro* studies, and also several clinical trials. Bosco looked into how the time of HBOT and administration of gemcitabine affected the PANC-1 cell line's *in vitro* death and discovered that the two together caused the most cytotoxicity [75]. When treating sarcoma, Takiguchi and coworkers coupled HBO with 5-fluorouracil. During the duration of the 17-week treatment period, the combined administration of 5-fluorouracil injections plus subsequent HBO therapy significantly slowed the growth of the tumor. Additionally, it was discovered that the combination group's 5-fluorouracil levels were notably greater as compared to those of the 5-fluorouracil-only group [76]. Similar conclusions were made by Moen *et al.* in 2009, who discovered that administering 5-fluorouracil intravenously concurrently with or just after HBOT significantly raised the medication concentration in tumor tissues [77]. Breast cancer caused by dimethylbenzanthracene (DMBA) was reported to have significantly decreased interstitial fluid pressure as well as collagen content after receiving many HBO treatments. For osteosarcoma adjuvant therapy, Kawasoe *et al.* used cisplatin and HBO [78]. Results showed that low-dose cisplatin-treated mice who received HBO treatment had their tumors develop far more slowly and lived significantly longer. All of these findings support the hypothesis that HBO might improve the effectiveness of cancer treatment [79, 80].

8.4.4 The Function of HBO in Photodynamic Therapies (PDT) System

Hyperbaric oxygen therapy plays a pivotal role in enhancing the efficacy of photodynamic therapy (PDT) systems, offering a synergistic approach to address the challenges associated with oxygen availability in targeted tissues. HBOT, involving the administration of pure oxygen under increased atmospheric pressure, significantly elevates systemic oxygen levels. In the context of PDT, where oxygen is a crucial component for the generation of reactive oxygen species, HBOT ensures an abundant supply of oxygen to the treated area. Overcoming tumor hypoxia, a common limitation in cancer therapy, HBOT contributes to the success of PDT by temporarily alleviating oxygen deficits within cancerous tissues. Additionally, HBOT aids in optimizing PDT outcomes by improving light penetration into tissues, particularly relevant for deeper or less vascularized tumors. In the tumor microenvironment (TME), photosensitizers (PS) in photodynamic treatment (PDT) for cancer convert photon energy into single-atom oxygen as well as reactive oxygen species (ROS) [47]. Thus, PDT's anticancer action depends on these three factors: PS, light, and molecular oxygen. Because PDT continually consumes oxygen in tumor tissue, and because hypoxia is a hallmark of solid tumors [81, 82], to maximize the therapeutic effectiveness of PDT, the amount of oxygen in the tumor area must be increased.

Therefore, PDT has been used in conjunction with HBO treatment to treat tumors for improved antitumor effectiveness since HBO is the most efficient approach to boost the oxygen supply of the body Dong *et al.* observed the first HBO to enhance the impacts of photodynamic therapy (PDT) on a mouse model of a transplanted tumor in 1987 [83]. Silva *et al.* found similar outcomes while studying fibrosarcoma in mice [84]. In clinical research done by Tomaselli *et al.* in 2001, they found that when HBO and PDT were used together to treat 30 patients with lung cancer, tumor size was decreased and patients' Karnofsky performance status was improved compared to the group treated with only PDT [52]. The modest patient sample size did not detract from the overwhelming evidence that combining HBO with PDT is safe, effective, and very straightforward. Another research using the same methodology found that combining HBO and PDT had a greater anticancer impact than PDT alone in treating malignant pleura tumors in 34 individuals [53]. These trials concurred in demonstrating the effectiveness of HBO as well as PDT in the therapy of cancer [85]. This integrated approach harnesses the combined benefits of HBO therapy and PDT, offering a promising avenue for advancing the precision and effectiveness of targeted therapies in various medical applications, notably in oncology. Ongoing research continues to refine the protocols and applications of this combined approach, further establishing its potential as a valuable treatment modality.

8.4.5 Enhancement of the Anticancer Efficacy of Nanomedicine via Hyperbaric Oxygenation

The enhancement of anticancer efficacy through the combination of nanomedicine and hyperbaric oxygenation (HBO) is an area of research that holds promise for improving cancer treatment outcomes. Both nanomedicine and hyperbaric oxygen therapy have shown potential benefits in cancer therapy, and their combination can offer synergistic effects. It is crucial to note that chemotherapy remains one of the three main techniques by which cancer is treated and that nanomedicine is playing an increasingly significant role in cancer chemotherapy. In 1995, the FDA greenlighted Doxil®, making it the first chemotherapeutic nanomedicine to enter clinical practice. The active ingredients in Doxil® are DOX and a long-circulating liposome. The amount of time that DOX spends in blood circulation is significantly increased by polyethylene glycol (PEG) coupling on the liposome's surface because it reduces the possibility that the liposome will be regulated by protein as well as absorbed by the reticuloendothelial system (RES) *in vivo*. The passive aggregation of liposomes near cancer tissue is made possible by their EPR action, which raises DOX levels. Thus, normal tissues and organs get less DOX, and fewer DOX-related adverse effects occur [54]. Doxil® was first licensed by the FDA in 1995 to treat Kaposi's sarcoma. By 1999, it had also been allowed to treat ovarian cancer, and in 2003, it had been approved to treat breast cancer. Doxil®, a combination treatment for multiple myeloma, was approved in Europe and Canada in 2007. Approval of the cancer drug Doxil® sparked widespread interest in nanomedicine [86–90].

Doxil®, however, shows underwhelming clinical efficacy. In a clinical efficacy study on Doxil® after 10 years on the market, the US Food and Drug Administration (FDA) as well as the European Medicines Evaluation Agency (EMA) discovered that it was marginally more effective than free

DOX in treating Kaposi's sarcoma as well as ovarian cancer, but did not significantly outperform free DOX in treating breast cancer as well as myeloma. Doxil®, however, has been shown in several tests to greatly lessen the severity of DOX's negative effects, particularly cardiotoxicity. As a result, Doxil® is solely useful for reducing the DOX-related negative effects and has no impact on the efficacy of the antitumor treatment. How to boost Doxilclinical®'s antitumor effectiveness is an important unresolved issue [91, 92].

As hyperbaric oxygen treatment may directly and efficiently raise the oxygen content, it has been utilized by complexing with radiation and photodynamic therapy to attack hypoxic solid tumors in the clinic [93, 94]. However, chemotherapeutic drugs that kill cancer cells by producing ROS are seldom coupled with HBO treatment. Consequently, the combination of DOX with HBO is uncommon in clinical practice. Based on the knowledge that Doxil® may dramatically lessen DOX-induced side effects, we logically integrated two clinically employed medicines, HBO and Doxil®, with the hope of increasing therapeutic effectiveness and decreasing adverse effects [95].

The use of HBO in conjunction with DOX is not possible due to the latter's serious adverse effects. Therefore, a toxicity test was the primary *in vivo* investigation conducted. By itself, hyperbaric oxygen treatment seems to not harm [96]. There was clear cardiotoxicity with both DOX and DOX + HBO. DOX with HBO was more harmful to cardiomyocytes than DOX alone. Histological damage was seen in nearly no one in the Doxil® and Doxil® + HBO groups, showing a reduction in cardiac toxicity. We also measured creatine kinase (CK) activity to demonstrate DOX's substantial cardiotoxicity. The value of CK after therapy with only DOX was considerably greater in comparison with the control group. The highest CK value was seen in patients who received both HBO and DOX, providing further evidence that HBO exacerbated the cardiac toxicity of DOX. Doxil® may help reduce DOX's negative effects since there was not any notable difference between the control group and Doxil® groups (Doxil® and Doxil® + HBO).

8.5 HYPERBARIC OXYGEN THERAPY FOR CANCER

The term "cancer" refers to a broad range of illnesses that share some characteristics. Tumor cells can avoid the immune system, promote tumor growth through inflammation, acquire immortality through genome instability, promote invasion and metastasis through activated signaling, and evade cell death and growth suppressors all while inducing angiogenesis and reprogramming metabolism [97]. Tumor-hypoxia may be the cause of several of these carcinogenic characteristics, which not only encourages an aggressive phenotype but also lessens the effectiveness of chemotherapy, radiation, as well as immunotherapy, giving cancer patients a worse prognosis [98–100]. In light of that, treatment strategies that aim to reduce tumoral hypoxia and the effectors it activates have been suggested for use in cancer therapy [101]. In the vein, growing data suggests that HBOT might reduce tumor development and improve the efficacy of treatment by influencing three key mechanisms: (1) reducing cancer-associated hypoxia, (2) generating ROS and RNS, as well as (3) restoring immunological functioning [102]. Breast cancer, brain tumors, head as well as neck cancer, prostate cancer, colorectal cancer, cervix cancer, leukemia, and bladder cancer are only some of the malignancies that have shown promise in clinical trials using HBOT [103]. There are potentially three major uses for HBOT in oncology: (a) as an integral element of treatment, (b) as a radiation adjuvant, as well as (c) as a chemotherapy adjuvant.

Although recent encouraging outcomes have emerged, HBOT has not yet been accepted for use in the therapy of cancer. Hypoxia is reduced to a greater extent under hyperbaric circumstances, as reported by Thews and Vaupel [104], who evaluated the performance of HBOT (2 atm) and NBOT (1 atm). Despite the high-pressure oxygenation, some hypoxia was still present in the tumor, demonstrating the limited effectiveness of HBOT alone. Even though HBOT has been linked to enhanced angiogenesis, the effects are insignificant in tumor cells [105], suggesting that the treatment may be useful in the control of cancer. In contrast, research by Pande and colleagues revealed that although

HBOT-treated mice first induced a reduction in tumor succession, a tumorigenic effect was noticed after the therapy. The tumorigenic effect was likely brought on by mutagenicity, impaired DNA repair, as well as chromosomal aneuploidies in addition to a modified blood supply as well as nutrients. Other authors contend, however, that HBOT may not be as effective as a therapy since it is difficult to create a hyperoxic environment within the tumor, also by combination of HBOT with other treatments, it may even be a cure for some cancers [106–107]. For the creation of a hyperoxic environment inside the tumor, which may result in DNA damage plus detention in the G2/M cycle, Lu *et al.* recommended combining HBOT with an ultrasound-guided transrectal prostate puncture in patients having prostate cancer [108]. Aerobic glycolysis also referred to as the "Warburg effect," is connected to the metabolic reprogramming of tumor cells, just like tumor hypoxia. Cancer cells, in that regard, turn to glycolysis and stop engaging in oxidative phosphorylation. The benefits of high-boiling-point oxygen therapy (HBOT) in conjunction with a ketogenic diet were documented by Wang *et al.* in a mouse model, where they successfully inhibited the spread of tumors and increased the animals' median survival time. Elevated formation of reactive oxygen species (ROS) and oxidative stress (OXS) is another way in which only HBOT or it in combination with low glucose as well as ketone supplementation, exerts various effects against late-stage metastatic malignancies [109, 110]. While these findings are promising, further study is needed to determine HBOT's effectiveness across cancer types and to determine the best way to use that treatment on a worldwide scale.

With up to 40% of cancers being cured with radiotherapy, it is clear that RT is an integral part of cancer care. Through the overproduction of ROS and RNS, which ultimately leads to double-strand breaks, chromosomal aberrations along with rearrangements, and finally death of the cell or its dysfunction, ionizing radiation delivers its antitumor effects. To ascertain whether and how HBOT affects human glioblastoma (GBM) (CHME-5) cells derived from patients as well as the cell biology of microglia [111]. HBO as well as RT together intelligibly demonstrated a radiosensitizing impact of HBO onto GBM cells [112]. Recurrent high-grade glioma (rHGG) seems to be treatable with hypo fractionated stereotactic radiotherapy (HSRT) following hyperbaric oxygen therapy (HBO-RT), as seen in a group of nine adult patients with rHGG. For individuals who are unable or unwilling to receive systemic medications, there may be a low-toxicity option [113]. However, radiation might also harm non-tumor cells, although to a lesser extent, by disrupting several cellular signaling pathways or triggering apoptosis, thereby explaining its plethora of negative consequences [114]. A variety of bioactive molecules, which include fibrogenic cytokines like TGF-, are dysregulated during irradiation, resulting in postradiation damage. [115], are one of the worst effects of irradiation. Similarly, obliterative endarteritis is a histological trait shared by almost all tissues suffering from delayed irradiation injury, ultimately leading to tissue destruction defined by hypoxia, hypo vascularity, and hypocellularity [116]. The therapeutic effectiveness of HBOT in treating radiation-induced damage has been acknowledged by both the UHMS [117] and the ECHM [8]. According to a Cochrane analysis released in 2016, the utilization of hyperbaric oxygen therapy has been associated with better outcomes and, to a lesser extent, with osteoradionecrosis along with the extraction of a tooth in an irradiated area [118]. The European Committee for Health Management (ECHM) suggests HBOT for treating mandibular osteoradionecrosis (type 1 recommendation, level B evidence), radiation proctitis (lype 1 recommendation, level A evidence), as well as hemorrhagic radiation cystitis (level B evidence), as well as for the prevention of mislaying of Osseointegrated implants in I (type 2 recommendation). Additionally, HBOT may be used to treat or prevent the central nervous system and laryngeal injuries caused by radiotherapy (type 3 recommendation, level C evidence) [119].

It has been demonstrated that using HBOT in addition to chemotherapy offers benefits. HBOT is effective in preventing chemotherapy-induced neuropathy *in vivo*, according to recent research by Brewer *et al.* This appears to be caused by the several ways that HBOT affects neuronal activity as well as signaling [120]. Additionally, Kawasoe and colleagues discovered that administering carboplatin along with hyperbaric oxygen therapy notably decreased mortality in C3H mice that had received injections of osteosarcoma cells. HBOT produced results that were equivalent to chemotherapeutic effects in lung cancer cell lines as well as animal models [78]. Paclitaxel and carboplatin, along with hyperthermia and HBOT, have been found to improve the state of patients having non-small cell lung cancer who have many metastases [121, 122]. Despite these findings, it might not be a good idea to combine HBOT and chemotherapy. For instance, utilization of HBOT with doxorubicin, cisplatin, or bleomycin may cause pulmonary toxicity, synergic cardiotoxicity, or inadequate healing of the wounds. That is a crucial issue to deal with when providing care for a cancer patient. To reduce the risk of side effects, it is best to space out chemotherapy treatments and only utilize HBOT when required. Physical activity is only one example of how hypoxia in tumors may be targeted and used as a therapeutic adjuvant [123]. In conclusion, further investigation into the efficacy of HBOT for cancer treatment has promise.

8.6 POTENTIAL ADVERSE REACTIONS AND SAFETY MEASURES

Despite HBOT's wide range of usefulness, the therapy is not without significant risks. Some difficulties arise from the use of that treatment due to the hyperoxia and hyperbaric atmosphere. Claustrophobia and barotrauma are the two most prevalent side effects of HBOT. Either may happen during either monoplace or multiplace chamber compression [124]. Barotrauma is described as damage sustained due to the body's failure to adapt to changes in air pressure outside the body. Although ear barotrauma, which is the most often described disorder influencing the middle ear, sinus/parasinasal, dental, and pulmonary barotrauma have also been documented [125]. Although the consequence is exceedingly uncommon [126], its severity must be taken into consideration when applying various techniques to avoid it [127], like antiepileptic medication, extended air brakes, or reducing the pressure of the treatment. The onset of seizures, which may have temporary but deleterious effects on cognitive performance and behavioral patterns, is linked to the emergence of the Paul Bert effect [128]. Most of these results come from oxygen's toxicity when it is present in excessive amounts. Although it may be crucial for critically ill patients, no threshold for accurately assessing pathological oxygen levels has been identified [129]. Toxic effects on the lungs are not seen with repeated hyperbaric oxygen treatments when standard procedures are followed [130]. One of the most typical HBOT-related ocular adverse effects, hyperbaric myopia, is frequently transient. Cataracts, keratoconus, and retinopathy of prematurity are all possible ophthalmological side effects for pregnant women who get HBOT [131]. A careful examination, the usage of certain instruments, and changing treatment practices may greatly lessen all these undesirable results [132, 133].

However, HBOT may be entirely contraindicated, or at least highly contraindicated, in certain circumstances. Untreated pneumothorax is the only example in the category since it has the potential to be fatal [134]. The remaining contraindications are a matter of degree, and whether or not, the treatment is needed. Other chemotherapeutic drugs, such as sulfation (Mafenide), may have a similar effect to cisplatin and prevent the wound-healing benefits of HBOT; thus, they too should be discontinued before treatment with HBOT [45]. If a patient has a pacemaker or other implanted device, the device's compatibility with high pressure or oxygen purity must be confirmed. Hyperbaric oxygen may produce severe hemolysis, making it unsafe for those with hereditary spherocytosis [43]. Apart from carbon monoxide poisoning, pregnancy is another possible contraindication for the treatment [135]. It is vital to check the blood glucose levels of non-diabetic individuals before HBOT because the procedure has the potential to exacerbate their hypoglycemic profile and they may experience hypoglycemia during the procedure. HBOT is contraindicated in patients having underlying respiratory-related pathologies like asthma, upper respiratory infections, or chronic obstructive pulmonary disease (COPD) because it can exacerbate pulmonary barotrauma, hypercapnia, sinus or middle ear barotrauma, and other conditions. In addition, hyperbaric oxygen therapy raises blood pressure. Patients suffering from heart failure or diminished cardiac ejection fractions may be more susceptible to hyperbaric oxygen-induced pulmonary edema and cardiovascular problems [136]. Some medications, including penicillin and disulfiram, as well as a personal or family history of epilepsy, hypoglycemia, hyperthyroidism, fever, or both, may all contribute to a lowered seizure threshold during treatment. Patients with diabetes should be cautioned to limit their use of hyperbaric oxygen treatment to avoid the therapy's hypoglycemic impact. To sum up, despite HBOT's many uses, it is crucial to think about the risks that patients can encounter as a result of the treatment, such as its side effects and the presence of underlying disorders that prevent it from being effective.

8.7 CONCLUSION AND PROSPECTIVE STRATEGIES

Independent of Hb transport, hyperbaric oxygen therapy is an efficient means of increasing tissue and blood oxygen levels. From three perspectives—physical (hyperbaric 100% oxygen), physiological (hyperoxia and hypoxemia), as well as cellular/molecular—it can be said that its therapeutic cornerstone is hyperbaric 100% oxygen. All of these characteristics contribute to HBOT's effectiveness in treating hypoxia-related conditions as well as hypoxemia, along with its direct effects on infection-causing agents as well as immune cells and its modulation of an extensive range of cellular signaling pathways, cytokine production, tissue processes like angiogenesis. Here, we show that HBOT helps treat medical crises such as air embolism and gas poisoning, demonstrating that it has a wide variety of potential applications for treating pathologies like infections, inflammatory/systemic disorders, wound healing issues, and vascular issues. The general rule that HBOT should be ignored in patients having respiratory infections and diseases does not apply in the case of SARS-CoV-2. Numerous well-conducted clinical investigations conducted in recent years have produced results that justify the utilization of HBOT in COVID-19. In addition, the use of the method for various cancers provides crucial aid in delaying radiation harm. Similar effects have been shown when using HBOT as a therapeutic agent in conjunction with other established therapies, such as chemotherapy; moreover, recent studies have indicated significantly enhanced outcomes when using nanomedicine strategies in tandem with HBOT.

HBOT has many potential uses, but several obstacles must be solved before it can reach its full potential. Concerning the line of thought is the fact that HBOT-induced hyperoxia does not entirely remove tumor hypoxia in some situations, such as tumoral cells. HBOT in conjunction with another treatment method may be an appealing option for addressing the issue. However, it is just as crucial to identify and assess any risks associated with HBOT, as well as any medical conditions that may prevent a patient from benefiting from it. The creation of trustworthy techniques for the evaluation of the potential advantages and risks of HBOT for specific patients before undergoing the treatment requires more focus. Predictive model development or other creative methodologies are two examples of avenues that may be pursued along these lines.

There are just 14 conditions for which the therapy technique has been officially authorized. We advocate for further research to determine the full range of applications of that method, taking into account the unique needs of each patient. The integration of HBOT in future clinical studies may provide a further resource for the therapeutic care of many illnesses.

REFERENCES

1. Sen S, Sen S. Therapeutic effects of hyperbaric oxygen: integrated review. *Med Gas Res*. 2021 Jan-Mar;11(1):30–3.
2. Memar MY, Yekani M, Alizadeh N, Baghi HB. Hyperbaric oxygen therapy: antimicrobial mechanisms and clinical application for infections. *Biomed Pharmacother*. 2019 Jan 1;109:440–7.
3. Raizandha MA, Hidayatullah F, Kloping YP, Rahman IA, Djatisoesanto W, Rizaldi F. The role of hyperbaric oxygen therapy in Fournier's Gangrene: a systematic review and meta-analysis of observational studies. *Int Braz J Urol*. 2022 Sep-Oct;48(5):771–81.

4. Shannon AM, Bouchier-Hayes DJ, Condron CM, Toomey D. Tumour hypoxia, chemotherapeutic resistance, and hypoxia-related therapies. *Cancer Treat Rev*. 2003 Aug;29(4):297–307.
5. Rankin EB, Giaccia AJ. The role of hypoxia-inducible factors in tumorigenesis. *Cell Death Differ*. 2008 Apr;15(4):678–85.
6. Roy S, Kumaravel S, Sharma A, Duran CL, Bayless KJ, Chakraborty S. Hypoxic tumor microenvironment: implications for cancer therapy. *Exp Biol Med*. 2020 Jul;245(13):1073–86.
7. Yadav AS, Radharani NNV, Gorain M, Bulbule A, Shetti D, Roy G, Baby T, et al. RGD functionalized chitosan nanoparticle-mediated targeted delivery of raloxifene selectively suppresses angiogenesis and tumor growth in breast cancer. *Nanoscale*. 2020;12(19):10664–84.
8. Mathieu D, Marroni A, Kot J. Tenth European Consensus Conference on Hyperbaric Medicine: recommendations for accepted and non-accepted clinical indications and practice of hyperbaric oxygen treatment. *Diving Hyperb Med*. 2017 Mar;47(1):24–32.
9. Meng L, Cheng Y, Tong X, Gan S, Ding Y, Zhang Y, Wang C, Xu L, Zhu Y, Wu J, Hu Y, Yuan A. Tumor oxygenation and hypoxia inducible factor-1 functional inhibition via a reactive oxygen species responsive nanoplatform for enhancing radiation therapy and abscopal effects. *ACS Nano*. 2018 Aug 28;12(8):8308–22.
10. Fahmy SA, Azzazy HM, Schaefer J. Liposome photosensitizer formulations for effective cancer photodynamic therapy. *Pharmaceutics*. 2021 Aug 27;13(9):1345.
11. Blanco E, Shen H, Ferrari M. Principles of nanoparticle design for overcoming biological barriers to drug delivery. *Nat Biotechnol*. 2015 Sep;33(9):941–51.
12. Cheng YH, He C, Riviere JE, Monteiro-Riviere NA, Lin Z. Meta-analysis of nanoparticle delivery to tumors using a physiologically based pharmacokinetic modeling and simulation approach. *ACS Nano*. 2020 Mar 24;14(3):3075–95.
13. Ye M, Gao Y, Liang M, Qiu W, Ma X, Xu J, Hu J, Xue P, Kang Y, Xu Z. Microenvironment-responsive chemotherapeutic nanogels for enhancing tumor therapy via DNA damage and glutathione consumption. *Chinese Chem Lett*. 2022 Sep 1;33(9):4197–202.
14. Yong T, Zhang X, Bie N, Zhang H, Zhang X, Li F, Hakeem A, Hu J, Gan L, Santos HA, Yang X. Tumor exosome-based nanoparticles are efficient drug carriers for chemotherapy. *Nat Commun*. 2019 Aug 23;10(1):3838.
15. Li Y, Wu Y, Chen J, Wan J, Xiao C, Guan J, Song X, Li S, Zhang M, Cui H, Li T, Yang X, Li Z, Yang X. A simple glutathione-responsive turn-on theranostic nanoparticle for dual-modal imaging and chemo-photothermal combination therapy. *Nano Lett*. 2019;19:5806–17.
16. Liu WL, Liu T, Cao AM, Qin SY, Feng J, Zhang XZ. Coordination between anti-inflammation and antitumor actions for systematic tumor treatments with improved prognosis. *Chem Eng J*. 2022 Jul 1;439:135711.
17. Liang Q, Bie N, Yong T, Tang K, Shi X, Wei Z, Jia H, Zhang X, Zhao H, Huang W, Gan L, Huang B, Yang X. The softness of tumor-cell-derived microparticles regulates their drug-delivery efficiency. *Nat Biomed Eng*. 2019 Sep;3(9):729–40.
18. Plafki C, Peters P, Almeling M, Welslau W, Busch R. Complications and side effects of hyperbaric oxygen therapy. *Aviat Space Environ Med*. 2000 Feb;71(2):119–24.
19. Gill AL, Bell CN. Hyperbaric oxygen: its uses, mechanisms of action and outcomes. *QJM*. 2004 Jul;97(7):385–95.
20. Camporesi EM, Bosco G. Mechanisms of action of hyperbaric oxygen therapy. *Undersea Hyperb Med*. 2014 May 1;41(3):247–52.
21. Bitterman H. Bench-to-bedside review: oxygen as a drug. *Crit Care*. 2009;13(1):205.
22. Heyboer M 3rd, Sharma D, Santiago W, McCulloch N. Hyperbaric oxygen therapy: side effects defined and quantified. *Adv Wound Care (New Rochelle)*. 2017 Jun 1;6(6):210–24.
23. Wang J, Zhang B, Sun J, Wang Y, Wang H. Nanomedicine-enabled modulation of tumor hypoxic microenvironment for enhanced cancer therapy. *Adv Ther (Weinh)*. 2020 Jan;3(1):1900083.
24. Peng HS, Liao MB, Zhang MY, Xie Y, Xu L, Zhang YJ, Zheng XF, Wang HY, Chen YF. Synergistic inhibitory effect of hyperbaric oxygen combined with sorafenib on hepatoma cells. *PLoS One*. 2014 Jun 23;9(6):e100814.

25. Jäger S, Dickgiesser S, Tonillo J, Hecht S, Kolmar H, Schröter C. EGFR binding Fc domain-drug conjugates: stable and highly potent cytotoxic molecules mediate selective cell killing. *Biol Chem.* 2022 Apr 1;403(5–6):525–34.
26. Lind F. A pro/con review comparing the use of mono- and multi-place hyperbaric chambers for critical care. *Diving Hyperb Med.* 2015 Mar;45(1):56–60.
27. Song G, Liang C, Gong H, Li M, Zheng X, Cheng L, Yang K, Jiang X, Liu Z. Core-shell MnSe@Bi2 Se3 fabricated via a cation exchange method as novel nanotheranostics for multimodal imaging and synergistic thermoradiotherapy. *Adv Mater.* 2015 Oct 28;27(40):6110–7.
28. Wang H, Wang W, Liu L, Wang M, Li G, Li H, Li B, Yu S, Ma D, Xue W. Biodegradable hollow polydopamine@ manganese dioxide as an oxygen self-supplied nanoplatform for boosting chemo-photodynamic cancer therapy. *ACS Appl Mater Interfaces.* 2021 Nov 22;13(48):57009–22.
29. Ansiaux R, Dewever J, Grégoire V, Feron O, Jordan BF, Gallez B. Decrease in tumor cell oxygen consumption after treatment with vandetanib (ZACTIMA; ZD6474) and its effect on response to radiotherapy. *Radiat Res.* 2009 Nov;172(5):584–91.
30. Davis DD, Hanley ME, Cooper JS. Osteoradionecrosis. *Curr Otorhinolaryngol Rep.* 2021;6:285–91.
31. Wang J, Zhang Y, Zhang G, Xiang L, Pang H, Xiong K, Lu Y, et al. Radiotherapy-induced enrichment of EGF-modified doxorubicin nanoparticles enhances the therapeutic outcome of lung cancer. *Drug Deliv.* 2022;29(1):588–99.
32. Zhou X, Shi K, Hao Y, Yang C, Zha R, Yi C, Qian Z. Advances in nanotechnology-based delivery systems for EGFR tyrosine kinases inhibitors in cancer therapy. *Asian J Pharm Sci.* 2020 Jan 1;15(1):26–41.
33. Nan Y. Lung carcinoma therapy using epidermal growth factor receptor-targeted lipid polymeric nanoparticles co-loaded with cisplatin and doxorubicin. *Oncol Rep.* 2019;42(5):2087–96.
34. Kuo YC, Liang CT. Inhibition of human brain malignant glioblastoma cells using carmustine-loaded catanionic solid lipid nanoparticles with surface anti-epithelial growth factor receptor. *Biomaterials.* 2011;32(12):3340–50.
35. Xiao Y, Lin ZT, Chen Y, Wang H, Deng YL, Le DE, Bin J, Li M, Liao Y, Liu Y, Jiang G. High molecular weight chitosan derivative polymeric micelles encapsulating superparamagnetic iron oxide for tumor-targeted magnetic resonance imaging. *Int J Nanomed.* 2015 Feb 5;10:1155–72.
36. Kim IY, Kang YS, Lee DS, Park HJ, Choi EK, Oh YK, Son HJ, et al. Antitumor activity of EGFR targeted pH-sensitive immunoliposomes encapsulating gemcitabine in A549 xenograft nude mice. *J Control Release.* 2009;140(1):55–60.
37. Aggarwal S, Yadav S, Gupta S. EGFR targeted PLGA nanoparticles using gemcitabine for treatment of pancreatic cancer. *J Biomed Nanotechnol.* 2011;7(1):137–8.
38. Salehnia Z, Shahbazi-Gahrouei D, Akbarzadeh A, Baradaran B, Farajnia S, Naghibi M. Synthesis and characterization of iron oxide nanoparticles conjugated with epidermal growth factor receptor (EGFR) monoclonal antibody as MRI contrast agent for cancer detection. *IET Nanobiotechnol.* 2019;13(4):400–6.
39. Shahbazi-Gahrouei D, Abdi N, Shahbazi-Gahrouei S, Hejazi SH, Salehnia Z. In vivo study of anti-epidermal growth factor receptor antibody-based iron oxide nanoparticles (anti-EGFR-SPIONs) as a novel MR imaging contrast agent for lung cancer (LLC1) cell detection. *IET Nanobiotechnol.* 2020;14(5):369–74.
40. Růžička J, Dejmek J, Bolek L, Beneš J, Kuncova J. Hyperbaric oxygen influences chronic wound healing–a cellular level review. *Physiol Res.* 2021 Dec;70(Suppl 3):S261.
41. Xue EY, Yang C, Fong WP, Ng DKP. Site-specific displacement-driven activation of supramolecular photosensitizing nanoassemblies for antitumoral photodynamic therapy. *ACS Appl Mater Interfaces.* 2022;14(13):14903–15.
42. Ganthala PD, Alavala S, Chella N, Andugulapati SB, Bathini NB, Sistla R. Co-encapsulated nanoparticles of Erlotinib and Quercetin for targeting lung cancer through nuclear EGFR and PI3K/AKT inhibition. *Colloids Surf B Biointerfaces.* 2022;211:112305.
43. Wen L, Moser M, Ley K. Molecular mechanisms of leukocyte β2 integrin activation. *Blood.* 2022;139(24):3480–92.
44. Kadry YA, Calderwood DA. Structural and signaling functions of integrins. *Biochim Biophys Acta-Biomembran.* 2020 May 1;1862(5):183206.

45. Backer MV, Backer JM. Imaging key biomarkers of tumor angiogenesis. *Theranostics.* 2012;2(5):502–15.
46. Cabodi S, Di Stefano P, Leal Mdel P, Tinnirello A, Bisaro B, Morello V, Damiano L, et al. Integrins and signal transduction. *Adv Exp Med Biol.* 2010; 674:43–54.
47. Nel AE, Mei KC, Liao YP, Liu X. Multifunctional lipid bilayer nanocarriers for cancer immunotherapy in heterogeneous tumor microenvironments, combining immunogenic cell death stimuli with immune modulatory drugs. *ACS Nano.* 2022 Mar 29;16(4):5184–232.
48. Rios De La Rosa JM, Spadea A, Donno R, Lallana E, Lu Y, Puri S, Caswell P, et al. Microfluidic-assisted preparation of RGD-decorated nanoparticles: exploring integrin-facilitated uptake in cancer cell lines. *Sci Rep.* 2020;10(1):14505.
49. Zhan C, Gu B, Xie C, Li J, Liu Y, Lu W. Cyclic RGD conjugated poly(ethylene glycol)-co-poly(lactic acid) micelle enhances paclitaxel anti-glioblastoma effect. *J Control Release.* 2010;143(1):136–42.
50. Long Q, Zhu W, Guo L, Pu L. RGD-conjugated resveratrol HSA nanoparticles as a novel delivery system in ovarian cancer therapy. *Drug Des Devel Ther.* 2020;14:5747–56.
51. Faggiano S, Ronda L, Bruno S, Abbruzzetti S, Viappiani C, Bettati S, Mozzarelli A. From hemoglobin allostery to hemoglobin-based oxygen carriers. *Mol Aspects Med.* 2022 Apr 1;84:101050.
52. Tomaselli F, Maier A, Sankin O, Anegg U, Stranzl U, Pinter H, Kapp K, Smolle-Jüttner FM. Acute effects of combined photodynamic therapy and hyperbaric oxygenation in lung cancer--a clinical pilot study. *Lasers Surg Med.* 2001;28(5):399–403.
53. Gong H, Chao Y, Xiang J, Han X, Song G, Feng L, Liu J, Yang G, Chen Q, Liu Z. Hyaluronidase to enhance nanoparticle-based photodynamic tumor therapy. *Nano Lett.* 2016;16:2512–21.
54. Cong Y, Ji L, Gao YJ, Liu FH, Cheng DB, Hu Z, Qiao ZY, Wang H. Microenvironment-induced in situ self-assembly of polymer–peptide conjugates that attack solid tumors deeply. *Angew Chem.* 2019 Mar 26;131(14):4680–5.
55. Yang RQ, Wang PY, Lou KL, Dang YY, Tian HN, Li Y, Gao YY, Huang WH, Zhang YQ, Liu XL, Zhang GJ. Biodegradable nanoprobe for NIR-II fluorescence image-guided surgery and enhanced breast cancer radiotherapy efficacy. *Adv Sci.* 2022;9(12):e2104728.
56. Song X, Feng L, Liang C, Yang K, Liu Z. Ultrasound triggered tumor oxygenation with oxygen-shuttle nano perfluorocarbon to overcome hypoxia-associated resistance in cancer therapies. *Nano Lett.* 2016 Oct 12;16(10):6145–5
57. Huang X, Liang P, Jiang B, Zhang P, Yu W, Duan M, Guo L, Cui X, Huang M, Huang X. Hyperbaric oxygen potentiates diabetic wound healing by promoting fibroblast cell proliferation and endothelial cell angiogenesis. *Life Sci.* 2020 Oct 15;259:118246.
58. Sureda A, Batle JM, Martorell M, Capó X, Tejada S, Tur JA, Pons A. Antioxidant response of chronic wounds to hyperbaric oxygen therapy. *PLoS ONE.* 2016;11:e0163371.
59. Boykin JV, Baylis C. Hyperbaric oxygen therapy mediates increased nitric oxide production associated with wound healing. *Adv Ski Wound Care.* 2007;20:382–89.
60. Dulai PS, Buckey JC, Raffals LE, Swoger JM, Claus PL, O'Toole K, Ptak JA, Gleeson MW, Widjaja CE, Chang J, et al. Hyperbaric oxygen therapy is well tolerated and effective for ulcerative colitis patients hospitalized for moderate-severe flares: a phase 2A Pilot multi-center, randomized, double-blind, Sham-controlled trial. *Am J Gastroenterol.* 2018;113:1516–23.
61. Luo L, Qing L, Yao C, Liu D, Li Y, Li T, Feng P. Efficacy and safety of hyperbaric oxygen therapy for moderate-to-severe ulcerative colitis: a protocol for a systematic review and meta-analysis. *BMJ Open.* 2021;11(6):e047543.
62. Oliai C, Fisher B, Jani A, Wong M, Poli J, Brady LW, Komarnicky LT. Hyperbaric oxygen therapy for radiation-induced cystitis and proctitis. *Int J Radiat Oncol Biol Phys.* 2012;84: 733–40.
63. Gray L H, Conger AD, Ebert M, Hornsey S, Scott OC. The concentration of oxygen dissolved in tissues at the time of irradiation as a factor in radiotherapy. *Br J Radiol.* 1953;26:638–48.
64. Malone M, Bjarnsholt T, McBain AJ, James GA, Stoodley P, Leaper D, Tachi M, Schultz G, Swanson T, Wolcott RD. The prevalence of biofilms in chronic wounds: a systematic review and meta-analysis of published data. *J Wound Care.* 2017;26:20–25.
65. Bennett MH, Feldmeier J, Smee R, Milross C. Hyperbaric oxygenation for tumor sensitization to radiotherapy. *Cochrane Database Syst Rev.* 2018 Apr 11;4(4):CD005007.

66. Agier J, Efenberger M, Brzezińska-Błaszczyk E. Cathelicidin impact on inflammatory cells. *Central Eur J Immunol.* 2015 Apr 1;40(2):225–35.
67. Peyssonnaux C, Datta V, Cramer T, Doedens A, Theodorakis EA, Gallo RL, Hurtado-Ziola N, Nizet V, Johnson RS. HIF-1α expression regulates the bactericidal capacity of phagocytes. *J Clin Investig.* 2005;115:1806–15.
68. Peyssonnaux C, Datta V, Cramer T, Doedens A, Theodorakis EA, Gallo RL, Hurtado-Ziola N, Nizet V, Johnson RS. HIF-1α expression regulates the bactericidal capacity of phagocytes. *J Clin Investig.* 2005 Jul 1;115(7):1806–15.
69. Gaudreault É, Gosselin J. Leukotriene B4 induces release of antimicrobial peptides in lungs of virally infected mice. *J Immunol.* 2008;180:6211–21.
70. Polom W, Klejnotowska A, Matuszewski M, Sicko Z, Markuszewski M, Krajka K. Hyperbaric oxygen therapy (HBOT) in case of hemorrhagic cystitis after radiotherapy. *Cent European J Urol.* 2012;65(4):200–3.
71. Allen S, Kilian C, Phelps J, Whelan HT. The use of hyperbaric oxygen for treating delayed radiation injuries in gynecologic malignancies: a review of literature and report of radiation injury incidence. *Support Care Cancer.* 2012 Oct;20:2467–72.
72. Nedrebø T, Bruun T, Skjåstad R, Holmaas G, Skrede S. Hyperbaric oxygen treatment in three cases of necrotizing infection of the neck. *Infect Dis Rep.* 2012;4:73–6.
73. Ohguri T, Imada H, Narisada H, Yahara K, Morioka T, Nakano K, Miyaguni Y, Korogi Y. Systemic chemotherapy using paclitaxel and carboplatin plus regional hyperthermia and hyperbaric oxygen treatment for non-small cell lung cancer with multiple pulmonary metastases: preliminary results. *Int J Hyperthermia.* 2009 Mar;25(2):160–7.
74. Stępień K, Ostrowski RP, Matyja E. Hyperbaric oxygen as adjunctive therapy in the treatment of malignancies, including brain tumors. *Med Oncol.* 2016 Sep;33(9):101.
75. Haroon AT, Patel M. Al-Mehdi AB. Lung metastatic load limitation with hyperbaric oxygen. *Undersea Hyperbaric Med.* 2007 Mar 1;34(2):83.
76. Takiguchi N, Saito N, Nunomura M, Kouda K, Oda K, Furuyama N, Nakajima N. Use of 5-FU plus hyperbaric oxygen for treating malignant tumors: evaluation of antitumor effect and measurement of 5-FU in individual organs. *Cancer Chemother Pharmacol.* 2001;47(1):11–4.
77. Moen I, Stuhr LEB. Hyperbaric oxygen therapy and cancer – a review. *Target Oncol.* 2012;7:233–42.
78. Moen I, Stuhr LE. Hyperbaric oxygen therapy and cancer—a review. Target Oncol. 2012 Dec;7:233–42.
79. Muzumdar D, Jhawar S, Goel A. Brain abscess: an overview. *Int J Surg.* 2011;9:136–44.
80. Tomoye EO, Moon RE. Hyperbaric oxygen for intracranial abscess. *Undersea Hyperb Med.* 2021;48:97–102.
81. Mazzucchelli S, Truffi M, Fiandra L, Sorrentino L, Corsi FJWJoP. Targeted approaches for HER2 breast cancer therapy: news from nanomedicine? *World J Pharmacol.* 2014;3(4):72–85.
82. Clark AS, Yau C, Wolf DM, Petricoin EF, can't Veer LJ, Yee D, Moulder SL, Wallace AM, et al. Neoadjuvant T-DM1/pertuzumab and paclitaxel/trastuzumab/pertuzumab for HER2+ breast cancer in the adaptively randomized I-SPY2 trial. *Nat Commun.* 2021;12(1):6428.
83. Dong GC, Hu SX, Zhao GY, et al. Experimental study on cytotoxic effects of hyperbaric oxygen and photodynamic therapy on mouse transplanted tumor. *Chin Med J.* 1987;100:697–702..
84. Silva ZS Jr, Bussadori SK, Fernandes KP, Huang YY, Hamblin MR. Animal models for photodynamic therapy (PDT). *Biosci Rep.* 2015 Sep 28;35(6):e00265.
85. Hamilton KJ, Hewitt SC, Arao Y, Korach KS. Estrogen hormone biology. *Curr Top Dev Biol.* 2017;125:109–46.
86. de Almeida Chuffa LG, Lupi-Júnior LA, Costa AB, de Arruda Amorim JP, Seiva FR. The role of sex hormones and steroid receptors on female reproductive cancers. *Steroids.* 2017 Feb 1;118:93–108.
87. Thomas C, Gustafsson JÅ. The different roles of ER subtypes in cancer biology and therapy. *Nat Rev Cancer.* 2011;11(8):597–608.
88. Kurmi BD, Paliwal R, Paliwal SR. Dual cancer targeting using estrogen functionalized chitosan nanoparticles loaded with doxorubicin-estrone conjugate: a quality by design approach. *Int J Biol Macromol.* 2020;164:2881–94.
89. Kapara A, Brunton V, Graham D, Faulds K. Investigation of cellular uptake mechanism of functionalized gold nanoparticles into breast cancer using SERS. *Chem Sci.* 2020;11(22):5819–29.

90. Mirdamadian SZ, Varshosaz J, Minaiyan M, Taheri A. 3D printed tablets containing oxaliplatin loaded alginate nanoparticles for colon cancer targeted delivery. An in vitro/in vivo study. *Int J Biol Macromol.* 2022 Apr 30;205:90–109.
91. Zhu J, Guo M, Cui Y, Meng Y, Ding J, Zeng W, Zhou W. Surface coating of pulmonary siRNA delivery vectors enabling mucus penetration, cell targeting, and intracellular radical scavenging for enhanced acute lung injury therapy. *ACS Appl Mater Interfaces.* 2022;14(4):5090–100.
92. Zhang Z, Qin S, Chen Y, Zhou L, Yang M, Tang Y, Zuo J, Zhang J, et al. Inhibition of NPC1L1 disrupts adaptive responses of drug-tolerant persister cells to chemotherapy. *EMBO Mol Med.* 2022;14(2):e14903.
93. Montanari E, Di Meo C, Oates A, Coviello T, Matricardi P. Pursuing intracellular pathogens with hyaluronan from a "Pro-Infection" polymer to a biomaterial for "Trojan Horse" systems. *Molecules.* 2018;23(4):939.
94. Wang T, Niu K, Ni S, Zhang W, Liu Z, Zhang X. Hyaluronic acid-modified gold-polydopamine complex nanomedicine for tumor-targeting drug delivery and chemo-photothermal-therapy synergistic therapy. *ACS Sustain Chem Eng.* 2022 Jan 20;10(4):1585–94.
95. Lei C, Liu XR, Chen QB, Li Y, Zhou JL, Zhou LY, Zou T. Hyaluronic acid and albumin-based nanoparticles for drug delivery. *J Control Release.* 2021;331:416–33.
96. Zheng N, Liu W, Li B, Nie H, Liu J, Cheng Y, Wang J, et al. Co-delivery of sorafenib and mifepristone encapsulated by CXCR4-targeted PLGA-PEG nanoparticles overcomes hepatocellular carcinoma resistance to sorafenib. *J Exp Clin Cancer Res.* 2019;38(1):232.
97. Xiao K, Liu Q, Suby N, Xiao W, Agrawal R, Vu M, Zhang H, et al. LHRH-targeted redox-responsive crosslinked micelles impart selective drug delivery and effective chemotherapy in triple-negative breast cancer. *Adv Healthc Mater.* 2021;10(3):e2001196.
98. Tian H, Zhang J, Zhang H, Jiang Y, Song A, Luan Y. Low side-effect and heat-shock protein-inhibited chemo-phototherapy nano platform via a co-assembling strategy of biotin-tailored IR780 and quercetin. *Chem Eng J.* 2020;382:123043.
99. Setrerrahmane S, Xu H. Tumor-related interleukins: old validated targets for new anti-cancer drug development. *Mol Cancer.* 2017;16(1):153.
100. Fei L, Ren X, Yu H, Zhan Y. Targeting the CCL2/CCR2 axis in cancer immunotherapy: one stone, three birds? Front Immunol. 2021 Nov 3;12:771210.
101. De La Torre C, Casanova I, Acosta G, Coll C, Moreno MJ, Albericio F, Aznar E, et al. Gated mesoporous silica nanoparticles using a double-role circular peptide for the controlled and target-preferential release of doxorubicin in CXCR4-expressing lymphoma cells. *Adv Funct Mater.* 2015;25(5):687–95.
102. Di-Wen S, Pan G, Hao L, Zhang J, Xue Q, Wang P, Yuan Q. Improved antitumor activity of epirubicin-loaded CXCR4-targeted polymeric nanoparticles in liver cancers. *Int J Pharm.* 2016;500(1–2):54–61.
103. Chittasupho C, Kewsuwan P, Murakami T. CXCR4-targeted nanoparticles reduce cell viability, induce apoptosis, and inhibit SDF-1α induced BT-549-Luc cell migration in vitro. *Curr Drug Deliv.* 2017;14(8):1060–70.
104. Thews O, Vaupel P. Zeitliche Veränderungen der Tumoroxygenierung und-durchblutung während normo-und hyperbarer inspiratorischer Hyperoxie. *Strahlentherapie und Onkologie.* 2016 Mar;192:174–81.
105. Xue L, Mao X, Ren L, Chu X. Inhibition of CXCL12/CXCR4 axis as a potential targeted therapy of advanced gastric carcinoma. *Cancer Med.* 2017;6(6):1424–36.
106. Pande S, Sengupta A, Srivastava A, Gude RP, Ingle A. Re-evaluate the effect of hyperbaric oxygen therapy in cancer – a preclinical therapeutic small animal model study. *PLoS ONE.* 2012;7(11):e48432.
107. Kim SH, Cha YS, Lee Y, Kim H, Yoon IN. Successful treatment of central retinal artery occlusion using hyperbaric oxygen therapy. *Clin Exp Emerg Med.* 2018;5:278–81.
108. Lu QZ, Li X, Ouyang J, Li JQ, Chen G. Further application of hyperbaric oxygen in prostate cancer. *Med Gas Res.* 2019 Jan 9;8(4):167–171.
109. Wang J, Sun D, Huang L, Wang S, Jin Y. Targeting reactive oxygen species capacity of tumor cells with repurposed drug as an anticancer therapy. *Oxid Med Cell Longev.* 2021 Sep 7;2021: 8532940.
110. Lalieu RC, Brouwer RJ, Ubbink DT, Hoencamp R, Bol Raap R, van Hulst RA. Hyperbaric oxygen therapy for nonischemic diabetic ulcers: a systematic review. *Wound Repair Regen.* 2020 Mar;28(2):266–75.

111. Abidia A, Laden G, Kuhan G, Johnson BF, Wilkinson AR, Renwick PM, Masson EA, McCollum PT. The role of hyperbaric oxygen therapy in ischaemic diabetic lower extremity ulcers: a double-blind randomized-controlled trial. *Eur J Vasc Endovasc Surg.* 2003;25:513–18.
112. Nakamura, H, Makiguchi, T, Atomura, D, Yamatsu, Y, Shirabe, K, Yokoo, S. Changes in skin perfusion pressure after hyperbaric oxygen therapy following revascularization in patients with critical limb ischemia: a preliminary study. *Int J Low Extrem Wounds.* 2020;19:57–62.
113. Rose JJ, Wang L, Xu Q, McTiernan CF, Shiva S, Tejero J, Gladwin MT. Carbon monoxide poisoning: pathogenesis, management, and future directions of therapy. *Am J Respir Crit Care Med.* 2017;195:596–606.
114. Martani L, Cantadori L, Paganini M, Camporesi EM, Bosco G. Carbon monoxide intoxication: prehospital diagnosis and direct transfer to the hyperbaric chamber. Minerva Anestesiol. 2019 Apr 2;85(8):920–2.
115. Rose JJ, Nouraie M, Gauthier MC, Pizon AF, Saul MI, Donahoe MP, Gladwin MT. Clinical outcomes and mortality impact of hyperbaric oxygen therapy in patients with carbon monoxide poisoning. *Crit Care Med.* 2018;46:e649–55.
116. Weaver LK, Hopkins RO, Chan KJ, Churchill S, Elliott CG, Clemmer TP, Orme JF, Thomas FO, Morris AH. Hyperbaric oxygen for acute carbon monoxide poisoning. *N Engl J Med.* 2002;347:1057–67.
117. Hampson NB, Piantadosi CA, Thom SR, Weaver LK. Practice recommendations in the diagnosis, management, and prevention of carbon monoxide poisoning. *Am J Respir Crit Care Med.* 2012;186:1095–101.
118. Hanley ME, Murphy-Lavoie HM. *Hyperbaric, cyanide toxicity.* StatPearls Publishing, Treasure Island, FL, USA. 2019.
119. Hansen MB, Olsen NV, Hyldegaard O. Combined administration of hyperbaric oxygen and hydroxocobalamin improves cerebral metabolism after acute cyanide poisoning in rats. *J Appl Physiol.* 2013 Nov 1;115(9):1254–61.
120. Brewer AL, Shirachi DY, Quock RM, Craft RM. Effect of hyperbaric oxygen on chemotherapy-induced neuropathy in male and female rats. *Behav Pharmacol.* 2020 Feb;31(1):61–72.
121. Rhee TM, Hwang D, Lee JS, Park J, Lee JM. Addition of hyperbaric oxygen therapy vs. medical therapy alone for idiopathic sudden sensorineural hearing loss: a systematic review and meta-analysis. *JAMA Otolaryngol Head Neck Surg.* 2018;144:1153–61.
122. Bayoumy AB, de Ru JA. The use of hyperbaric oxygen therapy in acute hearing loss: a narrative review. *Eur Arch Oto-Rhino-Laryngol.* 2019;276:1859–80.
123. Paderno E, Zanon V, Vezzani G, Giacon T, Bernasek T, Camporesi E, Bosco, G. Evidence-supported HBO therapy in femoral head necrosis: a systematic review and meta-analysis. *Int J Environ Res Public Health* 2021;18: 2888.
124. Brenner I, Shephard RJ, Shek PN. Immune function in hyperbaric environments, diving, and decompression. *Undersea Hyperb Med.* 1999;26:27–39.
125. Xu X, Yi H, Kato M, Suzuki H, Kobayashi S, Takahashi H, Nakashima I. Differential sensitivities to hyperbaric oxygen of lymphocyte subpopulations of normal and autoimmune mice. *Immunol. Lett.* 1997;59:79–84.
126. Yang B, Chen Y, Shi J. Reactive oxygen species (ROS)-based nanomedicine. *Chem Rev.* 2019;119(8):4881–985.
127. Panieri E, Santoro M. ROS homeostasis and metabolism: a dangerous liaison in cancer cells. *Cell Death Dis.* 2016;7:e2253.
128. Htike TT, Moriya F, Miyaishi S. Cyanide concentrations in blood and tissues of fire victims. *Legal Med.* 2019 Nov 1;41:101628.
129. Walsh JC, Lebedev A, Aten E, Madsen K, Marciano L, Kolb HC. The clinical importance of assessing tumor hypoxia: relationship of tumor hypoxia to prognosis and therapeutic opportunities. *Antioxid Redox Signal.* 2014;21(10):1516–54.
130. Sahu A, Kwon I, Tae G. Improving cancer therapy through the nanomaterials-assisted alleviation of hypoxia. *Biomaterials.* 2020;228:119578.
131. Wen J, Luo Y, Gao H, Zhang L, Wang X, Huang J, Shang T, Zhou D, Wang D, Wang Z, Li P. Mitochondria-targeted nanoplatforms for enhanced photodynamic therapy against hypoxia tumor. *J Nanobiotechnol.* 2021 Dec;19(1):1–22.

132. Zhang R, Song X, Liang C, Yi X, Song G, Chao Y, Yang Y, Yang K, Feng L, Liu Z. Catalase-loaded cisplatin-prodrug-constructed liposomes to overcome tumor hypoxia for enhanced chemo-radiotherapy of cancer. *Biomaterials*. 2017;138:13–21.
133. Wen M, Ouyang J, Wei C, Li H, Chen W, Liu YN. Artificial enzyme catalyzed cascade reactions: antitumor immunotherapy reinforced by NIR-II light. *Angew Chem Int Ed Engl*. 2019;58(48):17425–32.
134. Chen S, Jia Q, Zheng X, Wen Y, Liu W, Zhang H, Ge J, Wang P. PEGylated carbon dot/MnO2 nanohybrid: a new pH/H2O2-driven, turn-on cancer nanotheranostics. *Sci China Mater*. 2018;61(10):1325–38.
135. Wang D, Xue B, Ohulchanskyy TY, Liu Y, Yakovliev A, Ziniuk R, Xu M, Song J, Qu J, Yuan Z. Inhibiting tumor oxygen metabolism and simultaneously generating oxygen by intelligent upconversion nanotherapeutics for enhanced photodynamic therapy. *Biomaterials*. 2020 Aug 1;251:120088.
136. Xu Q, Zhang Y, Yang Z, Jiang G, Lv M, Wang H, Liu C, Xie J, Wang C, Guo K, Gu Z. Tumor microenvironment-activated single-atom platinum nanozyme with H2O2 self-supplement and O2-evolving for tumor-specific cascade catalysis chemodynamic and chemoradiotherapy. *Theranostics*. 2022;12(11):5155.

9 Combo Nanomedicine

The Co-Delivery of Multimodal Therapies for Effective, Targeted Plus Secure Treatment of Cancer

9.1 INTRODUCTION

Patients diagnosed with cancer are provided with an extensive range of contemporary remedies, which is indicative of the progress made in the field of oncology [1]. Hormone therapy interferes with hormonal signals that fuel certain cancers; chemotherapy targets and destroys rapidly dividing cancer cells; radiation therapy eliminates or shrinks tumors [2]; immunological therapy uses the body's immune system to recognize and fight cancer cells; and surgery removes tumors or affected tissue [3–4]. More research and ground-breaking treatment alternatives are required to minimize the patient population and put the illness under control. While picking the most effective treatment is crucial, no avenue should be off-limits. Conventional treatment has its benefits and drawbacks [5]. Increases in patient survival rates are one advantage. Misdiagnosis, pharmaceutical resistance, too powerful outcomes, and unanticipated bad effects all contribute to the problem. Emerging nanotechnology-based cancer therapies [6] have great promise. Cancer researchers are using nanotechnology to improve detection, staging, and treatment. Figure 9.1 shows diagrammatic representation of radiotherapy-assisted tumor removal.

To sustain tumor development and progression, cancer biology requires angiogenesis, the formation of new blood vessels from existing ones. Tumor cells produce signaling molecules such as vascular endothelial growth factor (VEGF), which induces the nearest blood arteries to form new capillaries to the tumor site. This procedure facilitates the infiltration of tumors into the circulation, hence facilitating the transportation of essential nutrients and oxygen. However, increased vascularity allows cancer cells to infiltrate surrounding tissues and migrate to distant organs, ensuring the condition malignant. The molecular principles of angiogenesis have led to the development of antiangiogenic medicines such medications that target VEGF or its receptors to stop tumor growth [7, 8]. For cancer to spread, infiltrate, and proliferate, angiogenesis is necessary [7]. The ovary, uterus, and placenta all engage in physiological angiogenesis [7–10], in which proliferating endothelial cells generate new blood vessels. Several cell types, including macrophages, endothelial cells, and pericytes, collaborate to maintain a healthy ratio of pro- to antiangiogenic substances. However, extensive angiogenesis has been seen during tumor development and wound healing [9]. Arterioles that are twisted, enlarged, saccular, and highly permeable are shared by cancer cells and diabetic retinopathy [11]. Because of its crucial function, angiogenesis is required in both conditions. Vascular endothelial growth factor production progresses along defective vascular architecture, decreasing the effectiveness of cytotoxic therapy [8, 12]. In both healthy and malignant tissues, vascular endothelial growth factor is a crucial controller of migration of cells, proliferation of the cell, plus the creation of new blood vessels. Increased levels of vascular endothelial growth factor are linked to the formation of tumors and aberrant angiogenesis [12]. Angiogenesis, the creation of new blood vessels, is tightly controlled by a balance of pro- and antiangiogenic factors. Insufficient

DOI: 10.1201/9781003451020-9

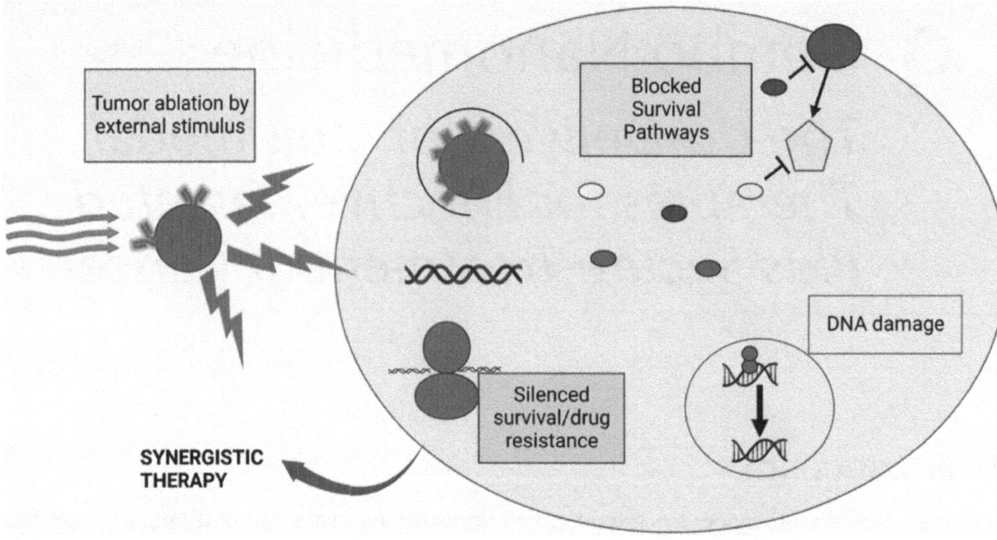

FIGURE 9.1 Diagrammatic representation of radiotherapy-assisted tumor removal.

synthesis of endostatin, thrombospondin-1 (TSP-1), and growth factors may cause tumor development and spread in dysregulated angiogenesis. Collagen XVIII precursor endostatin inhibits endothelial cell growth and migration, inhibiting angiogenesis. TSP-1, an endogenous protein, inhibits proangiogenic factors and promotes endothelial cell death to regulate angiogenesis [13–15]. Stimulating the body's natural process of vessel formation is vital to several cutting-edge therapies for cancer and diabetic retinopathy (angiogenesis). Anti-VEGF antibodies, such as bevacizumabas comparison to angiogenesis inhibitors, have been demonstrated to dramatically increase the overall survival rate in patients receiving conventional chemotherapy [16, 17] have been shown to destroy highly proliferative tumor cells by cutting off their supply of nutrients and oxygen [18, 19].

Death rates for many common malignancies have been rather stable over the last two decades, despite technological advances allowing for developments in cancer biology and anticancer drugs [20]. New approaches are needed immediately to boost the therapeutic index and effectiveness of cancer drugs [21]. Despite a seemingly permanent reduction in symptoms, the response to therapy may eventually fade since solid tumors develop resistance to treatment so quickly. The research demonstrates that combining NPs with a wide variety of therapeutic anticancer medications may be a successful treatment for malignancies that have developed resistance to regular therapy [22].

When treating cancer, a multimodal approach yields optimal pharmacokinetics and therapeutic payload distribution [21]. The use of medication combinations is a widespread practice in traditional chemotherapy because it can reduce the chance of drug resistance and boost the therapeutic effectiveness of the individual agents employed without significantly increasing the toxicity of the entire treatment. Most cancers do not react well to a single medication treatment (monotherapy). It is frequently required to combine two or more cancer treatments that target distinct genes, disease pathways, or checkpoints of cell-cycle in order to boost the likelihood of achieving complete remission [23]. Currently, the development stages of many potentially effective cancer therapies are underway. It is possible that the ideal synergistic drug ratio may be maintained until absorption by the target cancer cell if several therapeutic medicines with varied physicochemical and physiological properties are encapsulated into a single NP. Clinical and preclinical investigations have shown that the use of combination chemotherapy, sometimes known as the "two-in-one strategy," improves both response and survival [24]. Rapid advancements in nanotechnology since the early

2000s have made it possible to explore its medicinal applications. The use of nanoscale drug carriers, like liposomes as well as polymeric NPs, has improved the efficacy of many therapies [25, 26].

Because of tiny size as well as high penetrating power, nanoparticles (NPs) are desirable drug carriers and are the best vehicles for delivering hydrophobic/hydrophilic pharmaceutical chemicals, peptides, tiny molecule treatments, and antibodies onto the cancer site [27, 28]. For their potential anticancer properties as well as delivery, NPs like PMs, polymeric NPs, liposomes, carbon NPs, dendrimers, polymer–drug complexes, CNTs, quantum dots, nanoemulsions, as well as inorganic NPs have all been studied. Due to their adaptability in diseased tissue, theranostic nanocarriers have attracted considerable attention as a potential treatment for a wide range of disorders [29]. Health-related information may be sent using nanoparticles of metal or magnetite, a material utilized in nanomedicine. We have discussed the nanoparticles' execution mechanism and the several lethal chemicals they contained. Also, the mechanism of action of each cytotoxic medication, in addition to the combinatorial properties of the nanoparticles.

It is possible to prolong the effects of drugs by increasing their duration, plasma half-life, bioavailability, and biodistribution; decreasing toxicity and multidrug resistance; improving EPR; and postponing controlled release [25, 26, 27]. By selectively silencing genes of interest or decreasing the expression of treatment efficacy, RNA interference (RNAi)-based technologies may increase the efficacy of chemotherapeutic drugs. As a cancer therapeutic method, NPs have shown encouraging early outcomes [28].

Because it enables the utilization of chemotherapeutic medications and NPs at lower concentrations, minimizes undesirable cytotoxic effects, and increases efficacy, combination therapy is a desirable method for investigating cancer. The treatment of cancer using medication combinations has been found to be more effective than using any one medicine alone. The optimal synergistic medication ratio is maintained in a single carrier from the moment the nanoformulated drug is ingested by the targeted cancer cell until it is absorbed by the body for elimination (NPs). It has been shown that using a combination of drugs to treat cancer is both beneficial and feasible [30, 31]. Topics covered will include the follwing: (a) how nanoparticles target cancer cells during treatment; (b) the wide variety of nanoparticles used in cancer therapy; (c) global cancer incidence and mortality rates; (d), (e), (g), (f) how nanoparticles are created; and (g) both individually and in conjunction with other anticancer medications, how nanoparticles affect cancer.

9.2 POLYMERIC MICELLES FOR CANCER THERAPY: FEATURES AND ADVANTAGES

Polymeric micelles, and nanoscale amphiphilic block copolymer structures, are potential cancer medication delivery vehicles. Drug delivery to cancer cells while reducing tissue exposure is possible due to their particular permeability and retention [32]. The hydrophobic core encapsulates medicines, overcoming drug resistance. Engineering polymeric micelles to react to tumor microenvironment cues improves treatment effectiveness and reduces adverse effects [33]. Polymeric micelles have shown promise as a potential tool in cancer treatment, and it was initially suggested by Ringsdorf and colleagues in the 1980s [32–35]. Using biocompatible amphiphilic block copolymers, these nanoscale spherical particles (varying in size from 10 to 100 nm) self-assemble in water (Figure 9.1). When two components of a block copolymer are mixed together in water, the hydrophilic part forms an outside layer while the hydrophobic part hardens into a central core. Drug clearance is slowed by the hydrophilic exterior layer of micelles, while medications that do not dissolve in water are held by the hydrophobic interior layer [36]. Beyond biocompatibility and biodegradability, other desired qualities of the building blocks have also been investigated (for example, blocks that are sensitive to temperature or pH). Today, polyethylene glycol, which has a molecular weight ranging from 2 to 15 kD, is the polymer most frequently used to make coronas

(PEG). Polymers like poly(D,L-lactic acid), poly(propylene oxide), poly(-caprolactone), as well as poly(L-aspartic acid) are often found in the middle [37–40].

Drugs which are lipophilic, or insoluble in water, are frequently used in the treatment of cancer. Paclitaxel, a potent anticancer medication, may be dissolved in water at a concentration of around 0.0015 mg/mL. Paclitaxel binds to tubulin when it enters a cell, stopping it from building new microtubules. It is true that hydrophobic drugs may cross cell membranes rapidly, but intravenous administration carries the danger of rapid aggregation and the formation of capillary embolisms [41]. Putting the drug's hydrophobic core within a micelle has been shown to increase its apparent solubility. Paclitaxel's solubility was raised via micelle encapsulation from 0.0015–2 mg/mL [42–45]. Polymer micelles enable the administration of currently available drugs *in vivo* that were previously thought to have been either too poisonous or too hydrophobic for usage out of the laboratory [46].

When used *in vivo*, the hydrophilic micellar corona is crucial because it blocks opsonin proteins from accurately recognizing particles [47]. The reticuloendothelial system (RES) would quickly engulf the micelle through phagocytic processes and dispose of it if it did not have its bristle-like coating [14]. Polymeric micelles are insoluble in biological fluids despite their low concentration limits (usually on the order of 106–107 M) [48]. A number of additives that extend the drug's time in the bloodstream can increase bioavailability. Because of the tiny size as well as lengthy half-life, micelles preferentially gather in cancer tissue because of the increased permeability as well as retention (EPR) effect. As a result, fenestrations amongst endothelial cells within the angiogenic tumor vasculature can be passively targeted.

9.3 POLYMERIC MICELLES: ADVANTAGES OVER VARIOUS NANOTHERAPEUTIC SYSTEMS

Polymeric micelles are a viable substrate for drug administration in cancer treatment because of their unusual structure, which is made up of amphiphilic block copolymers that self-assemble into nanoscale structures. These micelles improve hydrophobic drug solubility and bioavailability, enabling the co-delivery of several treatments with different mechanisms. Due to their increased permeability and retention (EPR) effect, they preferentially accumulate in tumor tissues with leaky vasculature, reducing exposure to healthy tissues and boosting medication delivery to cancer cells [49, 50]. Polymeric micelles may be customized for active targeting, improving drug delivery selectivity and accuracy. In response to low pH or high temperatures, their stimuli-responsive properties limit medication release in the tumor microenvironment. Polymeric micelles excel in adaptability, passive and active targeting, and stimulus reactivity, making them a top nanomedicine system. Polymer–drug complexes, dendrimers, as well as liposomes are examples of polymer-based nanotherapeutic systems. Each of these systems has a unique chemical makeup and set of biological properties. The most promising results have come from liposome and polymer–drug conjugates in human trials. Liver cancer was the initial successfully treated with neocarzinostatin (NCS) as well as poly(styrene-co-maleic acid) (SMA) in the 1980s by Maeda *et al.* [51–55]. SMANCS, with a ten-fold longer half-life in circulation because of the EPR effect, might be utilized to more accurately target tumors. Hepatocellular carcinoma has been successfully treated recently, which may be due to improved stability and tumor selectivity. Polymer–drug conjugates including polyethylene glycol-camptothecin, dextran-doxorubicin, as well as polyglutamate-paclitaxel have shown promise in clinical trials. Although it has not been licenced for use in humans, methotrexate-containing polyamidoamine dendrimers have been shown to prevent carcinogenesis in the subcutaneous tissue of mice. In phase I/II clinical research, several doxorubicin (DOX) as well as paclitaxel micellar formulations are currently being evaluated [56]. A poly(ethylene glycol)-poly(L-aspartic acid) block copolymer was used in the manufacture of DOX micelles by Kataoka and coworkers to enhance their anticancer potential. Clearance was reduced and half-life was prolonged for NK911 (from 48 minutes to 2.3–2.8 hours) because of the use of micelles [57].

The covalent bond between drugs and carriers is essential for conjugated pharmaceuticals as well as dendrimer systems. Since the chemical groups that may be added to drug molecules are not always readily available, the scope of the method is limited. Only chemical mechanisms (such as enzymatic breakdown or acid-catalyzed hydrolysis) may be able to free drug molecules locked in chemically stable covalent bonds and transport them to tumor sites [58]. Glomeruli in the kidneys efficiently remove microbes from the bloodstream, especially those with a diameter of less than 10 nm.

Liposomes are cholesterol and phospholipids found in cell membranes that have self-assembled into nanovesicles. Liposomes' hydrophilic compartment allows them to carry water-soluble therapeutic proteins and DNAs. Medications intended to be entrapped by hydrophobic bilayer membranes have a low loading capacity because of the membrane's instability, which reduces the drugs' solubility [59, 60]. Numerous research demonstrate that combining lipid membranes with hydrophilic polymers like PEG creates stealth liposomes with extended circulation lengths and efficient passive targeting of solid tumors through the EPR effect. Liposomal particles larger than 90 nm in size may have trouble penetrating tumor tissues due to structural constraints. Particles that enter the body through extravasation [61–62]. Interstitial transmission is blocked by a physical barrier provided by collagen fibrils. When they reach malignant tissue, the conventional liposomal formulations deliver their drugs slowly. The effects of temperature and pH on the release of medications from liposomes have been studied.

Another nanoplatform for drug delivery, polymeric micelles are both unique and synergistic with the aforementioned nanosystems. Numerous poorly soluble anticancer drugs may be effectively transported by micelles due to their hydrophobic centers. In order to keep drugs in usable condition, non-covalent encapsulation is used instead of reactive chemical groups. Anticancer drugs like doxorubicin may form chemical interactions with these polymers due to their unique chemical compositions, leading to increased drug loading and less premature drug release after administration [63]. It is possible to adjust the size of the polymeric micelle produced by an amphiphilic copolymer by modifying its hydrophobic block, which typically lies in the 10–100 nm range [64]. Drugs in that size range may be able to bypass the kidneys' filtering systems, allowing them to reach tumors more efficiently than liposomes.

The utilization of polymer micelles for *in vivo* applications is widely studied, and much has been written about its potential advantages and limitations. The modest size of micelle systems (10–100 nm) restricts their drug loading capacity [64, 65]. The micelle's small size and low drug loading may cause it to release its contents prematurely, reducing the medication's effectiveness or causing it to miss its target entirely [66]. Options, including as chemical conjugation strategies, are being examined to improve micelle core compatibility with the target medication. As an additional note, the micelle stability of polymers has been questioned. It is promising that researchers are considering utilizing core-crosslinked micelles to increase *in vivo* stability [67]. There is scepticism about micelles' efficacy as a cancer therapy. To combat, several researchers have looked at methods of increasing micelle accumulation at tumor sites, followed by a controlled, prolonged release of their payload.

9.4 ACTIVE TARGETING SPECIFICALLY FOR MICELLES

Polymeric micelles' drug delivery techniques depend on active targeting. To activate cancer cell receptors, micelles are modified with targeted ligands like antibodies, peptides, or aptamers. Drug distribution is more selective and efficient, which benefits cancer treatment. Because polymeric micelles are adjustable, their surface characteristics may be tailored to different targeting ligands [68]. Cancer cell receptors are specifically recognized and bound by these ligands, facilitating receptor-mediated endocytosis. Active targeting increases micelle accumulation at the tumor location and cancer cell internalization, improving therapeutic payload to the target. Active targeting has shown promise in preclinical and clinical research for enhancing anticancer medication therapeutic index, enabling lower dosages, decreased toxicity, and better patient outcomes [69]. Therefore, active targeting strategies, such as adding a ligand to the micelle surface so that it may preferentially bind to tumor-specific receptors, have garnered significant attention. Accumulation at tumor locations and enhanced receptor-mediated endocytosis are other features of that phenomenon. Many other types of ligands are conceivable, including small chemical compounds, peptides, polysaccharides, monoclonal antibodies, DNA or RNA aptamers, and polysaccharides.

Folic acid is an example of a little chemical compound that may be utilized to selectively target cancer due to the high expression of its receptor (100–300 times) in many kinds of malignancies [70]. The addition of folic acid to DOX-containing PEG-PLGA micelles increased their bioavailability and cytotoxicity against KB cells, as shown by Hami *et al* [71]. Mice fed folate-labeled micelles showed considerably slower tumor growth compared to mice fed untargeted micelles in *in vivo* tests. Peptides' potential as ligands for the targeted administration of anticancer medications to tumors is another area of research. Recently, we have been investigating how to target v3 integrin, which is overexpressed on the outer surface of angiogenic tumor vessels, using a peptide known as cyclic(Arg-Gly-Asp-D-Phe-Lys) (cRGDfK) [72].

The addition of galactose and lactose has enhanced micelles. In hepatocellular carcinomas, the protein is overexpressed, and its target, the asialoglycoprotein receptor (ASGPR), is very selective [73]. Micelles constructed from a galactose-labeled poly(ethylene glycol)-co-poly(-benzyl L-glutamate) block copolymer have been shown to increase paclitaxel sensitivity in ASGPR cells by as much as 30%. Another important class of functional targeting ligands is the monoclonal antibody system. Using either the anticancer monoclonal antibody 2C5 or the antimyosin mAb 2G4, diacylglycerol-polyethylene glycol (PE-PEG) micelles have been proven to be selectively administered to cancer cells in lungs [74]. Tumors in the lungs of 2C5-expressing mice were more sensitive to the lethal effects of paclitaxel-carrying micelles after just 2 hours, with accumulation rising by a factor of 4. Aptamers are DNA or RNA oligonucleotides discovered via library screening; they are beginning to be beneficial as a targeted ligand for tumors. In a recent work, RNA aptamer technology was used to generate docetaxel-loaded PEG-PLGA micelles that selectively target prostate specific membrane antigen (PSMA) [51]. *In vivo* experiments with LNCaP xenografts showed more efficacy than with untargeted micelles, with complete tumor remission occurring in five of seven test animals.

9.4.1 Drug Release in Response to Stimuli

Micellar drug delivery methods for cancer therapy need precise drug release control. Micelles release their therapeutic payload in response to certain stimuli to kill cancer cells. Drug release may be induced by pH, temperature, or ultrasound, according to several theories. For optimum cancer cell payload delivery, pH-responsive micelles use the acidic tumor microenvironment to release drugs [75]. Tumors' higher temperatures trigger temperature-sensitive micelles to release drugs on demand [76]. Ultrasound-triggered drug release is non-invasive and allows spatiotemporal medication delivery. These stimuli-responsive techniques improve drug release accuracy, limiting off-target effects and boosting cancer cell therapy.

When compared to normal tissues, that consists a pH of 7.4, tumor tissues have a substantially lower pH (as low as 5.7), which is associated with the glycolysis metabolism of tumor cells. The mechanism is similar to endocytosis in that both require a pH range of vesicles (5.0–5.5). (such as late endosomes and strongly degradative lysosomes). After the medication has been injected into a patient's vein, the release of the drug may be expedited by exposing the micelles to various pH levels. There are two possible mechanisms by which drugs released from micelles in a pH-dependent way might be started. One non-covalent method is the usage of acid-labile bonds, while another is the selective protonation of pH-sensitive constituents within the micelle. The initial micelles were produced by Kataoka and colleagues by hydrazone bonding doxorubicin to a PEG-pAsp copolymer

[77]. The micelles formed with a high concentration of DOX (42.5% by weight), and the release of drug was found to be pH-dependent (3.0% after 48 hours at pH 7.4 and 25% at pH 5.5). In *in vivo* experiments, 50% of the mice examined exhibited better cancer development, tolerance, and regression. Some research organizations have explored pH-sensitive release using non-covalent technique [78]. Micelles are generated at higher pH (pH 8.0) in the triblock polymer created by Tang *et al.*, which comprises of poly(2-(dimethylamino) ethyl methacrylate, poly(ethylene glycol), as well as poly(2-diethylamino)ethyl acrylate. Dipyridamole drug release was proven to be pH dependent, with a 50% increase at a pH of 3.0 compared to a pH of 7.4.

The development of thermoresponsive polymer micelles has resulted from technological advances that allow for localised heating. Poly(N-isopropylacrylamide) (pNIPAM) is a wonderful polymer with a low critical solution temperature (LCST) of 32°C [79]. Okano and coworkers produced micelles, which are made up of a hydrophobic poly(butyl methacrylate) (PBMA) core and a thermosensitive poly(N-isopropylacrylamide) (pNIPAM) corona [80]. After 15 hours, it was determined that only 15 percent of the doxamethasone (DOX) placed into pNIPAM-b-PBMA micelles was released at 30°C, while 90% was released at 37°C. In cytotoxicity experiments, cell death was demonstrated to be less than 5% at 29°C and more than 65% at 37°C.

Several mechanisms, including a spike in local temperature, cavitation, that facilitates cellular membrane permeability, as well as the production of highly reactive species of free species, which hastens polymer breakdown, are used by current drug delivery systems to start the release of drugs [81]. Pluronic micelles sensitive to ultrasound were used by Ugarenko and colleagues to create a doxorubicin-loaded therapeutic nanocarrier [82]. In *in vivo* trials, tumor development was considerably postponed for longer when ultrasonic-treated micelles were compared to micelles without ultrasound, suggesting that both free DOX and DOX integrated into the micelles had enhanced anticancer action. PEG-phospholipid was used to keep micelles from breaking apart (PEG-DSPE) [83].

9.4.2 Imaging-Sensitive Polymer Microbubbles

Ultrasound, positron emission tomography, and computerized tomography are all examples of imaging methods used in medicine. Imaging techniques like positron emission tomography as well as magnetic resonance imaging are used to detect cancer and track its development throughout treatment. The development of nanomedicine and improvements in diagnostic imaging have allowed for the rapid and precise differentiation of healthy cells from cancerous ones [84–86].

Technology based on micelles is now often employed in magnetic resonance imaging. Medical imaging contrast agents, which are based on gadolinium, such as Magnevist®, have been shown to have therapeutic potential (Gd). When these substances are present, the proton T1 relaxation time of water decreases [87]. Polymeric micelles coated with Gd complex may significantly improve T1 relaxivity and detection sensitivity [88]. If the countless spin-orbits in the universe are useless, then what are they for? We have only reported on one formulation so far, and that is an SPIO nanoparticle wrapped in a polymeric micelle [89]. Hydrophobic SPIO nanoparticles inserted into the micelle core significantly enhanced T2 relaxivity. If the nanomolar levels can be formed into mousellar form, then MRI might detect them.

Polymeric micelles have been investigated for their possible utility in cancer diagnosis as an alternative imaging modality to computed tomography (CT) and single-photon emission computed tomography (SPECT) (SPECT). For usage as CT contrast agents, Torchilin *et al.* synthesized PLL-PEG polymer micelles containing iodine with a mean size of 100 nm and a concentration of 45% (w/w). Subcutaneous needle injections were given to the rabbits' rear legs, and then the animals' popliteal lymph nodes were scanned using CT scanners 2 hours later to assess the injection's effects. Micelles injected intravenously into rabbits for 30 minutes caused the veins in their livers to become opaque (IV) [89–92].

9.4.3 Polymeric Micelles with Multiple Functions

Known as modified micelles, these particles form when amphiphilic block copolymers or graft copolymers self-assemble into a core/shell structure (PMs). Injecting anticancer drugs directly into tumors using PMs with favorable thermodynamic and kinetic characteristics has been shown to increase drug efficacy [89]. Micelles were created by Bae *et al.* [90] in 2007 with a unimodal structure and a particle size of 100 nm for delivery to tumors. These micelles included the anticancer drugs doxorubicin (DOX) and wortmannin (WOR), an inhibitor of phosphatidylinositol-3 kinase. Cisplatin (CP) (II) may be released from cisplatin (IV) and paclitaxel (PTX) composite micelles by cellular reduction as well as acid hydrolysis. Together, the composite micelles reduced systemic toxicity and enhanced the effectiveness of cancer treatment [91, 92]. Zheng *et al.* synthesized caitic micelles from poly(ethylene glycol)-b-poly(l-lysine)-b-poly(l-leucine) to improve the solubility of DTX as well as siRNA-Bcl-2 in gene vectors (PEG-PLL-PLLeu). In a micelle combination, siRNA and Bcl-2 RNA rendered cells more susceptible to low concentrations of DTX. In a mouse MCF-7 xenograft model, it was discovered that the cationic micelles inhibited cancer progression more effectively than siRNA or DTX alone [92]. According to the research, Wang *et al.* hypothesize that combining nanoparticles (NPs) encasing micelles with landscape phage might boost the therapeutic index of cancer treatment. Cancer cells were killed by PTX in combination with an MCF-7-specific phage protein as well as PEG-PE micelles [93], whereas healthy cells were spared. Numerous *in vitro* as well as *in vivo* apoptotic studies proved that increasing doses of PTX significantly reduced tumor size and produced necrosis. Micelle-mediated combination treatment has showed promise as a potentially successful and tolerable chemotherapeutic option for persons with breast cancer [93]. PNP has the potential to facilitate the timed administration of numerous chemotherapy drugs. Docetaxel (DOX) administered intravenously in combination with platinum nanocarriers has shown clinical potential in cancer therapy (IV). Nanocarrier PCL-b-P (OEGMA-co-AzPMA) is its official chemical name (Pt[IV]). Recent research [94] reveals a dual-drug co-delivery method, whereby cells may absorb micelles and release drugs into the cells simultaneously.

The particles are formed when amphiphilic polymers dissolve in a fluid that promotes their spontaneous mixing. The process results in a net decrease in energy (PMs). Micelles are appealing because of their shell-core structure, compact size, and resistance to filtration, especially during the early stages of sterilization [95, 96]. pH-sensitive PMs were created by Taillefer *et al.* by combining methacrylic acid, N-isopropylacrylamide, and octadecyl acrylate [96]. Photoactive anticancer drug alu chlorophthalocyanine has been found to be translocated through micelles (AlClPc). AlClPc-loaded pH-responsive PMs outperformed a standard reference material. EMT-6 mouse mammary cancer cells were used to test the Cremophor EL formulation. To combat its low solubility in water, meso-tetraphenylporphine (MTP) is often encapsulated in pharmaceutic microemulsions (PMs) (TPP). In order to boost the effectiveness of photodynamic treatment (PDT) against murine (LLC, B16) as well as human (MCF-7, BT20) cancer cell lines, the use of polyethylene glycol (PEG) micelles or immunomicelles is recommended [97]. Female C57BL/6 mice with cancer can be treated with tumor-specific polyclonal 2C5 antibodies using TPP-loaded PEG-PE micelles under PDT settings. These EPR results were accomplished by the production of zinc protoporphyrin (ZnPP) polymer nanoparticles (PMs) encapsulated in the water-soluble, bio-compatible amphiphilic polymer PEG [98,99]. A SMA-ZnPP and PEG-ZnPP multicomponent micelle was treated with reactive singlet oxygen to enhance the death of tumor cells. It is seen that photodynamic therapy (PDT) medicines, which may include targeted chemotherapeutics such as water-soluble ZnPP PMs, have considerable therapeutic promise. PEG-block-PLA micelles may be useful for the effective transport of medicines with low water solubility, such as PTX, DTX, ETOP, as well as 17-AAG, at therapeutically acceptable dosages [100]. Combining 7-ethyl-10-hydroxycamptothecin (SN-38) in a polymeric micelle with the humanized monoclonal antibody bevacizumab (against vascular endothelial growth factor) against human lung cancer cells, demonstrated a considerable anticancer efficacy [101]. For improvement of therapeutic index and retention of intratumorally given chemotherapeutic medicines, poly(methyl)acrylamide (PMs) have been synthesized utilizing N-(2-hydroxypropyl) methacrylamide (HPMA). Results from *in vivo* experiments [102] indicate HPMA may enhance the synergistic effects of XRT and chemotherapy. Similar to the way cell-penetrating peptides work, deoxycholic acid (DA3) coupled to polyethylenimine (PEI) may promote extracellular macromolecule trafficking (PEI 1.8 kDa). When PTX is conjugated to a core–shell conjugation that is similar to a micelle, stable complexes (PTX/DA3/siRNA) are produced. The development of tumours was inhibited by PTX, DA3, and siRNA treatment in both cell culture as well as *in vivo* studies with tumor-bearing mice [103,104]. Paclitaxel-loaded N-octyl-O-sulfate chitosan micelles have been shown to be lethal to both wild-type and MDR mutant HepG2-P human HepG2 cells (PTX-M). By decreasing membrane fluidity and activating several pathways to increase P-gp ATPase activity, multidomain micelles may have substantial inhibitory effects on PTX binding to P-gp. Animal studies have shown that PTX-M is a more effective formulation of existing cancer medications due to increased cellular absorption and decreased cellular loss. To treat PXL-resistant ovarian cancer, Salzano *et al.* created self-assembling particles (anti-survivin siRNA/PXL PM) [105]. High-complexity micelles suppressed survivin expression in SKOV3-tr xenografted rat tumor tissues. Star-shaped amphiphilic polycarbonate/PEG copolymers have showed potential for directing treatment to tumors. When contrasted to their cholesterol-initiated diblock equivalent micelles, DOX-loaded NPs self-assembled from the star-like copolymer demonstrated significantly improved kinetic stability and DOX-loading capacity. Tumor growth in 4T1 mice was greatly inhibited by vesicles loaded with doxorubicin (DOX) [106,107] without leading to severe weight loss or cardiotoxicity. Some researchers believe that the EPR effect explains why tumor tissue has so many more vesicles than healthy tissue. To specifically target DTX, Kulhari *et al.* discovered a technique in 2015 for creating peptide-conjugated succinoyl-tocopheryl polyethylene glycol succinate nanomicelles. There is hope that the cRGDfK peptide may specifically target tumor cells due to their high expression of the integrin beta 3 (v3) receptor. Human umbilical vein endothelial cells and DU145 human prostate cancer cells both showed considerable suppression of angiogenesis when treated with peptide-conjugated doxorubicin (DTX) loaded nanomicelles. When given to breast cancer cells *in vitro* and *in vivo*, the PTX and honokiol combination in biodegradable PMs resulted in longer drug release, improved cellular uptake, and cytotoxicity. The medication was more effective when added to the PMs than when administered alone [108], where it was found at greater concentrations in tumor tissues. Ruttala *et al.* [109] developed crosslinked polypeptide-based micelles that react to changes in pH and redox state to increase the efficacy and lessen the toxicity of chemotherapy. When DTX and lonidamine (LND)-crosslinked micelles were employed instead of non-crosslinked micelles, oxidative stress, cellular component damage, and cell death were all significantly amplified. PMs may have a synergistic impact on tumor suppression when used with anticancer medicines [110–115].

9.5 LIMITATIONS AND THE STATE OF THE ART OF COMBINATION TREATMENT

Cancer is a major cause of mortality worldwide for both sexes despite therapeutic advancements. When it comes to fighting cancer, nanotechnology, namely nanomedicine, has demonstrated some very promising new discoveries [116]. The vast majority of currently available cancer medications were never intended for use against cancer. The use of nanotechnology in the area of oncology, for example, paves the way for more targeted nanomedicine, which has been shown to improve the success rate of standard cancer therapies and even help some patients overcome treatment resistance [117]. They anticipate that in the near future, therapeutic settings will make use of medications that are both safer and more effective. However, the employment of such cutting-edge methods requires the utmost caution. The increasing difficulty of nanoformulation necessitates rapid study [118].

The onus of proof rests on nanotechnology specialists to show that their wares are much better than their forebears, both in terms of clinical efficacy and durability/lower cost [119]. Nanomedicine operations need close coordination among specialists from a broad variety of fields, including pharmacokinetics, nanoformulation, toxicology, immunology, cell and molecular biology, as well as cancer.

Calcium phosphate nanoparticles (CaPN) as well as mesoporous silica nanoparticles (MSN) have many of the same desirable characteristics for delivery of thr drug to cancer cells, including high biocompatibility, pH sensitivity, bioactivity, as well as pore size. CaPN has a short half-life, a quick onset of action, and a similarly short duration of activity because of its low storage capacity. Since MSN's high permeability makes it ideal for storing large quantities of pharmaceuticals, it is likely that it might be the key to solving the problem with CaPN.

9.6 CONCLUSIONS

Polymeric micelles have shown efficacy in both diagnosing and treating cancer by selectively targeting tumors and enhancing the potency of antineoplastic drugs via a dose-dependent mechanism. Researchers often create micelles with inherent imaging capabilities to assess the efficacy of treatments. Cancer therapy is difficult and biochemically complicated, making multifunctional polymeric micelles attractive. It is difficult to discover an effective therapy for solid tumors due to the genetic and phenotypic variation. As more focused therapies become available, the selection of tumor cells that can tolerate the chosen technique will become clearer. The use of micellar nanomedicine to transport a broad variety of anticancer medications has the potential to dramatically enhance cancer treatment. Micelles, which are capable of identifying phenotypic manifestations inside solid tumors, have been proposed as a possible solution to the issue of cancer heterogeneity. Imaging may be used by doctors to evaluate and treat patients' adaptive resistance over time. The integration of personalized cancer treatment with theranostic micellar nanomedicine has the potential to significantly improve the efficacy and specificity of chemotherapy.

Current cancer treatment faces biodistribution, poor solubility, insufficient therapeutic agent targeting, poor oral bioavailability, dose-limiting toxicity to healthy tissues, low therapeutic indices, and emerging drug resistance. Nanoparticles (NPs) have been proposed as a means to enhance the efficacy of cancer drugs. The stability-maintaining qualities of NPs might potentially enhance the bioavailability, retention, and preferential accumulation of medicines at cancer sites, leading to enhanced permeability, decreased side effects, and an elevated therapeutic index. Nanoparticle technology has been used in direct anticancer medications and combinations of anticancer treatment, which has resulted in significant advancements in the targeting and destruction of cancer cells over the course of the last 10 years. Nanoparticles (NPs) can interfere with tumor development, invasion, metastasis, and treatment resistance when combined with traditional anticancer drugs. Nanoparticles (NPs) have the potential to enable significant progress in nanomedicine, allowing for the treatment of many diseases, such as cancer.

Research on nanocarriers may be carried out on a broad range of materials, such as fullerenes, nanoparticles, nanodisks, and carbon nanotubes (CNTs, NPs, and NDs, respectively). Graphene and related materials have shown promise as drug delivery systems for cancer therapy when exposed to photothermal or photothermal irradiation. Integrating carbon nanosystems into existing treatment approaches might potentially provide several beneficial therapeutic outcomes. However, the occurrence of aggregation and protein opsonization represents major challenges associated with carbon nanosystems. Through enhanced therapeutic advantages, efficacy, and medication resistance elimination, combination therapy improves cancer patients' chances of long-term remissions. However, nanoparticle-mediated combination treatment is presently hindered by some constraints, including the absence of appropriate preclinical models and insufficient collaboration among experimental and theoretical scientists, clinicians, engineers, and the pharmaceutical and biotechnology businesses. A multidisciplinary strategy is essential to guarantee nanocombination treatment delivers better outcomes, lower morbidity, and enhanced quality of life for cancer patients.

REFERENCES

1. Patel JD, Krilov L, Adams S, Aghajanian C, Basch E, Brose MS, Carroll WL, De Lima M, Gilbert MR, Kris MG, Marshall JL. Clinical cancer advances 2013: annual report on progress against cancer from the American Society of Clinical Oncology. *J Clin Oncol*. 2014 Jan 10;32(2):129–60.
2. Chandraprasad MS, Dey A, Swamy MK. 1 – Introduction to cancer and treatment approaches. In: Swamy MK, Pullaiah T, Chen Z-S (eds). *Paclitaxel*. 2022 Jan 1 (pp. 1–27). Academic Press, USA.
3. Pucci C, Martinelli C, Ciofani G. Innovative approaches for cancer treatment: current perspectives and new challenges. *Ecancermedicalscience*. 2019;13:961.
4. Kaliberov SA, Buchsbaum DJ. Chapter seven–cancer treatment with gene therapy and radiation therapy. *Adv Cancer Res*. 2012;115:221–63.
5. Chakraborty S, Rahman T. The difficulties in cancer treatment. *Ecancermedicalscience*. 2012 Nov 14;6:ed16.
6. Yadav P, Ambudkar SV, Rajendra Prasad N. Emerging nanotechnology-based therapeutics to combat multidrug-resistant cancer. *J Nanobiotechnol*. 2022 Dec;20(1):1–35.
7. Lugano R, Ramachandran M, Dimberg A. Tumor angiogenesis: causes, consequences, challenges and opportunities. *Cell Mol Life Sci*. 2020 May;77(9):1745–70.
8. Carmeliet P, Jain RK. Molecular mechanisms and clinical applications of angiogenesis. *Nature*. 2011 May 19;473(7347):298–307.
9. Kareva I, Abou-Slaybi A, Dodd O, Dashevsky O, Klement GL. Normal wound healing and tumor angiogenesis as a game of competitive inhibition. *PLoS One*. 2016 Dec 9;11(12):e0166655.
10. Reynolds LP, Grazul-Bilska AT, Redmer DA. Angiogenesis in the female reproductive organs: pathological implications. *Int J Exp Pathol*. 2002 Aug;83(4):151–63.
11. Jenkins AJ, Joglekar MV, Hardikar AA, Keech AC, O'Neal DN, Januszewski AS. Biomarkers in diabetic retinopathy. *Rev Diabet Stud*. 2015 Spring-Summer;12(1–2):159–95.
12. Amini A, Masoumi Moghaddam S, L Morris D, H Pourgholami M. The critical role of vascular endothelial growth factor in tumor angiogenesis. *Curr Cancer Drug Targets*. 2012 Jan 1;12(1):23–43.
13. O'Reilly MS, Boehm T, Shing Y, Fukai N, Vasios G, Lane WS, Flynn E, Birkhead JR, Olsen BR, Folkman J. Endostatin: an endogenous inhibitor of angiogenesis and tumor growth. *Cell*. 1997;88(2):277–5. https://doi.org/10.1016/s0092-8674(00)81848-6
14. Lawler J, Detmar M, Harrington EO. Role of thrombospondin-1 and -2 in regulating tumor progression. *Semin Cancer Biol*. 2001;12(2):97–106.
15. Sund M, Hamano Y, Sugimoto H, Sudhakar A, Soubasakos M, Yerramalla U, Benjamin LE, Lawler J, Kieran M, Shah A, et al. Function of endogenous inhibitors of angiogenesis as endothelium-specific tumor suppressors. *Proc Natl Acad Sci U S A*. 2005;102:2934–9.
16. Heath VL, Bicknell R. Anticancer strategies involving the vasculature. *Nat Rev Clin Oncol*. 2009;6:395–404.
17. Debela DT, Muzazu SG, Heraro KD, Ndalama MT, Mesele BW, Haile DC, Kitui SK, Manyazewal T. New approaches and procedures for cancer treatment: Current perspectives. *SAGE Open Med*. 2021 Aug 12;9:20503121211034366.
18. Rini BI, Tamaskar I, Shaheen P, Salas R, Garcia J, Wood L, Reddy S, Dreicer R, Bukowski RM. Hypothyroidism in patients with metastatic renal cell carcinoma treated with sunitinib. *J Natl Cancer Inst*. 2007;99:81–3.
19. Motzer RJ, Hutson TE, Tomczak P, Michaelson MD, Bukowski RM, Rixe O, Oudard S, Negrier S, Szczylik C, Kim ST, et al. Sunitinib versus interferon Alfa in metastatic renal-cell carcinoma. *N Engl J Med*. 2007;356:115–24.
20. Kawasaki ES, Player A. Nanotechnology, nanomedicine, and the development of new, effective therapies for cancer. *Nanomedicine*. 2005 Jun 1;1(2):101–9.
21. He Y, Lin J, Kong D, Huang M, Xu C, Kim T-K, Etheridge A, Luo Y, Ding Y, Wang K. Current state of circulating MicroRNAs as cancer biomarkers. *Clin Chem*. 2015;61:1138–55.

22. Hu CM, Zhang L. Therapeutic nanoparticles to combat cancer drug resistance. *Curr Drug Metabol.* 2009 Oct 1;10(8):836–41.
23. Xu JL, Jin B, Ren ZH, Lou YQ, Zhou ZR, Yang QZ, Han BH. Chemotherapy plus Erlotinib versus chemotherapy alone for treating advanced non-small cell lung cancer: a meta-analysis. *PLoS ONE.* 2015;10:e0131278.
24. Wang T, Suita Y, Miriyala S, Dean J, Tapinos N, Shen J. Advances in lipid-based nanoparticles for cancer chemoimmunotherapy. *Pharmaceutics.* 2021 Apr 9;13(4):520.
25. Parhi P, Mohanty C, Sahoo SK. Nanotechnology-based combinational drug delivery: an emerging approach for cancer therapy. *Drug Discov Today.* 2012;17:1044–52.
26. Surendiran A, Sandhiya S, Pradhan SC, Adithan C. Novel applications of nanotechnology in medicine. *Ind J Med Res.* 2009 Dec 1;130(6):689–701.
27. Gad A, Kydd J, Piel B, Rai P. Targeting cancer using polymeric nanoparticle mediated combination chemotherapy. *Int J Nanomed Nanosurg.* 2016;2:1–12.
28. Hiss DC, Gabriels GA, Folb PI. Combination of tunicamycin with anticancer drugs synergistically enhances their toxicity in multidrug-resistant human ovarian cystadenocarcinoma cells. *Cancer Cell Int.* 2007;7:1–14.
29. Siddhardha B, Parasuraman P. Theranostics application of nanomedicine in cancer detection and treatment. In *Nanomaterials for drug delivery and therapy.* (pp. 59–89). William Andrew Publishing. 2019 Jan 1.
30. Ning Xu, Haifeng Lin, Sheng Lin , Wanling Zhang, Shuang Han, Nakajima Hizuru, Mao Sifeng, Lin Jin-Ming. A fluidic isolation-assisted homogeneous-flow-pressure chip-solid phase extraction-mass spectrometry system for online dynamic monitoring of 25-hydroxyvitamin D3 biotransformation in cells. *Anal Chem.* 2021;93(4):2273–80.
31. Xu X, Ho W, Zhang X, Bertrand N, Farokhzad O. Cancer nanomedicine: From targeted delivery to combination therapy. *Trends Mol Med.* 2015;21:223–32.
32. Matsumura Y, Maeda H. A new concept for macromolecular therapeutics in cancer chemotherapy: mechanism of tumoritropic accumulation of proteins and the antitumor agent smancs. *Cancer Res.* 1986;46(12 Pt 1):6387–92.
33. Hu J, Wang J, Wang G, Yao Z, Dang X. Pharmacokinetics and antitumor efficacy of DSPE-PEG2000 polymeric liposomes loaded with quercetin and temozolomide: analysis of their effectiveness in enhancing the chemosensitization of drug-resistant glioma cells. *Int J Mol Med.* 2016;37:690–702.
34. Cabral H, Kataoka K. Progress of drug-loaded polymeric micelles into clinical studies. *J Control Release.* 2014;190:465–76.
35. Voinea M, Simionescu M. Designing of "intelligent" liposomes for efficient delivery of drugs. *J Cell Mol Med.* 2002;6:465–74.
36. Couvreur P, Vauthier C. Nanotechnology: intelligent design to treat complex disease. *Pharm Res.* 2006;23:1417–50.
37. Hubert A, Lyass O, Pode D, Gabizon A. Doxil (Caelyx): an exploratory study with pharmacokinetics in patients with hormone-refractory prostate cancer. *Anticancer Drugs.* 2000;11:123–7.
38. Croy SR, Kwon GS. Polymeric micelles for drug delivery. *Curr Pharm Design.* 2006 Dec 1;12(36):4669–84 .
39. Guaglianone P, Chan K, DelaFlor-Weiss E, Hanisch R, Jeffers S, Sharma D, Muggia F. Phase I and pharmacologie study of liposomal daunorubicin (DaunoXome). *Investig New Drugs.* 1994;12:103–10.
40. Forssen EA, Malé-Brune R, Adler-Moore JP, Lee MJ, Schmidt PG, Krasieva TB, Shimizu S, Tromberg BJ. Fluorescence imaging studies for the disposition of daunorubicin liposomes (DaunoXome) within tumor tissue. *Cancer Res.* 1996;56:2066–75.
41. Jun Chen, Feng Chen, Lei Zhang, Zhangyou Yang, Tao Deng, Yunfei Zhao, Tianye Zheng, Xuelan Gan, Hangtian Zhong, Yanqing Geng, Xinwei Fu, Yuanqiang Wang, Chao Yu. Self-assembling porphyrins as a single therapeutic agent for synergistic cancer therapy: a one stone three birds strategy. *ACS Appl Mater Interfaces.* 2021;13(24):27856–67.
42. Jinghua Sun, Liping Li, Wenwen Cai, Anqi Chen, Ruiping Zhang. Multifunctional hybrid nanoprobe for photoacoustic/PET/MR imaging-guided photothermal therapy of laryngeal cancer. *ACS Appl Bio Mater.* 2021;4(6):5312–23.

43. Biswas MC, Islam MT, Nandy PK, Hossain MM. Graphene quantum dots (GQDs) for bioimaging and drug delivery applications: a review. *ACS Mater Lett.* 2021;3(6):889–911.
44. Qiuhong Zhang, Junmin Zhang, Jun Song, Yizhen Liu, Xiangzhong Ren, Yanli Zhao. Protein-based nanomedicine for therapeutic benefits of cancer. *ACS Nano.* 2021;15(5):8001–38.
45. Cheng Tan, Jianqiang Wu, Zhi Wen. Doxorubicin-loaded MnO2@Zeolitic imidazolate framework-8 nanoparticles as a chemophotothermal system for lung cancer therapy. *ACS Omega.* 2021;6(20):12977–83.
46. Xiaotong Cheng, Hai-Dong Xu, Huan-Huan Ran, Gaolin Liang, Fu-Gen Wu. Glutathione-depleting nanomedicines for synergistic cancer therapy. *ACS Nano.* 2021;15(5):8039–68.
47. Yanyan Cui, Xi Chen, Yan Cheng, Xinyi Lu, Jiajia Meng, Ziwei Chen, Mengke Li, Chengcheng Lin, Yaling Wang, Jian Yang. CuWO4 nanodots for NIR-induced photodynamic and chemodynamic synergistic therapy. *ACS Appl Mater Interfaces.* 2021;13(19):22150–8.
48. Chavanpatil MD, Khdair A, Panyam J. Nanoparticles for cellular drug delivery: mechanisms and factors influencing delivery. *J Nanosci Nanotechnol.* 2006 Sep 1;6(9–10):2651–63.
49. Cabral H, Kataoka K. Progress of drug-loaded polymeric micelles into clinical studies. *J Control Release.* 2014;190:465–76.
50. Torchilin V. Tumor delivery of macromolecular drugs based on the EPR effect. *Adv Drug Deliv Rev.* 2007;63(3):131–5.
51. Maeda H. SMANCS and polymer-conjugated macromolecular drugs: advantages in cancer chemotherapy. *Adv Drug Deliv Rev.* 2001 Mar 1;46(1–3):169–85.
52. Genji Srinivasulu Y, Mozhi A, Goswami N, Yao Q, Xie J. Traceable nanocluster–prodrug conjugate for chemo-photodynamic combinatorial therapy of non-small cell lung cancer. *ACS Appl Bio Mater.* 2021;4(4): 3232–45.
53. Niculescu AG, Grumezescu AM. Polymer-based nanosystems—a versatile delivery approach. *Materials.* 2021 Nov 11;14(22):6812.
54. Yang Zou, Saran Long, Tao Xiong, Xueze Zhao, Wen Sun, Jianjun Du, Jiangli Fan, Xiaojun Peng. Single-molecule förster resonance energy transfer-based photosensitizer for synergistic photodynamic/photothermal therapy. *ACS Cent Sci.* 2021;7(2):327–34.
55. Prasad R, Jain NK, Yadav AS, Jadhav M, Radharani NNV, Gorain M, Kundu GC, Conde J, Srivastava R. Ultrahigh penetration and retention of graphene quantum dot mesoporous silica nanohybrids for image guided tumor regression. *ACS Appl Bio Mater.* 2021;4(2):1693–703.
56. Cagel M, Grotz E, Bernabeu E, Moretton MA, Chiappetta DA. Doxorubicin: nanotechnological overviews from bench to bedside. *Drug Discov Today.* 2017 Feb 1;22(2):270–81.
57. Xin Sun, Guihua He, Chuxiao Xiong, Chenyuan Wang, Xiang Lian, Liefeng Hu, Zhike Li, Scott J Dalgarno, Ying-Wei Yang, Jian Tian. One-pot fabrication of hollow porphyrinic MOF nanoparticles with ultrahigh drug loading toward controlled delivery and synergistic cancer therapy. *ACS Appl Mater Interfaces.* 2021;13(3):3679–93.
58. Chao Qi, Jin He, Lian-Hua Fu, Ting He, Nicholas Thomas Blum, Xikuang Yao, Jing Lin, Peng Huang. Tumor-specific activatable nanocarriers with gas-generation and signal amplification capabilities for tumor theranostics. *ACS Nano.* 2021;15(1):1627–39.
59. Ruijiao Sun, YongHao Ge, Hongxing Liu, Peng He, Weiling Song, Xiaoru Zhang. Erythrocyte membrane-encapsulated glucose oxidase and manganese/ferrite nanocomposite as a biomimetic "All in one" nanoplatform for cancer therapy. *ACS Appl Bio Mater.* 2021;4(1):701–10.
60. Bin Qiao, Yuanli Luo, Hong-Bo Cheng, Jianli Ren, Jin Cao, Chao Yang, Bing Liang, Anyu Yang, Xun Yuan, Jinrui Li, Liming Deng, Pan Li, Hai-Tao Ran, Lan Hao, Zhiyi Zhou, Maoping Li, Yuanyuan Zhang, Peter S Timashev, Xing-Jie Liang, Zhigang Wang. Artificial nanotargeted cells with stable photothermal performance for multimodal imaging-guided tumor-specific therapy. *ACS Nano.* 2020;14(10):12652–67.
61. Waite CL, Roth CM. Nanoscale drug delivery systems for enhanced drug penetration into solid tumors: current progress and opportunities. *Crit Rev Biomed Eng.* 2012;40(1):21–41.
62. Overchuk M, Harmatys KM, Sindhwani S, Rajora MA, Koebel A, Charron DM, Syed AM, Chen J, Pomper MG, Wilson BC, Chan WCW, Zheng G. Subtherapeutic photodynamic treatment facilitates tumor nanomedicine delivery and overcomes desmoplasia. *Nano Lett.* 2021;21(1):344–52.
63. Negut I, Bita B. Polymeric micellar systems—a special emphasis on "smart" drug delivery. *Pharmaceutics.* 2023 Mar 17;15(3):976.

64. Changchun Wen, Hua Chen, Xiaolu Guo, Zhaoxing Lin, Shuping Zhang, Xing-Can Shen, Hong Liang. Lysosome-targeted gold nanotheranostics for in situ SERS monitoring pH and multimodal imaging-guided phototherapy. *Langmuir*. 2021;37(1):569–77.
65. Zhihao Chen, Wanting Wang, Yusheng Li, Cui Wei, Ping Zhong, Dahua He, Huan Liu, Pengfei Wang, Zhenpeng Huang, Wanye Zhu, Yi Zhou, Linghao Qin. Folic acid-modified erythrocyte membrane loading dual drug for targeted and chemo-photothermal synergistic cancer therapy. *Mol Pharm.* 2021;18(1):386–402.
66. Jing Zhang, Yongtian Liu, Xiang Wang, Jun Du, Kang Song, Bing Li, Haizhou Chang, Ruizhuo Ouyang, Yuqing Miao, Yun Sun, Yuhao Li. Nanozyme-incorporated biodegradable bismuth mesoporous radiosensitizer for tumor microenvironment-modulated hypoxic tumor thermoradiotherapy. *ACS Appl Mater Interfaces.* 2020;12(52):57768–81.
67. Lu Y, Park K. Polymeric micelles and alternative nanonized delivery vehicles for poorly soluble drugs. *Int J Pharm.* 2013 Aug 30;453(1):198–214.
68. Shuyue Ye, Chaoxiang Cui, Xiaju Cheng, Meng Zhao, Qiulian Mao, Yuqi Zhang, Anna Wang, Jing Fang, Yan Zhao, Haibin Shi. Red light-initiated cross-linking of NIR probes to cytoplasmic RNA: an innovative strategy for prolonged imaging and unexpected tumor suppression. *J Am Chem Soc.* 2020;142(51):21502–12.
69. Danhier F, Feron O, Préat V. To exploit the tumor microenvironment: Passive and active tumor targeting of nanocarriers for anti-cancer drug delivery. *J Control Release.* 2010;148(2):135–46.
70. Cabral H, Kataoka K. Progress of drug-loaded polymeric micelles into clinical studies. *JControl Release.* 2014;190:465–76.
71. Hami Z, Amini M, Ghazi-Khansari M, Rezayat SM, Gilani K. Doxorubicin-conjugated PLA-PEG-folate based polymeric micelle for tumor-targeted delivery: synthesis and in vitro evaluation. *Daru.* 2014 Mar 6;22(1):30.
72. Yijian Gao, Qianqian Li, Chunli Li, Leyi Gao, Huan Chen, Tingting Liu, Yongwei Huang, Zhonghua Liu, Shengliang Li. Terselenophene regioisomer conjugated polymer materials for high-performance cancer phototheranostics. *ACS Appl Mater Interfaces.* 2020;12(50):55605–13.
73. Marin-Valencia I, Yang C, Mashimo T, Cho S, Baek H, Yang X-L, Rajagopalan KN, Maddie M, Vemireddy V, Zhao Z, et al. Analysis of tumor metabolism reveals mitochondrial glucose oxidation in genetically diverse human glioblastomas in the mouse brain in vivo. *Cell Metab.* 2012;15:827–37.
74. Li YL, Zhu XM, Liang H, Orvig C, Chen ZF. Recent advances in asialoglycoprotein receptor and glycyrrhetinic acid receptor-mediated and/or pH-responsive hepatocellular carcinoma-targeted drug delivery. Curr Med Chem. 2021 Mar 1;28(8):1508–34.
75. Zhiliang Gao, Zhonghe Zhang, Jianman Guo, Jingcheng Hao, Peiyu Zhang, Jiwei Cui. Polypeptide nanoparticles with pH-sheddable PEGylation for improved drug delivery. *Langmuir.* 2020;36(45):13656–62.
76. Lee ES, Gao Z, Bae YH. Recent progress in tumor pH targeting nanotechnology. *J Control Release.* 2008;132(3):164–70. https://doi.org/10.1016/j.jconrel.2008.05.013
77. Torchilin VP. Targeted polymeric micelles for delivery of poorly soluble drugs. *Cell Mol Life Sci.* 2004;61(19–20):2549–59.
78. Yongxin Li, Roy C. H. Wong, Xuehai Yan, Dennis K. P. Ng, Pui-Chi Lo. Self-assembled nanophotosensitizing systems with Zinc(II) phthalocyanine-peptide conjugates as building blocks for targeted chemo-photodynamic therapy. *ACS Appl Bio Mater.* 2020;3(9):5463–73.
79. Zhu C, Xiao J, Tang M, Feng H, Chen W, Du M. Platinum covalent shell cross-linked micelles designed to deliver doxorubicin for synergistic combination cancer therapy. *Int J Nanomed.* 2017;12:3697–710.
80. Dongdong Wang, Conghui Liu, Shiquan You, Kai Zhang, Meng Li, Yu Cao, Changtao Wang, Haifeng Dong, Xueji Zhang. Bacterial vesicle-cancer cell hybrid membrane-coated nanoparticles for tumor specific immune activation and photothermal therapy. *ACS Appl Mater Interfaces.* 2020;12(37):41138–47.
81. Yi Zhao, Biao-Qi Chen, Ranjith Kumar Kankala, Shi-Bin Wang, Ai-Zheng Chen. Recent advances in combination of copper chalcogenide-based photothermal and reactive oxygen species-related therapies. *ACS Biomater Sci Eng.* 2020;6(9):4799–815.
82. Ugarenko M, Chan CK, Nudelman A, Rephaeli A, Cutts SM, Phillips DR. Development of pluronic micelle-encapsulated doxorubicin and formaldehyde-releasing prodrugs for localized anticancer chemotherapy. *Oncol Res.* 2009;17(7):283–99.

83. Yan Ma, Dong-Yang Zhang, Zhuo Peng, Shixia Guan, Junqiu Zhai. Delivery of platinum (IV) prodrugs via Bi2Te3 nanoparticles for photothermal–chemotherapy and photothermal/photoacoustic imaging. *Mol Pharm.* 2020;17(9):3403–11.
84. Lei Ding, Xiao Lin, Ziguo Lin, Yanni Wu, Xiaolong Liu, Jingfeng Liu, Ming Wu, Xiaolong Zhang, Yongyi Zeng. Cancer cell-targeted photosensitizer and therapeutic protein co-delivery nanoplatform based on a metal–organic framework for enhanced synergistic photodynamic and protein therapy. *ACS Appl Mater Interfaces.* 2020;12(33):36906–16.
85. Katiyar SS, Muntimadugu E, Rafeeqi TA, Domb AJ, Khan W. Co-delivery of rapamycin- and piperine-loaded polymeric nanoparticles for breast cancer treatment. *Drug Deliv.* 2015;23:2608–16.
86. Khan MA, Zafaryab M, Mehdi SH, Ahmad I, Rizvi MMA. Characterization and anti-proliferative activity of curcumin loaded chitosan nanoparticles in cervical cancer. *Int J Biol Macromol.* 2016;93:242–53.
87. Surnar B, Jayakannan M. Triple block nanocarrier platform for synergistic cancer therapy of antagonistic drugs. *Biomacromolecules.* 2016;17:4075–85.
88. Kumar P, Wasim L, Chopra M, Chhikara A. Co-delivery of vorinostat and etoposide via disulfide cross-linked biodegradable polymeric nanogels: synthesis, characterization, biodegradation, and anticancer activity. *AAPS Pharm Sci Tech.* 2018;19:634–47.
89. Torchilin VP. PEG-based micelles as carriers of contrast agents for different imaging modalities. Adv Drug Deliv Rev. 2002 Feb 21;54(2):235–52.
90. Bae Y, Diezi TA, Zhao A, Kwon GS. Mixed polymeric micelles for combination cancer chemotherapy through the concurrent delivery of multiple chemotherapeutic agents. *J Control Release.* 2007;122:324–30.
91. Xiao H, Song H, Yang Q, Cai H, Qi R, Yan L, Liu S, Zheng Y, Huang Y, Liu T, et al. A prodrug strategy to deliver cisplatin(IV) and paclitaxel in nanomicelles to improve efficacy and tolerance. *Biomaterials.* 2012;33:6507–19.
92. Zheng C, Zheng M, Gong P, Deng J, Yi H, Zhang P, Zhang Y, Liu P, Ma Y, Cai L. Polypeptide cationic micelles mediated co-delivery of docetaxel and siRNA for synergistic tumor therapy. *Biomaterials.* 2013;34:3431–8.
93. Wang T, Yang S, Mei LA, Parmar CK, Gillespie JW, Praveen KP, Petrenko VA, Torchilin VP. Paclitaxel-loaded PEG-PE-based micellar nanopreparations targeted with tumor-specific landscape phage fusion protein enhance apoptosis and efficiently reduce tumors. *Mol Cancer Ther.* 2014;13:2864–75.
94. Huang X, Liao W, Zhang G, Kang S, Zhang CY. pH-sensitive micelles self-assembled from polymer brush (PAE-*g*-cholesterol)-*b*-PEG-*b*-(PAE-*g*-cholesterol) for anticancer drug delivery and controlled release. *Int J Nanomedicine.* 2017 Mar 21;12 :2215–26.
95. Djordjevic J, Del Rosario LS, Wang J, Uhrich KE. Amphiphilic scorpion-like macromolecules as micellar nanocarriers. *J Bioact Compat Polym.* 2008;23:532–51.
96. Taillefer J, Jones M-C, Brasseur N, van Lier JE, Leroux J-C. Preparation and characterization of pH-responsive polymeric micelles for the delivery of photosensitizing anticancer drugs. *J Pharm Sci.* 2000;89:52–62.
97. Roby A, Erdogan S, Torchilin VP. Solubilization of poorly soluble PDT agent, meso-tetraphenylporphin, in plain or immunotargeted PEG-PE micelles results in dramatically improved cancer cell killing in vitro. *Eur J Pharm Biopharm.* 2006;62:235–40.
98. Roby A, Erdogan S, Torchilin VP. Enhanced in vivo antitumor efficacy of poorly soluble PDT agent, meso-tetraphenylporphine, in PEG-PE-based tumor-targeted immunomicelles. *Cancer Biol Ther.* 2007;6:1136–42.
99. Iyer AK, Greish K, Seki T, Okazaki S, Fang J, Takeshita K, Maeda H. Polymeric micelles of zinc protoporphyrin for tumor targeted delivery based on EPR effect and singlet oxygen generation. *J Drug Target.* 2007;15:496–506.
100. Shin H-C, Alani AWG, Rao DA, Rockich NC, Kwon GS. Multi-drug loaded polymeric micelles for simultaneous delivery of poorly soluble anticancer drugs. *J Control Release.* 2009;140:294–300.
101. Kenmotsu H, Yasunaga M, Goto K, Nagano T, Kuroda J, Koga Y, Takahashi A, Nishiwaki Y, Matsumura Y. The antitumor activity of NK012, an SN-38-incorporating micelle, in combination with bevacizumab against lung cancer xenografts. *Cancer.* 2010;116:4597–604.
102. Lammers, T, Storm G, Kiessling F. Nanomedicine formulations for combination therapies. *Nano Rev.* 2010;1 :1–3.

103. Jang YL, Yun UJ, Lee MS, Kim MG, Son S, Lee K, Chae SY, Lim DW, Kim HT, Kim SH, et al. Cell-penetrating peptide mimicking polymer-based combined delivery of paclitaxel and siRNA for enhanced tumor growth suppression. *Int J Pharm.* 2012;434:488–93.
104. Jin X, Mo R, Ding Y, Zheng W, Zhang C. Paclitaxel-loaded N-Octyl-O-sulfate Chitosan micelles for superior cancer therapeutic efficacy and overcoming drug resistance. *Mol Pharm.* 2014;11:145–57.
105. Salzano G, Navarro G, Trivedi MS, De Rosa G, Torchilin VP. Multifunctional polymeric micelles co-loaded with anti-survivin siRNA and paclitaxel overcome drug resistance in an animal model of ovarian cancer. *Mol Cancer Ther.* 2015;14:1075–84.
106. Yang C, Liu SQ, Venkataraman S, Gao SJ, Ke X, Chia XT, Hedrick JL, Yang YY. Structure-directing star-shaped block copolymers: supramolecular vesicles for the delivery of anticancer drugs. *J Control Release.* 2015;208:93–105.
107. Wang N, Wang Z, Nie S, Song L, He T, Yang S, Yang X, Yi C, Wu Q, Gong C. Biodegradable polymeric micelles coencapsulating paclitaxel and honokiol: a strategy for breast cancer therapy in vitro and in vivo. *Int J Nanomed.* 2017;12:1499–514.
108. Kulhari H, Pooja D, Shrivastava S, Telukutala SR, Barui AK, Patra CR, Naidu Vegi GM, Adams DJ, Sistla R. Cyclic-RGDfK peptide conjugated succinoyl-TPGS nanomicelles for targeted delivery of docetaxel to integrin receptor over-expressing angiogenic tumours. *Nanomed Nanotechnol Biol Med.* 2015;11:1511–20.
109. Ruttala HB, Chitrapriya N, Kaliraj K, Ramasamy T, Shin WH, Jeong J-H, Kim JR, Ku SK, Choi H-G, Yong CS, et al. Facile construction of bioreducible crosslinked polypeptide micelles for enhanced cancer combination therapy. *Acta Biomater.* 2017;63:135–49.
110. Tomalia DA, Fréchet JMJ. Discovery of dendrimers and dendritic polymers: a brief historical perspective*. *J Polym Sci Part A Polym Chem.* 2002;40:2719–28.
111. Abbasi E, Aval S, Akbarzadeh A, Milani M, Nasrabadi H, Joo S, Hanifehpour Y, Nejati-Koshki K, Pashaei-Asl R. Dendrimers: synthesis, applications, and properties. *Nanoscale Res Lett.* 2014;9:247.
112. Clementi C, Miller K, Mero A, Satchi-Fainaro R, Pasut G. Dendritic poly (ethylene glycol) bearing paclitaxel and alendronate for targeting bone neoplasms. *Mol Pharm.* 2011;8:1063–72.
113. Duncan R, Izzo L. Dendrimer biocompatibility and toxicity. *Adv Drug Deliv Rev.* 2005;57:2215–37.
114. Patel HN, Patel PM. Dendrimer applications—a review. *Int J Pharma Bio Sci.* 2013;4:454–63.
115. Lai P-S, Lou P-J, Peng C-L, Pai C-L, Yen W-N, Huang M-Y, Young T-H, Shieh M-J. Doxorubicin delivery by polyamidoamine dendrimer conjugation and photochemical internalization for cancer therapy. *J Control Release.* 2007;122:39–46.
116. Gardikis K, Hatziantoniou S, Bucos M, Fessas D, Signorelli M, Felekis T, Zervou M, Screttas CG Steele BR, Ionov M, et al. New drug delivery nanosystem combining liposomal and dendrimeric technology (Liposomal locked-in dendrimers) for cancer therapy. *J Pharm Sci.* 2010;99:3561–71.
117. Thomas TP, Joice M, Sumit M, Silpe JE, Kotlyar A, Bharathi S, Kukowska-Latallo J, Baker JR, Choi SK, Choi SK. Design and in vitro validation of multivalent dendrimer methotrexates as a folate-targeting anticancer therapeutic. *Curr Pharm Des.* 2013;19:6594–605.
118. Kala S, Mak ASC, Liu X, Posocco P, Pricl S, Peng L, Wong AST. Combination of dendrimer-nanovector-mediated small interfering RNA delivery to target Akt with the clinical anticancer drug paclitaxel for effective and potent anticancer activity in treating ovarian cancer. *J Med Chem.* 2014; 57:2634–42.
119. Taratula O, Schumann C, Duong T, Taylor KL, Taratula O. Dendrimer-encapsulated naphthalocyanine as a single agent-based theranostic nanoplatform for near-infrared fluorescence imaging and combinatorial anticancer phototherapy. *Nanoscale.* 2015;7:3888–902.

10 Multipurpose Micellar Nanomedicine for the Treatment of Cancer

10.1 INTRODUCTION

Over 10 million new cases of cancer are diagnosed with the disease each year, making it one of the leading causes of death globally. Radiation, chemotherapy, and surgical resection are the available treatment options at this time. However, despite the FDA having approved more than 90 chemotherapeutic medications for clinical use, dose-limiting toxicity and patient morbidity have significantly impeded these medications' effectiveness [1]. Supramolecular core–shell nanoparticles called polymeric micelles have several benefits for cancer treatment and detection. Their spherical particles are supramolecular constructs that self-assemble into biocompatible, amphiphilic block copolymers in aqueous environments. These particles are nanosized, usually falling between 10 and 100 nm. The block copolymer's hydrophilic segment forms a coronal layer in water, while the hydrophobic portion self-associates into a semi-solid core. Because the outer shell shields the micelle from quick clearance and the hydrophobic core can serve as a reservoir for drugs that are insoluble in water, the resulting core–shell architecture is significant for drug delivery [2–4]. Rapid cell proliferation, the potential to induce angiogenesis, and the facilitation of invasion and metastasis make cancer the "most dreaded illness." It is challenging to design an effective treatment approach for cancer since there is no unique defining characteristic shared by the great majority of tumors [5]. Cancer is a disease that can strike anywhere in the body, although it is most commonly seen in the lungs, the breasts of women, the prostate, and the liver. Malignant tumors, the primary cause of death in humans, are the outcome of cancer's rapid and unregulated cell growth in a variety of internal organs. Physical agents like ultraviolet (UV) light and ionizing radiation, chemical agents like asbestos, cigarettes, and arsenic, and biological agents like viruses, bacteria, and parasites can all lead to cancer in humans [6].

Better education, clinical diagnostic tools, and treatment may avert 30–50% of cancer-related fatalities, according to the World Health Organization. In the last 10 years, cancer therapy has made tremendous strides forward. There are benefits and drawbacks to using tried-and-true methods like surgery, chemotherapy, and radiation to treat cancer [7, 8]. Although traditional chemotherapy is effective against cancer, it has several limitations, including its inability to target specific cancer cells, the rapid clearance of many anticancer agents, resistance to the drug, plus the toxicity generated from chemotherapeutics themselves often or at higher dosages after its administration [9]. Figure 10.1 describes the nanoscale supramolecular structures made of biocompatible amphiphilic block copolymers.

In patients with stage IV cancer, chemotherapy has demonstrated some benefit when administered alone. It has also demonstrated some benefits when combined with radiotherapy in patients with locally advanced cancer and the preoperative period in patients with early-stage non-small cell lung cancer. Based on clinical trials and meta-analyses, platinum drugs are still deemed to be of

DOI: 10.1201/9781003451020-10

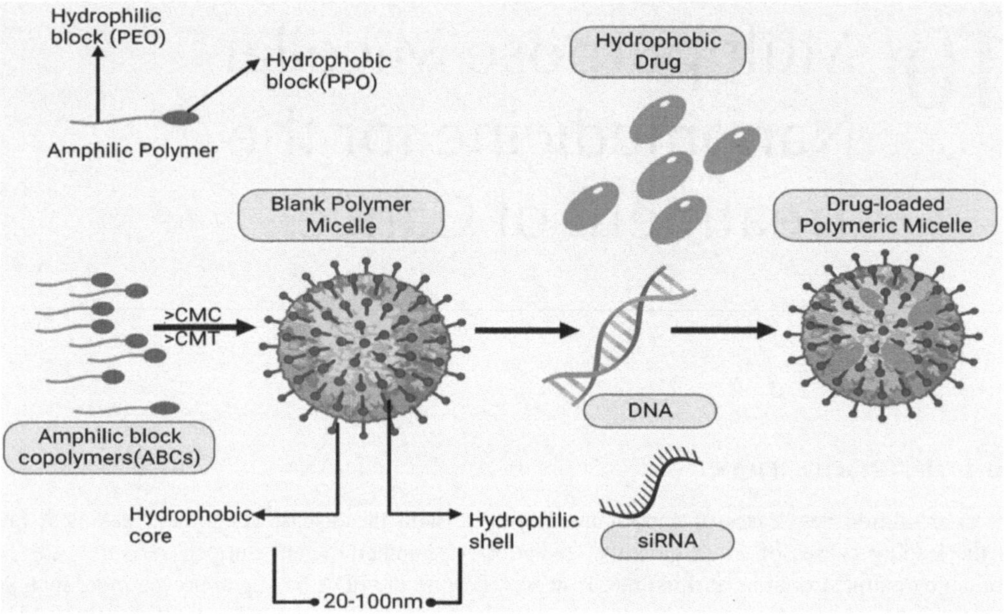

FIGURE 10.1 Diagrammatic illustration of nanoscale supramolecular structures made of biocompatible amphiphilic block copolymers.

significant interest. Their observed toxicity and intrinsic resistance are a drawback. Chemotherapy's low effectiveness and significant toxicity have contributed to years of widespread pessimism about the treatment due to the lack of discernible improvement in survival rates [10, 11]. As a result of their electronegative surfaces as well as zeta potential, the majority of anticancer medications are unable to enter their target cells. Because the negative charge at the cytomembranes drives the medicines back [12]. As a result, doctors often prescribe excessively high doses of the drug in the hope that the effects would last longer than they would otherwise. Customized drug delivery carriers are currently increasingly appealing for application in cancer therapy because they may increase therapeutic and diagnostic efficacy while decreasing undesirable effects [13]. For this reason, research has focused on developing chemotherapeutics that target cancer cells while sparing healthy tissue. Because of the need to maintain therapeutic drug concentrations over extended periods, regulated drug delivery systems must be carefully crafted.

The advantages of organic and inorganic drug delivery are extremely promising candidates that have already shown success in clinical applications for the development of drug delivery systems for cancer therapy. Because they can limit the systemic side effects that patients must endure during traditional chemotherapy by ensuring that the cytotoxic levels of the drugs are only present at the tumor sites, drug delivery systems based on nanoparticles are superior to conventional anticancer drugs [14].

10.2 POLYMERIC MICELLES FOR CANCER THERAPY: FEATURES AND ADVANTAGES

Among the earliest polymeric self-assemblies are PMs. Since they offer several physicochemical and biological advantages over other types of nanoassemblies, such as easy preparation, simple architecture, drug solubilization, improved biocompatibility, pharmacokinetics, and biodistribution, as well as more opportunities for further engineering, they have drawn a great deal of attention in the biomedical sciences over the past few decades, particularly as drug carriers. The biocompatible amphiphilic block copolymers create nanoscaled (usually between 10 and 100 nm) supramolecular structures in water (Figure 10.1) [15]. When a block copolymer's hydrophobic and hydrophilic components are mixed in water, the hydrophobic component produces a coronal layer, and the hydrophilic component a semisolid core. The hydrophobic center of the micelle can store drugs that are insoluble in water, and the micelle's outermost layer will prevent the drug from being expelled too fast [16–20]. PEG with a molecular weight of 2–15 kDa is the most widely used hydrophilic block. Conversely, polyesters, polyethers, or polyamino acids, such as poly(l-aspartic acid), PLA, poly(ε-caprolactone) (PCL), and poly(propylene oxide) (PPO), are usually used as hydrophobic blocks. The ability of polymers to spontaneously self-assemble into nanoscale aggregates is what distinguishes PMs. The hydrophilic segments form a corona or shell around the semisolid core of the hydrophobic blocks when they self-associate in aqueous solutions. The body's longer circulation time is caused by the hydrophilic shell, which also minimizes non-specific uptake by the reticuloendothelial system (RES) and offers steric stability [21–23]. Polymer micelles enable the *in vivo* application of medicines that would have been too hydrophobic or poisonous in the past without altering the drug's chemical structure. Due to its protected location within the polymer core, the medication is less likely to be broken down or rendered ineffective by digestive enzymes. The hydrophilic micellar corona is essential for biomedical applications because it blocks opsonin proteins from recognizing particles. Lacking its bristle-like covering, the micelle would be rapidly absorbed by the reticuloendothelial system (RES) [24]. Because of their low critical micelle concentration (CMC, the concentration limit of polymers at which micelles are generated, frequently in the range of 106–107 M), micelles are durable structures that do not disintegrate easily *in vivo* [25]. Furthermore, the stimuli-sensitive breakdown gives the micelles a useful way to transfer the medicinal material. The microenvironmental stimuli of tumors include elevated enzymes, hypoxia, and pH. Temperature, light, and ultrasonic stimulation are external stimuli that cause micellar disassembly to be destroyed and release the payload [26, 27].

10.3 THE CONTROL OF CANCER DRUG RELEASE BY NANOCARRIERS

Because of their many intriguing benefits, therapeutic drug delivery systems based on nanocarriers are favored over conventional drug delivery methods. First off, a higher surface-to-volume ratio of the nanocarriers may enable a greater drug contact area with the body under the same drug concentration conditions, improving drug delivery at the same dosage. The drug's toxicity problems and adverse effects will consequently be lessened by the lower dosage. Second, the surface chemistry of nanocarriers can be tuned to target different molecules and drugs. For instance, because it lacks tumor-specific cytotoxicity, the highly effective medication doxorubicin (DOX), which is used to treat a variety of tumor types, also has a significant side effect that can cause serious cardiotoxicity. The potential for prolonged and sustained drug release is made possible by the tuneable surface chemistry, which enhances the drug's bioavailability to the targeted location and time and prolongs its period of circulation beyond that of the drug alone [28–30]. It is important to note that nanocarriers can be either organic or inorganic. Dendrimers, micro/nanogels, polymeric micelles, liposomes, electrospun scaffolds, and nanoassemblies based on block or graft copolymers are all examples of organic nanocarriers [31, 32]. Getting drug delivery mechanisms within the cytoplasm in the cell is one of the primary obstacles to increasing the effectiveness of cancer treatment. Cancerous tissues generally exhibit faulty vascular architecture as well as poor lymphatic drainage because of the significant intercellular gap between the epithelial cells lining the blood vessels. Enhanced permeability, as well as retention (EPR), occurs when nanocarriers extravasate via these crevices and consolidate in tumor tissue. By modifying molecular weight and structure, for instance, with techniques like ATRP RAFT, NMO, and ROMP, the range of uses for polymers is greatly increased. Polymers, a form of flexible material, are becoming commonplace today [32,33].

There are certain benefits to employing solely pure drug administration, but drug delivery using nanoparticulate-based devices expands the range of options available for cancer treatment. By enhancing the medication's stability and solubility, these nanocarriers enhance the pharmacokinetics and therapeutic indices of the implanted chemotherapeutic drugs in comparison to traditional drug delivery systems. By maintaining stable therapeutic levels for longer, they reduce the drug's toxicity [34]. As a result, multifunctional targeted theranostic nanoparticles that effectively combine diagnosis and treatment are in development. Concurrent delivery and diagnosis make it possible to treat and monitor cancer simultaneously, which is a critical advancement toward the realization of personalized medicine. By revealing the true nature of cancer and its side effects in each patient, theranostics for non-invasive cancer screening during treatment can spot new conditions that might benefit from treatment [35]. Because they mostly affect cancer cells while barely affecting healthy cells, nanocarriers loaded with chemotherapeutic drugs minimize the development of chemoresistance [36]. Here is an overview of some of the available organic and inorganic carriers.

10.4 GRAFT POLYMERIC MATERIALS

Polymeric amphiphiles comprising hydrophilic and hydrophobic sections have received increasing attention for their potential to improve the efficacy of anticancer drugs owing to their small size, extended circulation time, and sustained drug release profile. The hydrophilic outer shells of polymeric nanoparticles envelop their hydrophobic cores in the aqueous phase. Hydrophobic anticancer medications can therefore be placed inside the inner core as a nanocontainer [37,38]. By analyzing and applying research on such polymers, we have gained exciting new insights, such as the potential to adjust chemical characteristics by design. Often referred to by the term "block copolymers," graft polymers are a type of polymer in which the side chains are chemically linked to the polymer's backbone in a straight line [39, 40]. Poly(L-lactic acid) (PLLA) has been chosen as the biocompatible biomedical polymer material to be grafted onto the cellulose backbones.

The benefits of both PLLA and cellulose will be combined in copolymers, including amphiphilic and biocompatibility properties. We successfully synthesized the cellulose graft-poly (L-lactic acid) (CE-g-PLLA) in the previous study, and we were able to control the degree of polymerization of poly(L-lactic acid) (DPPLLA), with different DPPLLA of the polymer exhibiting different degradabilities [41]. One of three methods—grafting through, grafting, and grafting onto—has been used so far to produce graft copolymers [42,43]. The promise of densely grafted molecular structures, and in particular brush polymers, for drug administration has prompted a rise in the study of these materials in recent years. It has been researched if diblock grafts of amphiphilic poly(-caprolactone)-b-poly(ethylene glycol) brush polymers may be used to contain and release the chemotherapeutic drug doxorubicin (DOX). DOX was shown to be better delivered to the tumor site after being encapsulated in PEG as well as cholesterol consisting amphiphilic copolymers of diblock brush at higher weight percents [44, 45]. For the simultaneous administration of the chemotherapeutics hydrophobic paclitaxel (PTX) and hydrophilic gemcitabine (GEM), as well as a tumor imaging agent, a multipurpose biodegradable brush polymer–drug conjugate (BPDC) were created by Sun *et al.* [46–49]. Drug moieties attached via a branching point to a polynorbornene backbone as well as a PEG side chain selected for its water solubility make up bivalent macromonomers and bivalent–brush polymers. Nuclear magnetic resonance (NMR) and gel permeation chromatography have both been used to show that ROMP grafting is successful. Camptothecin (CT) and doxorubicin (DOX) are anticancer medicines that can be combined by utilizing a degradable linker to provide continuous release of the drug upon stimulation. The disclosed method, which makes use of the adaptability of graft-through ROMP, is a unique method for adding extra cleavable linkers to such polymers [50–55].

CHEK2-deficient HCT116 colorectal cancer cells can be killed selectively and more effectively with LCS-1 nanoparticle formulations by taking advantage of the synthetic lethal interaction between

CHEK2 and SOD1. The nanoparticles exhibited favorable characteristics, proved to release LCS-1 drug continuously in phosphate-buffered physiological conditions, and were efficiently absorbed by metabolically active cancer cells. These nanoparticles with LCS-1 loaded were hemocompatible, cytocompatible, and non-toxic. Additionally, compared to free LCS-1, the LCS-1-loaded PCL-AC nanoparticles demonstrated enhanced efficacy (240 times) in killing CHEK2-deficient colon cancer cells, lowering the effective dose of LCS-1 needed for the cancer cells to become lethal. The size of NPs increased due to the formation of protein corona, but they still showed cytocompatibility and cellular uptake. As a result, our created nanocarriers for encapsulating LCS-1 may be utilized in preclinical research and may have translational value in treating cancer patients with CHEK2 gene abnormalities.

10.5 MICELLES

Polymeric micelles are nanoparticles generated by the self-assembly of amphiphilic block copolymers in specific solvents above concentrations termed critical micelle concentration (CMC). Micelles, or hydrophobic block domains of amphiphilic molecules (di-, tri-, or graft copolymers with hydrophobic and hydrophilic block domains) form when this concentration is exceeded because the hydrophobic block domains of the molecules orient themselves into a state of minimum energy [61–64]. It is at that crucial concentration that micelles begin to form (CMC). Drying of the hydrophobic tails causes micelles to form exceeding their critical micelle concentration (CMC), which provides an entropically favorable environment. Furthermore, the micelle core is formed when hydrophobic polymers link together through van der Waals forces. As a result, the hydrophilic shell reforms, creating new hydrogen bond networks along with the surrounding water [65]. Figure 10.2 depicts the micellar core to release the drug.

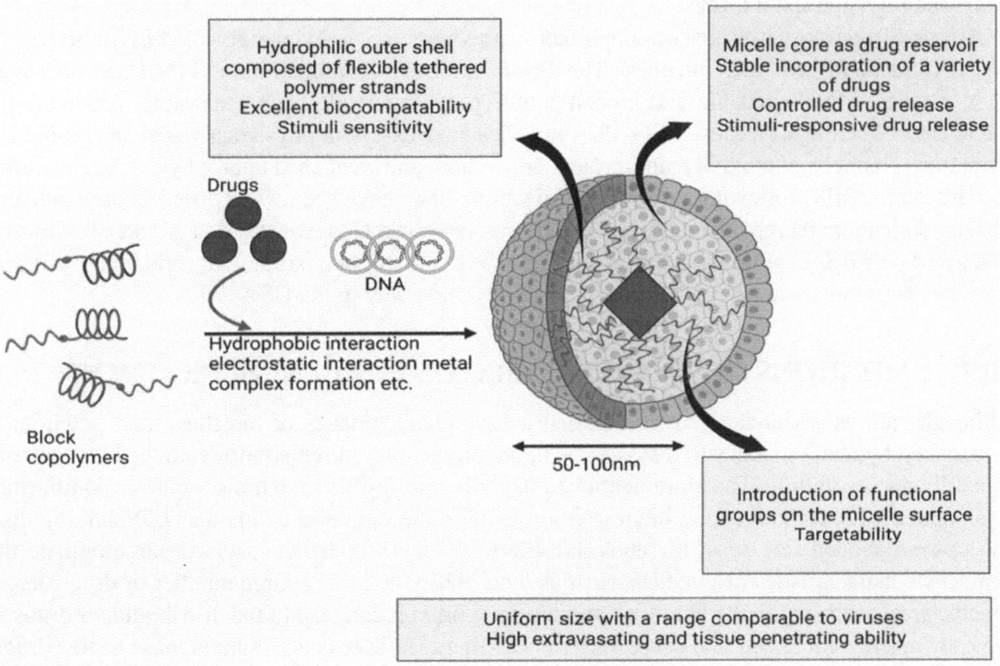

FIGURE 10.2 Drug release from the micellar core is shown schematically.

The EPR effect plays a major role in the tumor targeting of micelles. Recent years have seen the modification of polymeric micelles to actively target the desired site, make them stimuli-responsive, and address issues with early drug leakage and poor *in vivo* stability. To achieve targeted delivery of the micelles in addition to the EPR effect, active targeting primarily entails conjugating targeting moieties on the surface of the micelles.

10.6 CASE STUDIES OF POLYMERIC MICELLES' DRUG DELIVERY

As one of the most well-known amphipathic polymers, polyethylene glycol (PEG)-polylactide (PLA) is ideal for creating micelles. The Food and Drug Administration (FDA) has approved PLA, a type of biodegradable and biocompatible polyester made from renewable resources, for use in clinical settings. Because PEG–PLA micelles have excellent physicochemical and biological properties—namely, non-toxicity, non-protein adsorption, and weakened uptake by the reticuloendothelial system (RES) following intravenous injection—they have been widely used as drug delivery systems for cancer therapy. Notably, in 2007 Korea approved Genexol®-PM, a paclitaxel formulation based on PEG–PLA copolymer micelles, for the treatment of ovarian, lung, and breast cancers. Additionally, clinical development for it is presently underway in the USA [67, 68]. Micelles self-assemble from a combination of hydrophilic and hydrophobic block-copolymers, forming a hydrophobic core enveloped by a hydrophilic shell. Other possible arrangements for these blocks include grafted copolymers, A-B type of copolymers (diblock copolymer), and A-B-A type of copolymers (triblock copolymer) [69]. The hydrophobicity or hydrophilicity of the underlying polymer backbone in grafted polymers is a design choice that is made in light of the desired properties.

Micelle polymers are selected based on their hydrophilic and hydrophobic properties. Careful selection of hydrophilic micelle shells provides steric stability and reduces the likelihood of fast absorption by the reticuloendothelial system (RES), extending the half-life of the drug in circulation [70]. Most hydrophilic polymers use poly(ethylene glycol), or PEG, as their monomer of choice. PEG is a safe steric barrier due to its low toxicity, chemical inertness, biocompatibility, water solubility, and high hydration levels.

As one of the most well-known amphipathic polymers, polyethylene glycol (PEG)-polylactide (PLA) is ideal for creating micelles. The Food and Drug Administration (FDA) has approved PLA, a type of biodegradable and biocompatible polyester made from renewable resources, for use in clinical settings. Because PEG–PLA micelles have excellent physicochemical and biological properties—namely, nontoxicity, non-protein adsorption, and weakened uptake by the reticuloendothelial system (RES) following intravenous injection—they have been widely used as drug delivery systems for cancer therapy. Notably, in 2007 Korea approved Genexol®-PM, a paclitaxel formulation based on PEG–PLA copolymer micelles, for the treatment of ovarian, lung, and breast cancers. Additionally, clinical development for it is presently underway in the USA [75].

10.7 LIMITATIONS OF POLYMERIC MICELLES FOR CANCER TREATMENT

Although various researchers have identified unique characteristics of micelles, their potential is constrained by their tendency to disassociate upon intravenous administration into the bloodstream, primarily due to dilution. The aforementioned factor is responsible for a transition from equilibrium to a unimer state, as well as the binding of proteins to the unimeric components. Protein binding can cause a sudden release of the enclosed drugs into the bloodstream, which can eliminate the distinctive characteristics of micelles, such as their ability to carry a large number of drugs, target specific areas, and stay in the bloodstream for a long time. It can lead to the distribution of drugs in the body in a favorable way and cause toxicity with therapeutic effects similar to those of free drugs. The micellar formulation of Taxotere® exhibited diminished therapeutic efficacy following intravenous administration due to its rapid clearance from the bloodstream [76, 77].

The integrity of micelles is influenced by the physiological milieu. The introduction of micelles into the bloodstream leads to various alterations, such as the breakdown of the micellar structure through hydrolysis of the linkers, among other changes [78–80]. The disturbance of the micellar structure leads to an early liberation of the enclosed medication and the absorption of the medication in healthy tissues/organs, thereby triggering. The loaded drug may experience significant adverse reactions and a decrease in its therapeutic effectiveness [81–85]. One effective method to enhance the stability of micelles is by crosslinking them, which results in the formation of a rigid micellar structure and prolongs their circulation in the bloodstream. Micelles made of mPEG-PDLA were found to have a hydrophilic surface that was composed of a PEG chain. This enhances the micelles' ability to escape from the reticuloendothelial system, which ultimately results in a slower clearance. Enhanced permeability and prolonged circulation time led to a significant accumulation of the formulation in the tumors, which was a preferential accumulation of the formulation. Several studies have reported instances in which substantial optimization of the chemical structures and chain lengths of the block copolymers was essential for successful drug targeting. This is in addition to the problem that was mentioned earlier [86, 87]. The results of this study suggest that a significant amount of polymer chemistry is required to successfully synthesize the controlled chemical structures and chain lengths. An additional drawback of the polymeric micelle systems is that the technology for drug incorporation in a physical manner is still in its infancy. According to the findings of some researchers, the efficiency of drug incorporation processes was dependent on the physical incorporation processes. Therefore, it would appear that there is no universal incorporation method that can be applied to any polymer at this time. In light of this, researchers are required to conduct trial and error to discover an appropriate incorporation method for each unique drug. In addition, the incorporation of the drug may be challenging in certain methods when executed on a large industrial scale, but it is simple and effective when carried out on a smaller scale in the laboratory [88, 89]. When it comes to drug incorporation processes, such as solvent exchange through a dialysis membrane, the scale problem is more significant than the polymer synthesis matter. This is because physical factors, such as diffusion and the rate at which solvents are exchanged, are strongly influenced by the scales. As a result, additional research needs to be conducted in the fields of science and engineering to make significant progress in the field of incorporation technology.

In comparison to the chemical conjugation type of polymeric micelle, the physical entrapment type of micelle has been the subject of a greater number of studies. This is because the chemical conjugation type is more difficult to study. The drug incorporation process does not involve conjugation chemistry. To achieve an appropriate release rate in every drug case, however, the knowledge and technologies that are currently available are not sufficient enough to be obtained at this stage [90–93]. Polymer micelles' durability has also been called into question. Several research groups are hoping to boost *in vivo* stability and address these problems by using core-crosslinked micelles.

The therapeutic value of micelles as anticancer agents has also been questioned. Several research facilities have looked into ways to boost micelle accumulation at the tumor site, to release their contents in a controlled and predictable fashion. Learn how to accomplish micelle multifunctionalization for applications like cancer imaging that take advantage of their increased sensitivity, quicker drug release, and more active targeting

10.8 DIFFERENT APPROACHES OF POLYMERIC MICELLES FOR DRUG DELIVERY FOR CANCER TREATMENT

10.8.1 Active Micelle Targeting

Cancer cells and the vasculature of tumors frequently display increased expression of particular antigens or receptors in comparison to the expression of these molecules in normal cells and tissues. By actively targeting polymeric micelles, one can take advantage of this characteristic of cancer cells to selectively accumulate anticancer drugs within the tissue of the tumor. The surface of polymeric micelles is chemically modified by targeting ligands that have a strong binding for antigens or receptors that are over-expressed on cancer cells. This is done to prepare polymeric micelles for active targeting. Several different ligands have been investigated up to this point for their potential to actively target polymeric micelles. The majority of the targeting ligands for polymeric micelles have been antibodies because of their wide range of applications and high degree of specificity. In their study, Jin and colleagues prepared PEG-PLGA micelles that were conjugated with the bivalent fragment HAb18 F(ab′)2. This particular fragment has a strong affinity for hepatocellular carcinoma (HCC) cells. When compared to non-targeted micelles (DOX-loaded PEG-PLGA micelles), the cancer cells (Huh7 and HepG2) that were incubated with targeted micelles (DOX-loaded HAb18 F(ab′)2-PEG-PLGA micelles) demonstrated cellular uptake that was nearly 1.5 times higher [94, 95].

Active targeting ligands are more common, and monoclonal antibodies are only one example. To selectively target lung cancer cells, Recently, Torchilin [96] revealed the use of diacyllipid-PEG (PE-PEG) micelles coupled to either an antimyosin (mAb) (2G4) or an anticancer (mAb) 2C5. After 2 hours, the amount of paclitaxel accumulated in 2C5-encoded micelles was four times larger compared to that of control micelles, and the cytotoxicity of these micelles against lung tumors was likewise much higher. Growth in the utilization of aptamers, which are oligonucleotides of DNA or RNA, can be attributed to the practice of library screening. Docetaxel-loaded PEG-PLGA micelles containing an RNA aptamer targeting prostate-specific membrane antigen (PSMA) have recently shown promise in the treatment of prostate cancer [97]. After being given the targeted micelles, five out of seven rats with LNCaP xenografts completely regressed their tumors, demonstrating higher antitumor activity and reduced systemic toxicity in comparison to the non-targeted micelles.

10.8.2 Release of Stimulus-Responsive Drugs

A highly hydrophilic outer shell, which is necessary to extend the amount of time that micelles are in circulation, may make it more difficult for them to be taken up by tumor cells [98]. When compared to conventional micelles, stimuli-responsive micelles show greater promise in terms of their ability to control drug release.

Throughout the development and progression of a tumor, the cells that make up the tumor undergo several changes. The rapid proliferation of tumor cells and the accumulation of acid metabolites are two factors that contribute to the low extracellular pH of tumors (6.0–7.0), which is slightly lower than the pH of normal tissues [99]. To prepare pH-responsive polymeric micelles that are stable in circulation and rapidly depolymerized upon arrival at the tumor sites, two primary strategies can be utilized. The first method is based on the hydrolysis of micellar materials, while the second method is based on the protonation and deprotonation of proton donor groups [100, 101]. Endosomes, which have a pH ranging from 5.5 to 6.0, and lysosomes, which have a pH ranging from 4.5 to 5.0, each have completely different acidic environments [102]. For the treatment of cancer, Pitt and colleagues developed ultrasound-responsive pluronic micelles loaded with doxorubicin [58, 59]. After stabilizing these pluronic micelles with PEG-phospholipid (PEG-DSPE), *in vivo*, studies showed that ultrasound increased the anticancer activity of both free DOX and micelle-integrated DOX. Ultrasound significantly reduced tumor growth as well, though for a lot longer than with micelles by themselves.

10.8.3 Imaging-Sensitive Polymer Micelles

Ultrasound, single-photon emission computed tomography, positron emission tomography, magnetic resonance imaging, computed tomography as well as other imaging modalities are essential for diagnosis as well as monitoring of patients with cancer who are receiving therapy [103]. The fields of nanomedicine and medical imaging are merging to improve the ability to differentiate between normal as well as malignant tissues.

The field of magnetic resonance imaging (MRI) has seen the emergence of a plethora of micellar platforms. The T1 relaxation period of water protons may be shortened by using gadolinium (Gd)-based contrast agents (like Magnevistt), which may improve picture contrast [104]. After the Gd complex has been added to the surface of polymeric micelles, T1 relaxivity, and detection sensitivity are dramatically improved. Sensitivity is improved by using T2/T2 * agents such as superparamagnetic iron oxide (SPIO) instead of Gd-based T1 agents. Polymeric micelles have been used by the group to enclose SPIO nanoparticles, and we just published an article on the topic. Because of the clumping of hydrophobic SPIO nanoparticles within the micelle core, T2 relaxivity was dramatically increased. Results from MRI studies have shown that the micellar formulation can detect concentrations as low as a few nanomolars [105]. The potential of polymeric micelles involved in cancer imaging is investigated using several imaging modalities, including computed tomography (CT) and single-photon emission computed tomography (SPECT). CT scans were able to pinpoint the location of the popliteal lymph nodes 2 hours after injecting iodine-containing PLL-PEG polymer micelles subcutaneously into the rabbits' posterior thighs. After infusing the micelles IV into rabbits, scientists saw opacification liver as well as the spleen, with arteries in the liver becoming delineated within 30 minutes.

10.9 CONCLUSIONS AND PROSPECTS

Cancer is a major global health concern, with over 10 million new cases diagnosed each year. Treatment options include radiation, chemotherapy, and surgical resection. However, chemotherapeutic medications are limited by toxicity and patient morbidity. Polymeric micelles, supramolecular core–shell nanoparticles, have potential benefits for cancer treatment and detection. These nanosized particles self-assemble into biocompatible, amphiphilic block copolymers, enhancing drug bioavailability and prolonging circulation. Nanoparticulate-based devices improve drug stability, solubility, and pharmacokinetics, reducing toxicity and enabling simultaneous treatment and diagnosis.

Polymeric amphiphiles, including graft polymers and micelles, have been studied for their potential to improve anticancer drug efficacy due to their small size, extended circulation time, and sustained drug release profile. Graft polymers, such as poly(L-lactic acid) (PLLA) and cellulose, can contain and release chemotherapeutic drugs like doxorubicin. Micelles, made from hydrophilic and hydrophobic block-copolymers, have been used for drug delivery in cancer treatment, with active targeting ligands like antibodies being the most common. Therefore, they want to go forward with micellar nanomedicine, which can transport many medications to target different oncogenic pathways. To overcome the challenge of cancer heterogeneity, the development of micelles with imaging capabilities to detect phenotypic manifestations within solid tumors would be essential. Furthermore, imaging features allow for tracking of treatment results and, in light of adaptive resistance, possible alterations to therapy. The development of such theranostic micellar nanomedicine is crucial for improving the specificity and effectiveness of chemotherapy and enabling individualized cancer treatment.

REFERENCES

1. Blanco E, Kessinger CW, Sumer BD, Gao J. Multifunctional micellar nanomedicine for cancer therapy. *Exp Biol Med.* 2009 Feb;234(2):123–31.
2. Gros L, Ringsdorf H, Schupp H. Polymeric anti-tumor agents on a molecular and on a cellular-level. *Angew Chem Int Ed Engl.* 1981;20:305–25.
3. Jones M, Leroux J. Polymeric micelles—a new generation of colloidal drug carriers. *Eur J Pharm Biopharm.* 1999;48:101–11.

4. Torchilin VP. Structure and design of polymeric surfactant-based drug delivery systems. *J Control Release*. 2001;73:137–72.
5. Nishiyama N, Kataoka K. Current state, achievements, and future prospects of polymeric micelles as nanocarriers for drug and gene delivery. *Pharmacol Ther*. 2006;112:630–48.
6. Parsa N. Environmental factors inducing human cancers. *Iran J Public Health*. 2012;41(11):1–9.
7. Torchilin VP. Micellar nanocarriers: pharmaceutical perspectives. *Pharm Res*. 2007;24:1–16.
8. Liu J, Zeng F, Allen C. In vivo fate of unimers and micelles of a poly(ethylene glycol)-block-poly(caprolactone) copolymer in mice following intravenous administration. *Eur J Pharm Biopharm*. 2007;65:309–19.
9. Jones M, Leroux J. Polymeric micelles – a new generation of colloidal drug carriers. *Eur J Pharm Biopharm*. 1999;48:101–11.
10. Schiller JH, Harrington D, Belani CP, Langer C, Sandler A, Krook J, et al. Comparison of four chemotherapy regimens for advanced non-small-cell lung cancer. *N Engl J Med*. 2002;346:92–8.
11. Huang CY, Ju DT, Chang CF, Reddy PM, Velmurugan BK. A review on the effects of current chemotherapy drugs and natural agents in treating non–small cell lung cancer. *Biomedicine*. 2017 Dec;7(4):1–23.
12. Cheng X, Li D, Xu J, Wei B, Fang Q, Yang L, Xue Y, Wang X, Tang R. Self-assembled ternary hybrid nanodrugs for overcoming tumor resistance and metastasis. *Acta Pharm Sin B*. 2021 Nov;11(11):3595–607.
13. Moghimi SM, Hunter AC. Recognition by macrophages and liver cells of opsonized phospholipid vesicles and phospholipid headgroups. *Pharm Res*. 2001;18:1–8.
14. Grigore ME. Organic and inorganic nano-systems used in cancer treatment. *J Med Res Health Educ*. 2017;1(3):1–8.
15. Gros L, Ringsdorf H, Schupp H. Polymeric anti-tumor agents on a molecular and on a cellular-level. *Angew Chem Int Edit*. 1981;20:305–25.
16. Hashizume H, Baluk P, Morikawa S, McLean JW, Thurston G, Roberge S, Jain RK, McDonald DM. Openings between defective endothelial cells explain tumor vessel leakiness. *Am J Pathol*. 2000;156:1363–80.
17. Maeda H. The enhanced permeability and retention (EPR) effect in tumor vasculature: the key role of tumor-selective macromolecular drug targeting. *Adv Enzyme Regul*. 2001;41:189–207.
18. Senapati S, Mahanta AK, Kumar S, Maiti P. Controlled drug delivery vehicles for cancer treatment and their performance. *Signal Transduct Target Ther*. 2018 Mar 16;3:7.
19. Lee CC, MacKay JA, Frechet JM, Szoka FC. Designing dendrimers for biological applications. *Nat Biotechnol*. 2005;23:1517–26.
20. Torchilin VP. Recent advances with liposomes as pharmaceutical carriers. *Nat Rev Drug Discov*. 2005;4:145–60.
21. Sutton D, Nasongkla N, Blanco E, Gao J. Functionalized micellar systems for cancer targeted drug delivery. *Pharm Res*. 2007;24(6):1029–46.
22. Torchilin VP. Structure and design of polymeric surfactant-based drug delivery systems. *J Control Release*. 2001;73(2–3):137–72.
23. Torchilin VP. Micellar nanocarriers: pharmaceutical perspectives. *Pharm Res*. 2007;24(1):1–16.
24. Haider MS, Lübtow MM, Endres S, Forster S, Flegler VJ, Böttcher B, Aseyev V, Pöppler AC, Luxenhofer R. Think beyond the core: impact of the hydrophilic corona on drug solubilization using polymer micelles. *ACS Appl Mater Interfaces*. 2020 Jun 3;12(22):24531–43.
25. Li M, Gao M, Fu Y, et al. Acetal-linked polymeric prodrug micelles for enhanced curcumin delivery. *Colloids Surf B Biointerfaces*. 2016;140:11–8.
26. Kale AA, Torchilin VP. Design, synthesis, and characterization of pH-sensitive PEG-PE conjugates for stimuli-sensitive pharmaceutical nanocarriers: the effect of substitutes at the hydrazone linkage on the ph stability of PEG-PE conjugates. *Bioconjug. Chem*. 2007;18:363–70.
27. Ghosh B, Biswas S. Polymeric micelles in cancer therapy: state of the art. *J Control Release*. 2021;332:127–47.
28. Liu M, Du H, Zhang W, Zhai G. Internal stimuli-responsive nanocarriers for drug delivery: design strategies and applications. *Mater Sci Eng C*. 2017 Feb 1;71:1267–80.

29. Li Z, Tan BH. Towards the development of polycaprolactone based amphiphilic block copolymers: molecular design, self-assembly and biomedical applications. *Mater Sci Eng C*. 2014 Dec 1;45:620–34.
30. Zhang H, Zhai Y, Wang J, Zhai G. New progress and prospects: the application of nanogel in drug delivery. *Mater Sci Eng C*. 2016 Mar 1;60:560–8.
31. Yang CC, Yang SY, Chieh JJ, et al. Biofunctionalized magnetic nanoparticles for specifically detecting biomarkers of Alzheimer's disease in vitro. *ACS Chem Neurosci*. 2011;2(9):500–5.
32. Rahman MM, Islam F, Anwar Parvez MA, Ashraf GM, Ullah MF, Ahmed M. Citrus limon L.(lemon) seed extract shows neuro-modulatory activity in an in vivo thiopental-sodium sleep model by reducing the sleep onset and enhancing the sleep duration. *J Integr Neurosci*. 2022;21(1):042–9.
33. Wu J. the enhanced permeability and retention (EPR) effect: the significance of the concept and methods to enhance its application. *J Pers Med*. 2021 Aug 6;11(8):1–8. doi: 10.3390/jpm11080771. PMID: 34442415; PMCID: PMC8402171.
34. Cevenini E, Caruso C, Candore G, et al. Age-related inflammation: the contribution of different organs, tissues and systems. How to face it for therapeutic approaches. *Curr Pharm Design*. 2010;16(6):609–18.
35. Kashkooli FM, Soltani M, Souri M. Controlled anti-cancer drug release through advanced nano-drug delivery systems: Static and dynamic targeting strategies. *J Control Release*. 2020 Nov 10;327:316–49.
36. Yao Y, Zhou Y, Liu L, Xu Y, Chen Q, Wang Y, Wu S, Deng Y, Zhang J, Shao A. Nanoparticle-based drug delivery in cancer therapy and its role in overcoming drug resistance. *Front Mol Biosci*. 2020 Aug 20;7:193.
37. Endres TK, Beck-Broichsitter M, Samsonova O, Renette T, Kissel TH. Self-assembled biodegradable amphiphilic PEG-PCL-lPEI triblock copolymers at the borderline between micelles and nanoparticles designed for drug and gene delivery. *Biomaterials*. 2011;32:7721–31.
38. Ghosh Chaudhuri R, Paria S. Core/shell nanoparticles: classes, properties, synthesis mechanisms, characterization, and applications. *Chem Rev*. 2011;112:2373–433.
39. Campisi J, di Fagagna FDA. Cellular senescence: when bad things happen to good cells. Nat Rev *Mol Cell Biol*. 2007;8(9):729–40.
40. Krtolica A, Parrinello S, Lockett S, Desprez PY, Campisi J. Senescent fibroblasts promote epithelial cell growth and tumorigenesis: a link between cancer and aging. *Proc Natl Acad Sci U S A*. 2001;98(2):12072–7.
41. Dai L, Li D, He J. Degradation of graft polymer and blend based on cellulose and poly (L-lactide). *J Appl Polymer Sci*. 2013 Nov 15;130(4):2257–64.
42. Purohit P, Bhatt A, Mittal RK, Abdellattif MH, Farghaly TA. Polymer Grafting and its chemical reactions. *Front Bioeng Biotechnol*. 2023 Jan 11;10:1044927.
43. Pribluda A, Elyada E, Wiener Z, et al. A senescence-inflammatory switch from cancer-inhibitory to cancer-promoting mechanism. *Cancer Cel*. 2015;27(6):877–78.
44. Dall'Olio F, Vanhooren V, Chen CC, Slagboom PE, Wuhrer M, Franceschi C. N-Glycomic biomarkers of biological aging and longevity: a link with inflammaging. *Ageing Res Rev*. 2013;12(2):685–98.
45. Feldman N, Rotter-Maskowitz A, Okun E. DAMPs as mediators of sterile inflammation in aging-related pathologies. *Ageing Res Rev*. 2015;24(A):29–39.
46. Sun H, Yan L, Chang MYZ, Carter KA, Zhang R, Slyker L, Lovell JF, Wu Y, Cheng C. A multifunctional biodegradable brush polymer-drug conjugate for paclitaxel/gemcitabine co-delivery and tumor imaging. *Nanoscale Adv*. 2019;1(7):2761–71.
47. Zou J, Yu Y, Li Y, Ji W, Chen CK, Law WC, Prasad PN, Cheng C. Well-defined diblock brush polymer-drug conjugates for sustained delivery of paclitaxel. *Biomater Sci*. 2015 Jul;3(7):1078–84.
48. Shukla A, Maiti P. Nanomedicine and versatile therapies for cancer treatment. *Med Commun*. 2022;3:e163.
49. Noverr MC, Huffnagle GB. Does the microbiota regulate immune responses outside the gut? *Trends Microbiol*. 2004;12(12):562–8.
50. Kashtanova DA, et al. Gut microbiota and aging. In: Moskalev, A. (Eds.) Biomarkers of Human Aging. Healthy Ageing and Longevity (vol 10, pp 263–278). Springer, Gewerbestrasse, Cham. 2019. https://doi.org/10.1007/978-3-030-24970-0_17.

51. Farokhzad OC, Cheng J, Teply BA, Sherifi I, Jon S, Kantoff PW, Richie JP, Langer R. Targeted nanoparticle-aptamer bioconjugates for cancer chemotherapy in vivo. *Proc Natl Acad Sci U S A*. 2006;103:6315–20.
52. Potineni A, Lynn DM, Langer R, Amiji MM. Poly(ethylene oxide)-modified poly(beta-amino ester) nanoparticles as a pH-sensitive biodegradable system for paclitaxel delivery. *J Control Release*. 2003;86:223–34.
53. Stapert HR, Nishiyama N, Jiang DL, Aida T, Kataoka K. Polyion complex micelles encapsulating light-harvesting ionic dendrimer zinc porphyrins. *Langmuir*. 2000;16:8182–88.
54. Johnson JA, Lu YY, Burts AO, Xia Y, Durrell AC, Tirrell DA, Grubbs RH. Drug-loaded, bivalent-bottle-brush polymers by graft-through ROMP. *Macromolecules*. 2010 Dec 28;43(24):10326–35.
55. Liu SQ, Tong YW, Yang YY. Thermally sensitive micelles self-assembled from poly(N-isopropylacrylamide-co-N,N-dimethylacrylamide)-b-poly(D,L-lactide-c o-glycolide) for controlled delivery of paclitaxel. *Mol Biosyst*. 2005;1:158–65.
56. Zhu D, Yan H, Zhou Z, Tang J, Liu X, Hartmann R, Parak W. J, Feliu N, Shen Y. Detailed investigation on how the protein corona modulates the physicochemical properties and gene delivery of Polyethylenimine (PEI) polyplexes. *Biomater Sci*. 2018;6:1800–17.
57. García-Á lvarez R, Hadjidemetriou M, Sánchez-Iglesias A, Liz-Marzán LM, Kostarelos K. In vivo formation of protein corona on gold nanoparticles. The effect of their size and shape. *Nanoscale*. 2018;10:1256–64.
58. Yeo ELL, Thong PSP, Soo KC, Kah JCY. Protein corona in drug delivery for multimodal cancer therapy in vivo. *Nanoscale*. 2018;10:2461–72.
59. Yang J, Wang B, You Y, Chang W.-J, Tang K, Wang Y.- C, Zhang W, Ding F, Gunasekaran S. Probing the modulated formation of gold nanoparticles–beta-lactoglobulin corona complexes and their applications. *Nanoscale*. 2017;9:17758–69.
60. Walkey CD, Olsen JB, Song F, Liu R, Guo H, Olsen DWH, Cohen Y, Emili A, ChanWCW. Protein corona fingerprinting predicts the cellular interaction of gold and silver nanoparticles. *ACS Nano*. 2014;8:2439–55.
61. Torchilin VP. Structure and design of polymeric surfactant-based drug delivery systems. *J Control Release*. 2001; 73(2–3):137–72.
62. Tyrrell ZL, Shen Y, Radosz M. Fabrication of micellar nanoparticles for drug delivery through the self-assembly of block copolymers. *Prog Polym Sci*. 2010;35:1128–43.
63. Jin C, Qian N, Zhao W, et al. Improved therapeutic effect of DOXPLGA-PEG micelles decorated with bivalent fragment HAb18 F(ab')(2) for hepatocellular carcinoma. *Biomacromolecules*. 2010;11(9):2422–31.
64. Abouzeid AH, Patel NR, Torchilin VP. Polyethylene glycolphosphatidylethanolamine (PEG-PE)/ vitamin E micelles for codelivery of paclitaxel and curcumin to overcome multi-drug resistance in ovarian cancer. *Int J Pharm*. 2014;464(1–2):178–84.
65. Trubetskoy VS, Gazelle GS, Wolf GL, Torchilin VP. Block-copolymer of polyethylene glycol and polylysine as a carrier of organic iodine: design of long-circulating particulate contrast medium for X-ray computed tomography. *J Drug Target*. 1997;4:381–8.
66. Hussein YHA, Youssry M. Polymeric micelles of biodegradable diblock copolymers: enhanced encapsulation of hydrophobic drugs. *Materials (Basel)*. 2018 Apr 27;11(5):688.
67. Wang J, Xu W, Ding J, Lu S, Wang X, Wang C, et al. Cholesterol-enhanced polylactide-based stereocomplex micelle for effective delivery of doxorubicin. *Materials*. 2015;8:216–30.
68. Wang X, He C, Yang Q, Tan L, Liu B, Zhu Z, et al. Dynamic covalent linked triblock copolymer micelles for glutathione-mediated intracellular drug delivery. *Mater Sci Eng C*. 2017;77:34–44.
69. Rapoport N, Gao Z, Kennedy A. Multifunctional nanoparticles for combining ultrasonic tumor imaging and targeted chemotherapy. *J Natl Cancer Inst*. 2007;99:1095–106.
70. Nasongkla N, Bey E, Ren J, Ai H, Khemtong C, Guthi JS, Chin SF, Sherry AD, Boothman DA, Gao J. Multifunctional polymeric micelles as cancer-targeted, MRI-ultrasensitive drug delivery systems. *Nano Lett*. 2006;6:2427–30.
71. Li X, Yang X, Lin Z, Wang D, Mei D, He B, et al. A folate modified pH sensitive targeted polymeric micelle alleviated systemic toxicity of doxorubicin (DOX) in multi-drug resistant tumor bearing mice. *Eur J Pharm Sci*. 2015;76:95–101.

72. Gerweck LE, Vijayappa S, Kozin S. Tumor pH controls the in vivo efficacy of weak acid and base chemotherapeutics. *Mol Cancer Ther*. 2006;5:1275–9.
73. Hubbell JA. Enhancing drug function. *Science*. 2003;300:595–6.
74. Schmaljohann D. Thermo-and pH-responsive polymers in drug delivery. *Adv Drug Deliver Rev*. 2006;58:1655–70.
75. Wang Z, Li X, Wang D, et al. Concurrently suppressing multidrug resistance and metastasis of breast cancer by co-delivery of paclitaxel and honokiol with pH-sensitive polymeric micelles. *Acta Biomater*. 2017;62:144–56.
76. van Nostrum CF. Covalently cross-linked amphiphilic block copolymer micelles. *Soft Matter*. 2011;7:3246–59.
77. Blanco E, Shen HF, Ferrari M. Principles of nanoparticle design for overcoming biological barriers to drug delivery. *Nat Biotechnol*. 2015;33:941–51.
78. Lu Y, Zhang E, Yang J, Cao Z. Strategies to improve micelle stability for drug delivery. *Nano Res*. 2018;11:4985–98.
79. Wakaskar R. Polymeric micelles and their properties. *J Nanomed Nanotechnol*. 2017;8(2):1–3.
80. Talelli M, Barz M, Rijcken C.J, Kiessling F, Hennink W.E, Lammers T. Core-crosslinked polymeric micelles: principles, preparation. *Biomed Appl Clin Transl Nano Today*. 2015;10:93–117.
81. Guo X, Zhao Z, Chen D, Qiao M, Wan F, Cun D, Sun Y, Yang M. Co-delivery of resveratrol and docetaxel via polymeric micelles to improve the treatment of drug-resistant tumors. *Asian J Pharm Sci*. 2019;14:78–85.
82. Chen T, Tu L, Wang G, Qi N, Wu W, Zhang W, Feng J. Multi-functional chitosan polymeric micelles as oral paclitaxel delivery systems for enhanced bioavailability and anti-tumor e fficacy. *Intern J Pharm*. 2020;578:119105.
83. Wang W, Zhao B, Meng X, She P, Zhang P, Cao Y, Zhang X. Preparation of dual-drug conjugated polymeric micelles with synergistic anti-cancer efficacy in vitro. *J Drug Deliv Sci Technol*. 2018;43:388–96.
84. Wei X, Liu L, Li X, Wang Y, Guo X, Zhao J, Zhou S. Selectively targeting tumor-associated macrophages and tumor cells with polymeric micelles for enhanced cancer chemo-immunotherapy. *J Control Release*. 2019;313:42–53.
85. Senevirathne SA, Washington KE, Biewer MC, Stefan MC. PEG based anti-cancer drug conjugated prodrug micelles for the delivery of anti-cancer agents. *J Mater Chem B*. 2016;4:360–70.
86. Yokoyama M, Opanasopit P, Okano T. Polymer design and incorporation method for polymeric micelle carrier system containing water-insoluble anti-cancer agent camptothecin. *J Drug Target*. 2004;12:373–84
87. Opanasopit P, Yokoyama M, Okano T. Block copolymer design for camptothecin incorporation into polymeric micelles for passive tumor targeting. *Pharm Res*. 2004;21:2003–10.
88. Yokoyama M, Kwon GS, Kataoka K. Preparation of micelle-forming polymer-drug conjugates. *Bioconjugate Chem*. 1992;3:295–301.
89. Yamamoto T, Yokoyama M, Maitani Y, et al. What are determining factors for stable drug incorporation into polymeric micelle carriers? Consideration on physical and chemical characters of the micelle inner core. *J Control Release*. 2007;123:11–8.
90. Koizumi F, Kitagawa M, Negishi T, et al. Novel SN38-incorporating polymeric micelles, NK012, eradicate vascular endothelial growth factor-secreting bulky tumors. *Cancer Res*. 2006; 66:10048–56.
91. Yokoyama M, Kwon GS, Okano T, et al. Influencing factors on in vitro micelle stability of adriamycin-block copolymer conjugates. *J Control Release*. 1994;28:59–65.
92. Akiba I, Terada N, Hashida S, et al. Encapsulation of a hydrophobic drug into a polymer-micelle core explored with synchrotron SAXS. *Langmuir*. 2010;26:7544–51.
93. Yokoyama M. Polymeric micelles as drug carriers: their lights and shadows. *J Drug Target*. 2014;22(7):576–83.
94. Prabhakar U, Hiroshi M, Rakesh KJ, Eva MS-M, William Z, Omid CF, Simon TB, Alberto G, Piotr G, David CB. Challenges and key considerations of the enhanced permeability and retention effect for nanomedicine drug delivery in oncology; EPR Effect and Nanomedicine Drug Delivery in Oncology. *Cancer Res*. 2013;73:2412–17.
95. Jin C, Yang W, Bai L, Wang J, Dou K. Preparation and characterization of targeted DOX-PLGA-PEG micelles decorated with bivalent fragment HAb18 F(ab')2 for treatment of hepatocellular carcinoma. *J Control Release*. 2011;152(Suppl. 1):e14–e15.

96. Torchilin VP. PEG-based micelles as carriers of contrast agents for different imaging modalities. *Adv Drug Deliv Rev*. 2002;54:235–52.
97. Ko NR, Oh JK. Glutathione-triggered disassembly of dual disulfide located degradable nanocarriers of polylactide-based block copolymers for rapid drug release. *Biomacromolecules*. 2014;15:3180–9.
98. Xu W, Wang H, Dong L, Zhang P, Mu Y, Cui X, Zhou J, Huo M, Yin T. Hyaluronic acid-decorated redox-sensitive chitosan micelles for tumor-specific intracellular delivery of gambogic acid. *Int J Nanomed*. 2019; 14:4649–66.
99. Xu C, Song RJ, Lu P, Chen JC, Zhou YQ, Shen G, Jiang MJ, Zhang W. pHtriggered charge-reversal and redox-sensitive drug-release polymer micelles codeliver doxorubicin and triptolide for prostate tumor therapy. *Int J Nanomed*. 2018;13:7229–49.
100. Zeng Y, Ma J, Zhan Y, Xu X, Zeng Q, Liang J, Chen X. Hypoxia-activated prodrugs and redox-responsive nanocarriers. *Int J Nanomed*. 2018;13:6551–74.
101. Liu B, Thayumanavan S. Substituent effects on the pH sensitivity of acetals and ketals and their correlation with encapsulation stability in polymeric nanogels. *J Am Chem Soc*. 2017;139:2306–17.
102. Liu H, Chen H, Cao F, Peng D, Chen W, Zhang C. Amphiphilic block copolymer poly (acrylic acid)-B-polycaprolactone as a novel pH-sensitive nanocarrier for anticancer drugs delivery: in-vitro and in-vivo evaluation. *Polymers*. 2019;11:820.
103. Xie C, Powell C, Yao M, et al. Ubiquitin-conjugating enzyme E2C: a potential cancer biomarker. *Int J Biochem Cell Biol*. 2014;47:113–7.
104. Jayatilaka H, Umanzor FG, Shah V, et al. Tumor cell density regulates matrix metalloproteinases for enhanced migration. *Oncotarget*. 2018; 9:32556–69.
105. Guthi JS, Yang SG, Huang G, Li S, Khemtong C, Kessinger CW, Peyton M, Minna JD, Brown KC, Gao J. MRI-visible micellar nanomedicine for targeted drug delivery to lung cancer cells. *Mol Pharm*. 2010 Feb 1;7(1):32–40.

11 Cellular Targeting of Nanoparticles for Targeted Cancer Therapy

11.1 INTRODUCTION

Cancer is defined by unregulated cell proliferation and the lack of planned cell death, which results in the growth of an aberrant cell mass known as a tumor. Abnormal cells are responsible for disrupting the strictly controlled systems of cell development and death, which are essential to maintain the delicate balance of the body's biological functions. The unregulated multiplication of neoplastic cells progressively impairs the proper functioning of non-malignant cells, causing damage to the delicate equilibrium of homeostasis that is vital for the general health of the organism. Tumor cells struggle for resources and change the microenvironment to promote growth and survival when they invade neighboring tissues. This instability of cellular dynamics and interactions accelerates cancer, highlighting cancer's complex alterations to the body's natural balance [1]. The primary malignant tumor develops, eventually reaching metastatic potential, and disseminates to other proximal or distal body sites, in contrast to benign or non-cancerous tumors. A metastatic lesion forms after growth begins in the secondary site and could ultimately result in death [2].

The development of tactics to specifically target cancer cells while minimizing damage to healthy tissues has been the main focus of recent developments in cancer therapy. Targeted therapy using nanoparticles has become one of these methods and is showing promise [3]. Advantageous characteristics of nanoparticles include their tiny size, high surface area, and capacity to contain medicinal ingredients [4]. Personalizing nanoparticle surface characteristics improves targeting and allows cancer cells to receive precise therapeutic payloads. Nanoparticles may interact selectively with cancer cell receptors or biomolecules by adding targeted ligands or changing charge and hydrophobicity [5]. This surface change allows cancer cells to recognize and ingest drugs more precisely while limiting off-target effects on healthy tissues. The capacity to precisely control the surface characteristics of nanoparticles is an example of a flexible strategy in cancer nanomedicine, maximizing the therapeutic effect and advancing the development of individualized and targeted therapeutic approaches.

Achieving effective cellular targeting is crucial for nanoparticle-based targeted cancer therapy. Nanoparticles can preferentially attach to cancer cells through particular ligand–receptor interactions or physical features, allowing internalization and subsequent release of therapeutic drugs within the tumor microenvironment [6]. The focused strategy has a great deal of potential to improve treatment results while reducing the off-target side effects connected with traditional chemotherapy [7].

A thorough comprehension of the intricate interactions between nanoparticles and cancer cells is necessary for efficient cellular targeting. The creation of tailored nanoparticles necessitates the interdisciplinary integration of several fields, such as materials science, chemistry, biology, and medicine [8]. Numerous methods, including surface modifications, ligand conjugation, and stimuli-responsive systems, have been investigated to improve cellular targeting [9]. These methods seek

DOI: 10.1201/9781003451020-11

to increase the cellular internalization rates, stability, and binding affinity of nanoparticles, hence increasing therapeutic efficacy [10]. In-depth information on cellular targeting of nanoparticles for targeted cancer therapy is provided in this book chapter, which also goes over how to construct and optimize nanoparticle-based systems, emphasizing their potential for therapeutic application.

11.2 PASSIVE AND ACTIVE CELLULAR TARGETING

Cancer nanomedicine utilizes both passive and active targeting techniques to improve the transport of therapeutic medicines to cancerous cells. Passive targeting is based on the different physiological characteristics of tumors, including the presence of permeable blood arteries and compromised lymphatic drainage. These characteristics can be used by nanoparticles that are the right size, and form, and have the right surface properties. This enables them to carefully build up in the tumor through the increased permeability and retention (EPR) effect [11]. This method enhances the concentration of drugs specifically at the tumor's site while reducing the exposure to healthy tissues. Nanoparticle-based cancer treatment uses passive and active cellular targeting. These methods aim to promote nanoparticle accumulation in cancer cells by exploiting tumor tissue properties and engaging with specific receptors [12]. The efficacy and selectivity of cancer treatments have been proven to be greatly improved by recent developments in these tactics.

The enhanced permeability and retention (EPR) effect, which is a phenomenon seen in tumor tissues and is characterized by leaky blood arteries and restricted lymphatic outflow, is the foundation of passive targeting. Nanoparticles can make use of the EPR effect to collect preferentially in tumor tissues if they have the right physicochemical characteristics, such as small size, extended circulation duration, and surface changes to minimize opsonization [13]. Numerous formulations of nanoparticles, including liposomes, polymeric nanoparticles, and inorganic nanoparticles, have been created for passive targeting as a result of extensive research [14]. Nanoparticle surfaces may be modified with particular ligands to engage with receptors overexpressed on cancer cells, a process known as active targeting. This modification improves nanoparticle uptake and internalization by precisely recognizing and binding to cancer cells [15]. Active targeting offers a more selective and efficient delivery method, ensuring that medicinal payloads reach their intended site. To maximize passive accumulation in tumors and enhance therapeutic effects, recent research has concentrated on optimizing nanoparticle features, such as size, surface charge, and surface coating [16].

On the other hand, active cellular targeting entails conjugating targeting ligands to the surface of nanoparticles. To facilitate receptor-mediated endocytosis and internalization of nanoparticles, these ligands specifically identify and bind to overexpressed receptors on cancer cells [17]. For active targeting, a variety of ligands have been investigated, including antibodies, peptides, aptamers, and small molecules [18]. Active targeting enables the targeted delivery of nanoparticles to cancer cells while limiting the uptake by healthy cells. The creation of multifunctional nanoparticles that can combine targeting ligands with other functions, including imaging agents or therapeutic payloads, for synergistic effects has recently received attention in active targeting strategy research [19]. In addition, the development of new ligands with high selectivity and affinity for cancer cells has been made possible by the application of sophisticated ligand engineering techniques, including phage display and combinatorial chemistry [20].

The effectiveness of cellular targeting can be increased, and therapeutic results enhanced by combining passive and active targeting procedures. Dual-targeting strategies combine passive and active targeting mechanisms into a single system of nanoparticles. For instance, nanoparticles may be made to carry targeted ligands that will aggressively bind to particular cancer cell receptors while also utilizing the EPR effect to passively accumulate in tumor tissues [21]. The dual-targeting technique is provided by a synergistic approach that boosts nanoparticle accumulation inside the tumor and makes it easier to distribute therapeutic drugs selectively [22].

11.3 CELLULAR AND SUBCELLULAR TARGETING

Recent developments in nanoparticle-based targeted cancer therapy have concentrated on obtaining precise subcellular targeting in addition to effective cellular targeting. Researchers want to improve treatment efficacy and reduce off-target effects by targeting nanoparticles to particular cellular compartments or organelles.

Cellular targeting involves the development of nanoparticles that specifically interface with and transport therapeutic payloads to cancer cells. Nanoparticles surface-enhanced with targeting ligands that bind to receptors overexpressed on cancer cell membranes are a common method to accomplish this. Optimizing treatment results while minimizing damage to healthy tissues is achieved by ensuring a greater concentration of therapeutic drugs at the tumor site [23]. Cellular targeting is directing nanoparticles to particular cancer cell types, such as those that express particular receptors excessively or have unique metabolic profiles. Utilizing ligands that selectively bind to receptors on the surface of cancer cells is one method for achieving cellular targeting [24]. To help with receptor-mediated internalization, for instance, antibodies, peptides, or aptamers can be attached to nanoparticles [25]. Recent studies have concentrated on finding and perfecting new ligands that have high specificity and affinity for cancer cell receptors, allowing for precise cellular targeting [26].

To transport nanoparticles to particular organelles or intracellular spaces within cancer cells, such as the nucleus, mitochondria, or endosomes/lysosomes, subcellular targeting is used. Subcellular targeting can be accomplished using a variety of techniques, such as taking advantage of organelle-specific transport processes, utilizing pH or redox gradients, or using peptides or proteins that specifically target particular organelles [27]. For instance, nanoparticles can be created to effectively release drugs into endosomes and lysosomes by taking advantage of the acidic pH of these organelles [28]. Nanoparticles can release their cargo exclusively in the acidic environment of endosomes and lysosomes by utilizing pH-responsive materials or pH-sensitive linkers, maximizing therapeutic efficacy while lowering systemic toxicity. In addition, scientists have created mitochondria-targeting nanoparticles to deliver therapeutic drugs directly to mitochondria, taking advantage of these organelles' special characteristics and roles in cancer cells [29].

Nanotechnology has recently made it possible to address subcellular structures at the molecular level. The visualization and monitoring of particular molecules or signaling pathways within cancer cells have been made possible by developments in nanoscale imaging and sensing. To monitor cellular activities in real-time and facilitate targeted drug delivery, nanoprobes or nanosensors can be made to selectively interact with target molecules [30]. For instance, the visualization of protein expression, enzyme activity, or gene expression within cancer cells using quantum dots, gold nanoparticles, or fluorescent nanosensors can be used to provide important insights for diagnosis and treatment [31].

The combination of subcellular and cellular targeting techniques has enormous potential for improving the accuracy and efficacy of cancer therapy. Researchers want to maximize therapeutic outcomes while minimizing off-target effects by targeting nanoparticles to particular cancer cell types and delivering them to precise subcellular compartments. It is anticipated that these developments in cellular and subcellular targeting will lead to more individualized and effective cancer treatments.

11.4 FACTORS AND STRATEGIES FOR CELLULAR TARGETING

For nanoparticle-based targeted cancer therapy to be successful, several variables and tactics are essential.

11.4.1 Surface Modifications

Nanoparticle surface changes are crucial for increasing the effectiveness of cellular targeting. The affinity and selectivity of nanoparticles for cancer cells can be improved by functionalizing the surface of the particles with certain ligands, such as antibodies, peptides, or aptamers [32]. Surface modifications include the modification of nanoparticle exteriors by attaching different molecules, such as ligands, antibodies, or peptides, that identify and bind to particular receptors on the surface of target cells. These modifications allow for both improved cellular absorption and active targeting of nanoparticles to certain cell types, including cancer cells. To provide a precise and customized interaction, ligands or targeting moieties may be chosen according to the overexpression of certain receptors on the target cells [33]. To decrease non-specific interactions and lengthen circulation duration, stealth coatings like polyethylene glycol (PEG) can be added using surface engineering techniques [34]. To achieve the best targeting performance, recent developments in surface modification methods have concentrated on optimizing ligand density, orientation, and spacing [35].

11.4.2 Ligand Selection

Ligand-based targeting is an important method in cellular targeting, in which nanoparticle surfaces are functionalized with ligands that bind to particular receptors or biomarkers [36]. This increases the precision of nanoparticle interactions and promotes the uptake of nanoparticles into certain cell types. Ligands include a variety of compounds, including antibodies, peptides, aptamers, and small molecules, which are selected for their unique binding and selectivity toward the target receptors [37]. These interactions stimulate receptor-mediated endocytosis, which increases the absorption of nanoparticles into specific cells and guarantees efficient drug delivery [38]. Discovering ligands that specifically target receptors that are overexpressed on the surface of cancer cells has been the focus of recent research [39]. Ligand-based targeting is a flexible and applicable approach that may be used for a broad range of disorders and cell types, making it very adaptable in the field of nanomedicine. To achieve selective cellular targeting, it is essential to choose the right ligands. These ligands may be created to recognize particular receptors or cell surface indicators connected to oncogenic signaling pathways. The finding of ligands with high affinity and specificity for cancer cells has been made easier by advancements in ligand discovery approaches, such as phage display or combinatorial chemistry [40]. Additionally, receptor-mediated endocytosis and intracellular distribution of nanoparticles are made possible by the application of ligands that target internalizing receptors [41].

11.4.3 Nanoparticle Size and Shape

The effectiveness of cellular absorption and targeting of nanoparticles is substantially influenced by their size and shape. For efficient cellular targeting, nanoparticles with diameters between tens and hundreds of nanometers are typically favored because they can extravasate from leaky tumor vasculature and accumulate in the tumor tissue through the EPR effect [42]. Furthermore, research has demonstrated that the form of nanoparticles might affect their targeting and uptake by cells. In comparison to spherical nanoparticles, non-spherical nanoparticles like rods, discs, or branched shapes have shown superior cellular internalization [43]. Recent developments in nanoparticle production methods have made it possible to precisely manipulate size, shape, and surface characteristics, improving the ability to target cells. How NPs can enhance the effectiveness of radiation therapy in cancer cells is shown in Figure 11.1.

11.4.4 Stimuli-Responsive Systems

The implementation of stimuli-responsive materials enables the regulation of drug release in particular cellular environments. These materials can react to parameters such as pH, temperature, or enzyme activity associated with the specific cells they are targeting, which improves the accuracy of drug delivery [44]. Cellular targeting strategies are paying more attention to stimuli-responsive

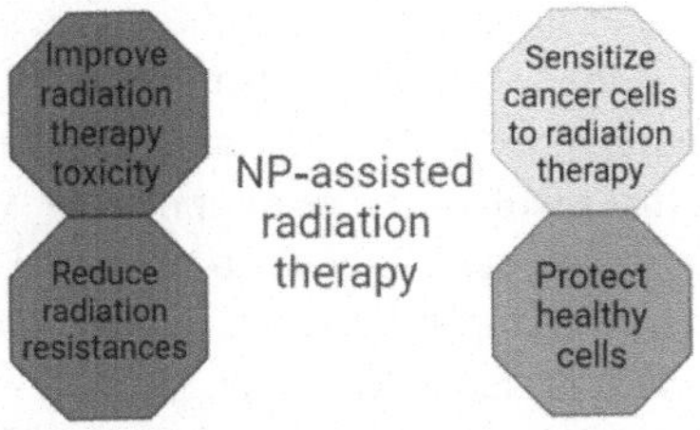

FIGURE 11.1 Diagram showing how NPs can enhance the effectiveness of radiation therapy in cancer cells.

systems. To activate nanoparticles or release their payloads in particular cellular conditions, these systems use internal or external stimuli, such as pH, temperature, light, or enzymes [45]. By reacting to particular features of the tumor microenvironment, such as an acidic pH or enhanced enzyme activity, stimuli-responsive devices can improve targeting efficiency [46]. The development of smart nanomaterials that react to particular stimuli for regulated and targeted medicine administration has recently received a lot of attention.

11.4.5 Combination Therapies

Combination therapy with targeted nanoparticle distribution has become a viable method for overcoming treatment resistance and enhancing therapeutic results. Researchers can generate synergistic effects and target several pathways involved in tumor development and survival by mixing various therapeutic agents, such as chemotherapeutic medicines, immunomodulators, or gene therapy designs, within a single nanoparticle system [47]. To maximize treatment efficacy, recent developments in combination medicines have brought attention to the significance of choosing complementary drugs and fine-tuning their release profiles.

11.5 IMPROVING CELLULAR UPTAKE OF THERAPEUTIC AGENTS

Enhancing the internalization of therapeutic substances by cells is an essential component in maximizing the effectiveness of drug delivery systems. Various techniques may be used to improve the incorporation of nanoparticles into certain cells. To improve cellular uptake efficiency and enable receptor-mediated endocytosis, one important strategy is to alter the surface of the cell in some way, such as for instance by attaching ligands. These ligands then bind preferentially to receptors that are overexpressed on the cell surface [48]. Nanoparticle size and form also matter, with smaller particles penetrating cell membranes and certain shapes increasing cellular uptake [49]. The effectiveness of targeted cancer therapy is greatly dependent on the cellular uptake of therapeutic chemicals delivered by nanoparticles. Recent research has concentrated on unraveling the intricate processes governing cellular uptake and formulating methods to speed up the internalization of nanoparticles and their payload into cancer cells.

11.5.1 Endocytic Pathways and Nanoparticle Design

The primary endocytic mechanisms for cellular uptake of nanoparticles include clathrin-mediated endocytosis, caveolae-mediated endocytosis, and macropinocytosis. Designing nanoparticles with optimized characteristics for effective uptake has been made possible by an understanding of these pathways and how they are regulated [50]. To encourage selective engagement with cell surface receptors and improve receptor-mediated endocytosis, scientists have created nanoparticles with specific surface modifications, such as ligand conjugation or charge manipulation [51]. Additionally, improvements in nanomaterial engineering have made it possible to precisely regulate the physicochemical characteristics of nanoparticles, such as size, shape, and surface charge, enabling customization for particular cellular absorption pathways [52]. Designing nanoparticles that can enter cells and deliver therapeutic payloads requires an understanding of endocytic mechanisms. Endocytosis is a cellular process that involves the development of vesicles to transport things from outside the cell. Various endocytic routes, such as clathrin-mediated endocytosis, caveolae-mediated endocytosis, and macropinocytosis, have specific functions in the process of cellular uptake [53]. The selection of the endocytic route is dependent upon variables such as the dimensions of the particle, its surface charge, and the presence of certain ligands. The design of nanoparticles may be customized to take advantage of these routes, via surface changes and the optimization of particle size and surface charge. Developing nanocarriers for efficient medicine delivery requires this understanding.

11.5.2 Targeting Intracellular Trafficking

Delivering therapeutic cargo to the intended subcellular compartments requires effective intracellular trafficking. Researchers have concentrated on creating nanoparticles that can successfully transit through the endosomal-lysosomal system, get past intracellular barriers, escape degradation, and promote cargo release into the cytoplasm or certain organelles [54]. To enable endosomal escape and intracellular release of cargo, strategies include integrating pH-responsive materials or membrane-disrupting agents into nanoparticles [55]. Additionally, the design of therapeutic compounds can be delivered precisely to the desired subcellular locations by utilizing organelle-targeting nanoparticles, such as those that are particularly tailored to accumulate in mitochondria or nuclei [56].

11.5.3 Active Cellular Uptake Strategies

Active cellular absorption techniques have drawn a lot of attention in addition to passive cellular uptake methods. For active targeting and improved uptake into cancer cells, scientists have created nanocarriers that take advantage of specific interactions with cell surface receptors, such as folate receptors or transferrin receptors [57]. Additionally, stimuli-responsive nanocarriers have been developed to take advantage of the special features of the tumor microenvironment, like low pH or high enzymatic activity, to cause active cellular absorption [58]. These techniques make use of the cancer cells' dynamic nature and their surroundings to effectively internalize medicinal medicines.

11.5.4 Co-Delivery Systems

To increase cellular absorption and therapeutic efficacy, the co-delivery of numerous therapeutic drugs within a single nanoparticle system has become a potent technique. Researchers can circumvent drug resistance mechanisms, target various pathways, and enhance therapeutic effects by concurrently administering synergistic medicines or combination therapy [59]. Co-delivery systems can be created by combining several techniques, such as layer-by-layer assembly, hybrid nanomaterials, and co-encapsulation, to precisely regulate the drug's release kinetics and spatial distribution inside cancer cells [60]. Further increasing cellular uptake and therapeutic response is the introduction of imaging agents or stimuli-responsive components in co-delivery systems, which allows for real-time monitoring and regulated release of therapeutic drugs.

11.5.5 Advanced Imaging Techniques

High-resolution imaging tools have greatly aided the understanding of cellular uptake processes. Super-resolution microscopy, intravital imaging, and live-cell imaging are examples of advanced imaging modalities that allow for the quantitative study and real-time visualization of nanoparticle uptake at the cellular and subcellular levels [61]. Researchers can now optimize nanoparticle design and create more potent methods to increase cellular uptake by the use of insights these techniques offer into nanoparticle–cell interactions, uptake kinetics, and intracellular trafficking dynamics.

11.6 LIGAND-BASED TARGETING OF NANOPARTICLES

Targeted cancer therapy now employs a potent tactic known as ligand-based targeting of nanoparticles. Researchers can improve the selectivity and effectiveness of drug delivery to cancer cells while minimizing off-target effects by adding particular ligands to the surface of nanoparticles.

11.6.1 Ligand Selection and Optimization

Effective cellular targeting depends heavily on the choice and refinement of ligands. Finding ligands that specifically bind to overexpressed receptors on cancer cells has been a research priority [62]. These ligands, which recognize and bind to particular cell surface indicators or receptor proteins linked to cancer growth, can be antibodies, peptides, aptamers, or small compounds [63]. The identification of ligands with high affinity and specificity for cancer cells has been made easier by recent developments in ligand screening methods, such as phage display or combinatorial chemistry. Affinity maturation and structure-guided design are two further ligand optimization procedures that have been used to increase ligand–receptor interactions and boost targeted effectiveness [64].

11.6.2 Multivalent Ligand Presentation

By displaying several ligands on nanoparticle surfaces, multivalent ligand presentation increases the avidity and binding affinity of nanoparticles for cancer cell receptors [65]. Utilizing multivalent interactions between ligands and receptors, the multivalent ligand presentation tactic enhances cellular uptake and targeting specificity [66]. Recent research has concentrated on creating nanoscale platforms, including dendrimers, polymersomes, or virus-like particles, that can deliver numerous ligands in a regulated manner [67]. These multivalent systems boost the effectiveness of cellular targeting by increasing ligand–receptor interactions, simulating the ligand clustering seen in cell–cell interactions naturally.

11.6.3 Ligand-Mediated Endocytosis

A crucial mechanism that ligand-targeted nanoparticles use for cellular uptake is ligand-mediated endocytosis. The internalization of nanoparticles into cancer cells can be caused by ligands having a high affinity for the receptors on cancer cells [68]. Understanding the intracellular trafficking pathways following ligand-mediated endocytosis has received a lot of attention recently, making it possible to design nanoparticles with optimized release mechanisms inside particular subcellular compartments [69]. By attaching endosmotic peptides or pH-responsive moieties to nanoparticles, endosomal escape, and cytoplasmic release are made possible, enhancing the intracellular transport of medicinal drugs [70].

11.6.4 Ligand-Mediated Targeting Beyond Cell Surface Receptors

In addition to cell surface receptors, various biomarkers or microenvironmental elements linked to tumor growth are also included in ligand-based targeted techniques. Ligands that recognize particular elements of the tumor microenvironment, such as hypoxia-inducible factors or enzymes that are overexpressed in the tumor stroma, have been studied by researchers [71]. Additionally, it has been studied whether blocking tumor angiogenesis or enhancing drug delivery to solid tumors can be accomplished by ligand-mediated targeting of tumor vasculature or lymphatic vessels [72]. These developments in ligand-based targeting techniques broaden the application of nanoparticle-based targeted cancer therapy beyond cell surface receptors, enabling a more thorough and efficient strategy.

11.6.5 Ligand-Mediated Therapeutic Combination Strategies

Ligand-based targeting can also be employed to achieve therapeutic combination strategies. Researchers have conjugated different ligands onto nanoparticles, each targeting a specific receptor or cellular component, to deliver multiple therapeutic agents simultaneously [73]. The ligand-mediated therapeutic combination strategies approach enables the synergistic delivery of different therapeutic modalities, such as chemotherapy drugs, small interfering RNA (siRNA), or immunomodulators, to target multiple signaling pathways or overcome drug resistance mechanisms [74]. Ligand-mediated therapeutic combination strategies hold great potential for improving treatment outcomes and addressing the heterogeneity of cancer cells.

11.7 UTILIZATION OF ANTIBODY FOR CELLULAR TARGETING

The field of targeted cancer therapy has undergone a revolution by using antibodies for cellular targeting. The precise delivery of therapeutic drugs to tumor cells is made possible by antibodies' high specificity and affinity for cancer cell surface antigens while reducing the likelihood of off-target effects.

11.7.1 Monoclonal Antibodies

Due to their high specificity and low immunogenicity, monoclonal antibodies (mAbs) have become essential tools for cellular targeting. Researchers can obtain selective binding to cancer cell surface indicators by attaching mAbs to the surface of nanoparticles, enabling tailored delivery of therapeutic drugs [75]. To increase tissue penetration and improve tumor targeting, recent developments have concentrated on designing antibody fragments, such as single-chain variable fragments (scFv) or bispecific antibodies [76]. Additionally, the creation of antibody–drug conjugates (ADCs), in which cytotoxic medications are coupled to antibodies, has made it possible to deliver strong anticancer agents to specific locations [77].

11.7.2 Antibody-Targeted Drug Delivery Systems

The design of medication delivery systems has extensively investigated antibody-based targeting techniques. Antibody-functionalized nanoparticles may recognize and bind to cancer cell surface markers with high specificity, facilitating cellular uptake and intracellular drug release [78]. When compared to non-targeted formulations, antibody-targeted drug delivery methods have demonstrated improved therapeutic efficacy and decreased systemic toxicity [79]. To improve antibody-mediated cellular targeting, recent developments have concentrated on optimizing nanoparticle features, such as size, shape, and surface chemistry [80]. Additionally, the precise control of drug release within the target cells is made possible by the insertion of stimuli-responsive components, such as pH or enzyme-responsive linkers [81].

11.7.3 Antibody-Conjugated Theranostic Nanoparticles

Therapeutic and diagnostic capabilities are combined in a single platform by theranostic nanoparticles. Targeted delivery of therapeutic medicines and imaging probes to cancer cells is made possible by antibody-conjugated theranostic nanoparticles [82]. Real-time monitoring of the biodistribution, cellular uptake, and therapeutic response of nanoparticles is made possible by conjugating antibodies to imaging agents like fluorescent dyes, magnetic nanoparticles, or radioactive tracers [83]. Multiple imaging modalities and theranostic functions have recently been integrated into a single nanoparticle system, enabling multimodal imaging and individualized treatment approaches [84].

11.7.4 Antibody-Coated Liposomes

Liposomes coated with antibodies have become adaptable drug delivery vehicles. The receptor-mediated endocytosis and subsequent intracellular drug release are triggered by the antibody-coated liposomes' ability to recognize and bind to cancer cell surface antigens [85]. Recent developments in liposome engineering have made it possible to create antibody-coated liposomes with increased tumor accumulation, longer circulation times, and greater stability [86]. Additionally, the intracellular distribution of liposomal cargos is improved by the addition of stimuli-responsive lipid bilayers or membrane fusion-promoting peptides [87].

11.7.5 Antibody-Mediated Immune Cell Targeting

For improved anticancer immune responses, antibodies can potentially be used to target immune cells. Immune cell activation, proliferation, and tumor infiltration can all be improved by targeting immune cells with antibodies, such as dendritic cells or T cells [88]. Researchers can improve the transport of immunomodulatory drugs or antigenic peptides to immune cells, thereby increasing the antitumor immune response [89] by conjugating antibodies specific to immune cell surface markers to nanoparticles. Recent research has focused on creating multifunctional nanoparticles that synergistically improve cancer immunotherapy by combining immune cell targeting with other functions like medication delivery or immune checkpoint inhibition [90].

11.8 STRATEGIES TO IMPROVE NANOPARTICLE–CELLULAR MEMBRANE INTERACTION

Strategies to improve nanoparticle–cellular membrane interactions are critical for increasing the effectiveness of medication delivery systems. Surface modifications are essential for incorporating certain ligands, peptides, or polymers that facilitate beneficial interactions with the cellular membrane. These changes may stabilize nanoparticles, inhibit premature clearance, and aid receptor-mediated endocytosis for cellular uptake [91]. Furthermore, modifying the physicochemical characteristics of nanoparticles, including their dimensions, morphology, and electrostatic charge, enables tailoring to specific cellular receptors and desired internalization routes. Furthermore, biomimetic techniques, such as covering nanoparticles with cell membrane components, increase biocompatibility and mirror natural cell interactions, resulting in better cellular adhesion and uptake [92]. Successful cellular targeting and internalization of nanoparticles in targeted cancer therapy depend on effective nanoparticle–cellular membrane interaction. The interface between nanoparticles and cellular membranes has been improved via the development of numerous techniques, increasing their cellular absorption and therapeutic effectiveness. An illustration of penetration barriers in tumors and techniques to increase barrier is shown in Figure 11.2.

11.8.1 Surface Engineering and Functionalization

To enhance the interaction of nanoparticles with biological membranes, surface engineering and functionalization have been extensively investigated. The interaction of nanoparticles with the cell membrane and cellular absorption can be improved by altering their surface features, such as charge,

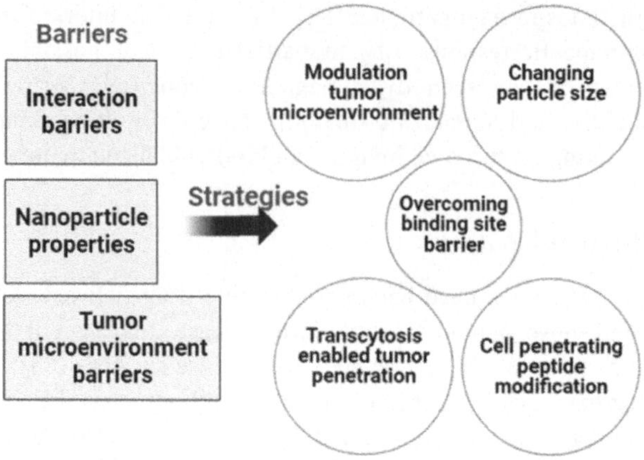

FIGURE 11.2 An illustration of tumor penetration barriers and the accompanying techniques to increase tumor penetration.

hydrophobicity, or surface chemistry [93]. Recent research has concentrated on creating biomimetic nanoparticles, where the surface is altered to replicate the characteristics of cell membranes, by integrating components obtained from cell membranes or covering nanoparticles with fragments of cell membranes [94]. These bioinspired strategies encourage beneficial interactions with biological membranes, which improves nanoparticle internalization.

11.8.2 Ligand–Receptor Interactions

Another efficient method to improve nanoparticle–cellular membrane connection is to use ligand–receptor interactions. Researchers can enable selective binding and absorption of nanoparticles by functionalizing them with ligands specific to receptors overexpressed on the surfaces of cancer cells [95]. The interaction between nanoparticles and biological membranes has been improved by the use of designed ligands with improved affinity and specificity, such as peptide mimetics or aptamers [96]. Additionally, the combination of several ligands or ligand clustering on the nanoparticle surface can boost targeting effectiveness and receptor-mediated internalization [97].

11.8.3 Membrane-Penetrating Peptides

Membrane-penetrating peptides (MPPs) have become effective tools for improving the interaction between nanoparticles and biological membranes. MPPs can pierce cell membranes, facilitating the internalization of nanoparticles effectively [98]. MPPs have recently undergone design and optimization to increase their capacity for endosomal escape and cellular absorption [99]. Additionally, MPPs can be added to nanoparticle formulations as surface modifications or as elements of coatings, which improves the interaction with cellular membranes and boosts intracellular transport and therapeutic efficacy [100].

11.8.4 Physical Methods

Physical techniques have been investigated to facilitate membrane breakdown or permeabilization to enhance the interaction between nanoparticles and biological membranes. To increase nanoparticle uptake, methods including sonoporation, electroporation, or photothermal effects have been used [101]. For instance, nanoparticle internalization can be improved by cell membrane rupture caused by ultrasonic [102]. To achieve precise and controlled nanoparticle–cellular membrane contact, minimize cellular damage, and enhance therapeutic effects, recent developments have concentrated on optimizing the parameters of these physical approaches.

11.8.5 Nanoparticle Physical Properties

The interaction of nanoparticles with biological membranes is highly dependent on the size and form of the particles. Recent research has shown that nanoparticles with particular size and shape properties have improved cellular uptake because of their positive interactions with cell membranes [103]. For instance, compared to bigger or spherical nanoparticles, smaller or elongated nanoparticles have demonstrated superior cellular internalization [104]. Improved cellular targeting efficiency can result from the rational design and manufacture of nanoparticles with certain sizes and shapes that optimize their interaction with cellular membranes.

11.9 CONCLUSION AND FUTURE PROSPECTIVE

Significant progress has been made in the field of cellular targeting of nanoparticles for targeted cancer therapy in recent years. A promising method for selectively delivering therapeutic medicines to cancer cells while minimizing off-target effects is the use of antibodies for cellular targeting. To increase the specificity and effectiveness of nanoparticle internalization, passive and active cellular targeting techniques have been investigated. To promote nanoparticle accumulation within cancer cells and particular cellular compartments, cellular and subcellular targeting techniques have been developed. To enhance the interaction of the nanoparticle with the cellular membrane and subsequent cellular uptake, factors such as nanoparticle size, surface changes, and ligand–receptor interactions have been optimized. To improve treatment outcomes, methods to increase the cellular absorption of therapeutic substances, such as drug-loaded nanoparticles, have been investigated. Modern ligand-based targeting techniques have shown improved specificity and selectivity in the delivery of nanoparticles to cancer cells. The creation of antibody-coated liposomes and antibody–conjugated nanoparticles has demonstrated potential for increasing tumor targeting and lowering systemic toxicity. Additionally, using antibodies to target immune cells has created opportunities for improving anticancer immune responses and utilizing synergistic methods in cancer immunotherapy.

Surface engineering, ligand–receptor interactions, membrane-penetrating peptides, physical methods, and optimization of nanoparticle size and shape have been the main approaches to enhance nanoparticle–cellular membrane contact. These methods have shown increased intracellular drug delivery and cellular uptake, which has improved therapeutic effects. To further strengthen the interface between nanoparticles and cellular membranes and to increase the effectiveness of targeting, future research should keep investigating novel methods and materials. In conclusion, for cancer therapy, cellular targeting of nanoparticles holds enormous promise for enhancing the efficacy and accuracy of treatments. The field has advanced greatly with the aid of, developments in passive and active targeting, cellular and subcellular targeting, factors and techniques for cellular targeting, ligand-based targeting, antibody utilization, and nanoparticle–cellular membrane interaction. The creation of precise targeting ligands, surmounting biological obstacles, enhancing the characteristics of nanoparticles, and resolving potential toxicity issues are still difficulties. These issues should be addressed in the next studies, along with the advancement of preclinical and clinical research and the application of results to the development of efficient and individualized cancer treatments. Researchers can revolutionize cancer therapy approaches by utilizing the potential of cellular targeting of nanoparticles, giving patients more precise, effective, and focused medicines while minimizing negative effects on healthy tissues. The implementation of cellular targeting of nanoparticles into standard clinical practice will be made possible by interdisciplinary collaborations and technical developments, which will ultimately improve patient outcomes and change the face of cancer therapy.

REFERENCES

1. Weinberg RA, Hanahan D. The hallmarks of cancer. *Cell.* 2000 Jan 7;100(1):57–70.
2. Gupta GP, Massague J. Cancer metastasis: building a framework. *Cell.* 2006;127:679–95.
3. Dreaden EC, Alkilany AM, Huang X, Murphy CJ, El-Sayed MA. The golden age: gold nanoparticles for biomedicine. *Chem Soc Rev.* 2012;41(7):2740–79.
4. Poon W, Zhang Y, Ouyang B, Kingston BR, Wu JLY, Wilhelm S, Chan WC. Elimination pathways of nanoparticles. *ACS Nano.* 2019;13(5):5785–98.
5. Yang DH, Nah H, Lee D, Min SJ, Park S, An SH, Wang J, He H, Choi KS, Ko WK, Lee JS, Kwon IK, Lee SJ, Heo DN. A review on gold nanoparticles as an innovative therapeutic cue in bone tissue engineering: Prospects and future clinical applications. *Mater Today Bio.* 2024;12(26):1–16. doi: 10.1016/j.mtbio.2024.101016.
6. Yang T, Zhai J, Hu D, Yang R, Wang G, Li Y, Liang G. "Targeting design" of nanoparticles in tumor therapy. *Pharmaceutics.* 2022 Sep 11;14(9):1919.
7. Wilhelm S, Tavares AJ, Dai Q, Ohta S, Audet J, Dvorak HF, Chan WC. Analysis of nanoparticle delivery to tumors. *Nat Rev Mater.* 2016;1(5):16014.
8. Ferrari M. Cancer nanotechnology: opportunities and challenges. *Nat RevCancer.* 2005;5(3):161–71.
9. Jokerst JV, Lobovkina T, Zare RN, Gambhir SS. Nanoparticle PEGylation for imaging and therapy. *Nanomedicine.* 2011;6(4):715–28.
10. Chauhan VP, Popović Z, Chen O. Nanoparticle vaccines against infectious diseases. *Front Immunol.* 2020;11:1–21.
11. Maeda H, Nakamura H, Fang J. The EPR effect for macromolecular drug delivery to solid tumors: improvement of tumor uptake, lowering of systemic toxicity, and distinct tumor imaging in vivo. *Adv Drug Deliv Rev.* 2013;65(1):71–9.
12. Elumalai K, Srinivasan S, Shanmugam A. Review of the efficacy of nanoparticle-based drug delivery systems for cancer treatment. *Biomed Technol.* 2024;5:109–s122, https://doi.org/10.1016/j.bmt.2023.09.001.
13. Chen J, Li Q, et al. Tumor-derived extracellular vesicle drug delivery system for chemo-photothermal-immune combination cancer treatment. *iScience.* 2024;27(2):1–15. doi:10.1016/j.isci.2024.108833.
14. Chauhan VP, Jain RK, Stylianopoulos T. Delivering nanomedicine to solid tumors. *Nat Rev Cancer.* 2013; 13(9):653–62.
15. Anarjan FS. Active targeting drug delivery nanocarriers: ligands. *Nano Struct Nano Objects.* 2019 Jul 1;19:100370.
16. Shi J, Kantoff PW. Nanomedicine in cancer therapy: challenges, opportunities, and clinical applications. *J Clin Investig.* 2017;127(3):971–81.
17. Master AM, Sen Gupta A. EGF receptor-targeted nanocarriers for enhanced cancer treatment. *Nanomedicine.* 2012 Dec;7(12):1895–906.
18. Li SD, Huang L. Nanoparticles evading the reticuloendothelial system: role of the supported bilayer. *Biochim Biophys Acta Biomembran.* 2010;1788(10):2259–66.
19. Jokerst JV, Lobovkina T, Zare RN, Gambhir SS. Nanoparticle PEGylation for imaging and therapy. *Nanomedicine.* 2011;6(4):715–28.
20. Jafari M, Molavi O, Kahani B, Saeednia L, Kazemi Oskuee R. Engineering of targeted nanoparticles for cancer therapy using internalizing aptamers. *Adv Pharm Bull.* 2019;9(2):210–20.
21. Torchilin VP. Multifunctional, stimuli-sensitive nanoparticulate systems for drug delivery. *Nat Rev Drug Discov.* 2011;10(9):627–48.
22. Cai L, Chen X, Hu J. Dual targeting of passive and active tumor homing for efficient tumor regression. *ACS Appl Mater Interfaces.* 2021;13(10):12154–73.
23. Ashfaq UA, Riaz M, Yasmeen E, Yousaf MZ. Recent advances in nanoparticle-based targeted drug-delivery systems against cancer and role of tumor microenvironment. *Crit Rev Ther Drug Carrier Syst.* 2017;34(4):317–53.
24. Raj S, Khurana S, Choudhari R, Kesari KK, Kamal MA, Garg N, Ruokolainen J, Das BC, Kumar D. Specific targeting cancer cells with nanoparticles and drug delivery in cancer therapy. In *Seminars in Cancer Biology.* 2021 Feb 1 (Vol. 69, pp. 166–177). Academic Press.
25. Xu S, Olenyuk BZ, Okamoto CT, Hamm-Alvarez SF. Targeting receptor-mediated endocytotic pathways with nanoparticles: rationale and advances. *Adv Drug Deliv Rev.* 2013 Jan 1;65(1):121–38.

26. Xiao Z, Levy-Nissenbaum E, Alexis F, Lupták A, Teply BA, Chan JM, Shi J, Digga E, Cheng J, Langer R, Farokhzad OC. Engineering of targeted nanoparticles for cancer therapy using internalizing aptamers isolated by cell-uptake selection. *ACS Nano*. 2012 Jan 24;6(1):696–704.
27. Li SD, Huang L. Nanoparticles evading the reticuloendothelial system: Role of the supported bilayer. *Biochim Biophys Acta Biomembran*. 2010;1788(10):2259–66.
28. Zhang L, Gu FX, Chan JM, Wang AZ, Langer RS, Farokhzad OC. Nanoparticles in medicine: therapeutic applications and developments. *Clin Pharmacol Ther*. 2008;83(5):761–769.
29. Chu S, Shi X, Tian Y, Gao F. pH-responsive polymer nanomaterials for tumor therapy. *Front Oncol*. 2022 Mar 22;12:855019.
30. Algar WR, Medintz IL. Proteolytic activity and quantification of cysteine protease enzymes using nanosensors. *Chem Commun*. 2011;47(9):2520–36.
31. Gao X, Nie S. Spectrally encoded beads for multiplexed optical coding of biomolecules. *Anal Chem*. 2003;75(8):2146–50.
32. Jokerst JV, Lobovkina T, Zare RN, Gambhir SS. Nanoparticle PEGylation for imaging and therapy. *Nanomedicine*. 2011;6(4):715–28.
33. Dreaden EC, Alkilany AM, Huang X, Murphy CJ, El-Sayed MA. The golden age: gold nanoparticles for biomedicine. *Chem Soc Rev*. 2012;41(7):2740–79.
34. Zhang L, Gu FX, Chan JM, Wang AZ, Langer RS, Farokhzad OC. Nanoparticles in medicine: Therapeutic applications and developments. *Clin Pharmacol Ther*. 2008;83(5):761–9.
35. Zhang X, Chen X, Liang Y, Wang X, Sun L, Dong S, Wang E. Recent advances in ligand-directed strategies for delivery of therapeutics using nanoparticles. *Chem Bio Chem*. 2020;21(18):2606–17.
36. Das M, Mohanty C, Sahoo SK. Ligand-based targeted therapy for cancer tissue. *Expert Opin Drug Deliv*. 2009 Mar 1;6(3):285–304.
37. Conner SD, Schmid SL. Regulated portals of entry into the cell. *Nature*. 2003;422(6927):37–44.
38. Danhier F, Feron O, Préat V. To exploit the tumor microenvironment: passive and active tumor targeting of nanocarriers for anti-cancer drug delivery. *J Control Release*. 2010;148(2):135–46.
39. Peer D, Karp JM, Hong S, Farokhzad OC, Margalit R, Langer R. Nanocarriers as an emerging platform for cancer therapy. *Nat Nanotechnol*. 2007;2(12):751–60.
40. Jafari M, Molavi O, Kahani B, Saeednia L, Kazemi Oskuee R. Engineering of targeted nanoparticles for cancer therapy using internalizing aptamers. *Adv Pharm Bull*. 2019;9(2):210–20.
41. Agemy L, Friedmann-Morvinski D, Kotamraju VR, Roth L, Sugahara KN, Girard OM, Ruoslahti E, et al. Targeted nanoparticle-enhanced proapoptotic peptide as potential therapy for glioblastoma. *Proc Natl Acad Sci*. 2011;108(42):17450–5.
42. Maeda H, Nakamura H, Fang J. The EPR effect for macromolecular drug delivery to solid tumors: improvement of tumor uptake, lowering of systemic toxicity, and distinct tumor imaging in vivo. *Adv Drug Deliv Rev*. 2013;65(1):71–9.
43. Niikura K, Matsunaga T, Suzuki T, Kobayashi S, Yamaguchi H. Orally active insulin delivery systems using self-assembled chitosan nanoparticles. *J Control Release*. 2011;152(1):54–61.
44. Torchilin VP. Multifunctional, stimuli-sensitive nanoparticulate systems for drug delivery. *Nat Rev Drug Discov*. 2014;13(11):813–27.
45. Torchilin VP. Multifunctional, stimuli-sensitive nanoparticulate systems for drug delivery. *Nat Rev Drug Discov*. 2011;10(9):627–48.
46. Li Z, Zhao R, Wu X, Sun Y, Yao M, Li J, Zhang, H. Stimuli-responsive nanomedicines for overcoming cancer multidrug resistance. *Theranostics*. 2020;10(17):7968–95.
47. Liu J, Liao S, Diop-Frimpong B, Chen W, Goel S, Naxerova K, Jain RK, et al. TGF-β blockade improves the distribution and efficacy of therapeutics in breast carcinoma by normalizing the tumor stroma. *Proc Natl Acad Sci*. 2015;109(41):16618–23.
48. Albanese A, Tang PS, Chan WC. The effect of nanoparticle size, shape, and surface chemistry on biological systems. *Annu Rev Biomed Eng*. 2012;14:1–16.
49. Gratton SE, Ropp PA, Pohlhaus PD, Luft JC, Madden VJ, Napier ME. The effect of particle design on cellular internalization pathways. *Proc Natl Acad Sci*. 2008;105(33):11613–18.
50. Sun W, Ji W, Hall JM, Hu Q, Wang C, Beisel CL, Gu Z, et al. Self-assembled DNA nanoclews for the efficient delivery of CRISPR-Cas9 for genome editing. *Angew Chem Int Ed*. 2014;53(41):1192–96.
51. Wang H, Wu J, Williams GR, Fan Q, Kang Y. Cell membrane biomimetic nanoparticles: a new biomimetic platform for tumor diagnosis and treatment. *Engineering*. 2021;7(5):598–611.

52. Li X, Chen Y. Overcoming endosomal barrier in nanoparticle-mediated drug delivery: current status and strategies. *ACS Nano*. 2018;12(9):8340–50.
53. Kaźmierczak Z, Szostak-Paluch K, Przybyło M, Langner M, Witkiewicz W, Jędruchniewicz N, Dąbrowska K. Endocytosis in cellular uptake of drug delivery vectors: molecular aspects in drug development. *Bioorg Med Chem*. 2020 Sep 15;28(18):115556.
54. Zhang L, Gu FX. Designing nanoparticles for targeted therapy: strategies for improving antitumor efficacy and minimizing side effects. *Curr Pharm Design*. 2015;21(20):2796–803.
55. Xu X, Saw PE, Tao W, Li Y, Ji X, Yu M, Farokhzad OC. Tumor microenvironment-responsive multistaged nanoplatform for systemic RNAi and cancer therapy. *Nano Lett*. 2017;17(7):4427–35.
56. Ma X, Gong N, Zhong L, Sun J, Liang XJ. Future of nanotherapeutics: targeting the cellular sub-organelles. *Biomaterials*. 2016 Aug 1;97:10–21.
57. Wang L, Li PC, Wang JC, Zhang JR, Shen Y, Liang WQ, Zhang Q, et al. Folate receptor-targeted mixed polysialic acid micelles for combinational delivery of paclitaxel and survivin shRNA in treating multidrug-resistant cancer. *Adv Funct Mater*. 2018;28(20):1–12.
58. Zhang Y, Wang F, Li M, Yu S, Zhao C, Zhang L, Huang X, et al. A smart nanoparticle-based system for intracellular mRNA delivery and gene silencing in cancer therapy. *Adv Funct Mater.* 2020;30(29):1–14.
59. Liu Y, Zhang P. The effects of curcumin on breast cancer cells. *J Breast Cancer*. 2016;19(1):1–11.
60. Li S, Chen Y, Liu F, Gu W, Wei Y. Co-delivery of nanomedicines for enhanced cancer therapy. *Adv Healthc Mater*. 2018;7(24):1–19.
61. Dai Q, Wilhelm S, Ding D, Syed AM, Sindhwani S, Zhang Y, Chen YY, MacMillan P, Chan WCW. Quantifying the ligand-coated nanoparticle delivery to cancer cells in solid tumors. *ACS Nano*. 2018 Aug 28;12(8):8423–35. doi: 10.1021/acsnano.8b03900. Epub 2018 Jul 26. PMID: 30016073.
62. Gray BP, Brown KC. Combinatorial peptide libraries: mining for cell-binding peptides. *Chem Rev*. 2014 Jan 22;114(2):1020–81.
63. Liu D, Yang F, Xiong F, Gu N. The smart drug delivery system and its clinical potential. *Theranostics*. 2019;9(11):2626–39.
64. Zhao RY, Wilhelm S, Wang HY, Xu ZR. Lipopeptide-based nanoparticles for targeted cancer therapy. *Adv Drug Deliv Rev.* 2020;156:41–55.
65. Sacchetti C, Liu-Bryan R, Magrini A. The potential role of nanotechnology in therapeutic approaches for rheumatoid arthritis. *Nanomedicine*. 2018;13(1):269–86.
66. Torchilin VP. Multifunctional, stimuli-sensitive nanoparticulate systems for drug delivery. *Nat Rev Mater.* 2020;5(5):1–21.
67. Wiogo HT, Lim M, Bulmus V. Toward development of highly modular protein-based nanoparticles. *Adv Healthc Mater*. 2014;3(7):975–91.
68. Agemy L, Friedmann-Morvinski D, Kotamraju VR, Roth L, Sugahara KN, Girard OM, Ruoslahti E, et al. Targeted nanoparticle enhanced proapoptotic peptide as potential therapy for glioblastoma. *Proc Natl Acad Sci*. 2011;108(42):17450–5.
69. Gilleron J, Querbes W, Zeigerer A, Borodovsky A, Marsico G, Schubert U, Bickle M, et al. Image-based analysis of lipid nanoparticle-mediated siRNA delivery, intracellular trafficking and endosomal escape. *Nat Biotechnol*. 2013;31(7):638–46.
70. Li W, Zhang J, Chen S, Hu R, Jin Y. pH-sensitive polymeric nanoparticles for tumor-targeted drug delivery. *Pharm Res* . 2020;37(3):1–19.
71. Mi P, Cabral H, Kataoka K. Ligand-installed nanocarriers toward precision therapy. *Adv Mater*. 2020;32(13):1–32.
72. Huang J, Yuan Y, Wang Y, Mu X, Deng R, Liu S, Liu X. Targeting tumor microenvironment for tumor therapy. *J Control Release*. 2021;333:1–24.
73. Ma X, Zhao Y, Liang XJ. Theranostic nanoparticles engineered for clinic and pharmaceutics. *Accounts Chem Res*. 2011;44(10):1114–22.
74. Hu Q, Sun W, Wang C, Gu Z. Recent advances in nanoparticle-based combination therapy for cancer treatment. *RSC Adv*. 2015;5(74):60687–705.
75. Scott AM, Wolchok JD, Old LJ. Antibody therapy of cancer. *Nat Rev Cancer*. 2012;12(4):278–87.
76. Maruani A, Smith MEB, Miranda E, Chester KA, Chudasama V. Cysteine-selective antibody conjugation for site-specific labeling of engineered antibodies. *Nat Protocols*. 2015;10(5):1453–68.

77. Chari RVJ, Miller ML. Antibody-drug conjugates: an emerging concept in cancer therapy. *Angew Chem Int Ed.* 2019;58(2):430–48.
78. Yang L, Cao Z, Sajja HK. Antibody-nanoparticle conjugates for targeted cancer therapy. Methods Mol Biol. 2019;1950:63–84.
79. Allen TM, Cullis PR. Liposomal drug delivery systems: from concept to clinical applications. *Adv Drug Deliv Rev*. 2013;65(1):36–48.
80. Wang X, Yang L. Antibody-mediated delivery of therapeutics for cancer therapy. *Adv Healthc Mater.* 2019;8(20):1–19.
81. He C, Hu Y, Yin L, Tang C, Yin C. Effects of particle size and surface charge on cellular uptake and biodistribution of polymeric nanoparticles. *Biomaterials*. 2010;31(13):3657–66.
82. Cheng L, Wang C, Ma X, Wang Q, Cheng Y. Multifunctional upconversion nanoparticles for dual-modal imaging-guided stem cell therapy under remote magnetic control. *Adv Funct Mater.* 2017;27(43):1–10.
83. Liu J, Yu M, Zhou C, Zheng J. Renal-clearable noble metal nanoparticles: photoluminescence, elimination, and biomedical applications. *Wiley Interdiscipl Rev*. 2017;9(5):1–23.
84. Li S, Chen Y. Co-delivery of nanomedicines for enhanced cancer therapy. *Adv Healthc Mater.* 2018;7(24):1–19.
85. Torchilin VP. Multifunctional, stimuli-sensitive nanoparticulate systems for drug delivery. *Nat Rev Drug Discov*. 2011;10(9):627–48.
86. Zou P, Yu M, Zheng J, Huang X. A new dawn for cancer therapy: perspectives on the convergence of biological therapy and nanomedicine. *Bioconjug Chem*. 2017;28(4):846–58.
87. Bozzuto G, Molinari A. Liposomes as nanomedical devices. *Int J Nanomed.* 2015;10:975–99.
88. Douglass J, Hynes RO. Immune cell targeting of therapeutic nanoparticles. *Nat Rev Immunol.* 2021;21(2):88–101.
89. Irvine DJ, Dane EL, Langer R. Harnessing biomaterials to engineer the lymph node microenvironment for immunity or tolerance. *AAPS J.* 2020;22(3):1–17.
90. Fan Y, Wang C, Cheng L, Wang Q, Cheng Y. Multifunctional nanoparticles for programmed cancer immunotherapy. *Curr Med Chem*. 2020;27(34):5770–95.
91. Poon Z, Hammond PT. Nanoparticle-Cell Membrane Interactions. *Small.* 2016;12(30):4056–62.
92. Hu CMJ, Fang RH, Wang KC, Luk BT, Thamphiwatana S, Dehaini D, Zhang L, et al. Nanoparticle biointerfacing by platelet membrane cloaking. *Nature*. 2015;526(7571):118–21. https://doi.org/10.1038/nature15373
93. Nel AE, Mädler L, Velegol D, Xia T, Hoek EM, Somasundaran P, Klaessig F, Castranova V, Thompson M. Understanding biophysicochemical interactions at the nano-bio interface. *Nat Mater.* 2009;8(7):543–57.
94. Hu CM, Fang RH, Wang KC, Zhang L. Biomimetic nanosponges for targeted delivery of therapeutics to suppress angiogenesis in pancreatic cancer. *Cancer Res*. 2015;75(18):3782–91.
95. Díez-Pascual AM. Surface engineering of nanomaterials with polymers, biomolecules, and small ligands for nanomedicine. *Materials*. 2022 Apr 30;15(9):3251.
96. Jafari M, Molavi O, Kahani B, Saeednia L, Kazemi Oskuee R. Engineering of targeted nanoparticles for cancer therapy using internalizing aptamers. *Adv Pharm Bull.* 2019;9(2):210–20.
97. Li SD, Huang L. Nanoparticles evading the reticuloendothelial system: role of the supported bilayer. *Biochim Biophys Acta Biomembran.* 2008;1788(10):2259–66.
98. Zaro JL, Shen WC. Cationic albumin conjugates for peptide and protein delivery. *Adv Drug Deliv Rev*. 2011;63(10–11):1013–23.
99. Veiga AS, Sinthuvanich C, Gaspar D, Franquelim HG, Castanho MA, Schneider JP. Arginine-rich self-assembling peptides as potent antibacterial gels. *Biomaterials*. 2012;33(35):8907–16.
100. Fan Y, Wang C, Cheng L, Wang Q, Cheng Y. Multifunctional nanoparticles for programmed cancer immunotherapy. *Curr Med Chem.* 2020;27(34):5770–95.
101. Zhang Y, Guan Y, Zhou L, Yu B, Yan Z, Zheng J, Zhang Y, Zhang D, Li Z. Nanoparticle size and surface property dependent cellular uptake behaviors of Prussian blue nanoparticles. *Int J Nanomed.* 2020;15:133–45.

102. Shpak O, Vereshchagina E, Leshansky A. Understanding the roles of acoustic cavitation in sonoporation and sonothrombolysis. *Phys Rep.* 2021;912:1–50.
103. Kulkarni SA, Feng SS. Effects of particle size and surface modification on cellular uptake and biodistribution of polymeric nanoparticles for drug delivery. *Pharm Res.* 2013 Oct;30:2512–22.
104. Chithrani BD, Ghazani AA, Chan WCW. Determining the size and shape dependence of gold nanoparticle uptake into mammalian cells. *Nano Lett.* 2006;6(4):662–68.

Index

T

V